*f*P

The
Invisible
People

How the U.S. Has Slept Through the Global AIDS Pandemic,
the Greatest Humanitarian Catastrophe of Our Time

Greg Behrman

FREE PRESS

NEW YORK   LONDON   TORONTO   SYDNEY

FREE PRESS
A Division of Simon & Schuster, Inc.
1230 Avenue of the Americas
New York, NY 10020

For information regarding special discounts for bulk purchases,
please contact Simon & Schuster Special Sales at 1-800-456-6798
or business@simonandschuster.com

Designed by Joseph Rutt

Manufactured in the United States of America

10 9 8 7 6 5 4 3 2 1

Library of Congress Cataloging-in-Publication Data

Behrman, Greg.
    The invisible people : how the United States has slept through the global AIDS
pandemic, the greatest humanitarian catastrophe of our time / Greg Behrman.
        p.   cm.
    Includes index.
    1. AIDS (Disease)—Government policy—United States.   I. Title.

RA643.83.B44   2004
362.196'9792'00973—dc22   2004040466

ISBN 0-7432-5755-3

To My Father, My Hero

with Eternal Devotion

Contents

I am an invisible man . . .
I am invisible, understand, simply because people refuse to see me.

Ralph Ellison,
The Invisible Man, 1952

Preface

Invisible graves line the fields of faraway lands. Therein lie invisible people—25 million of them—all laid to rest by one of the most lethal scourges in the history of mankind. Hundreds of millions of empty graves await those who may follow.

Over the past two decades, 65 million people have become infected with HIV, the virus that causes AIDS. Approximately 25 million people—more than the aggregate battle deaths of the twentieth century combined—have lost their lives to this plague. More than 40 million are currently infected. Every day, 8,000 people (nearly three times 9/11's death toll) die of AIDS.

Since the first century, the world's wars have exacted approximately 149 million deaths. It is projected that by 2010, more than 100 million will have been infected with HIV. There will be as many as 250 million new HIV infections by 2025.

Beyond the ineffable human toll, the pandemic is refashioning the social, economic, and geopolitical dimensions of our world.

Even as the virus's shadow looms, poised to explode on other continents, AIDS has been decimating sub-Saharan Africa, home to almost 70 percent of those infected worldwide. Approximately 40 percent of adults in Botswana are HIV positive. More than 20 percent of those in South Africa are infected. Life expectancy in Botswana has decreased from seventy-one to thirty-nine years, and in Zimbabwe, from seventy to thirty-eight years. Four other countries in the region have life expectancies below forty. By 2010, several African countries are expected to have life expectancies of thirty years or less. "We are threatened with extinction," Botswana's president, Festus Mogae, has said.

Most ominously, the pandemic is creating an entire generation of orphans. By 2010, Africa will be host to 20 million of the world's 25 million AIDS orphans. Reared in abject poverty and without moral guidance, Africa's AIDS orphans, it has been said, constitute an army in search of a leader.

Suffering almost endemic poverty, Africa's economies will be pulverized by the pandemic. It is commonplace for businesses to train two or three workers for every one job. Such are the chances that workers will become infected and die. AIDS will shrink many economies by 15 to 20 percent or more by decade's end. Within several generations, the World Bank predicts, economic collapse is a possibility.

The disease will have grave consequences for U.S. and global security. 9/11 demonstrated the danger of a failed state. In Africa, the world confronts nothing less than the potentiality of a failed continent. The disease is eviscerating national militaries (some have infection rates, it is believed, as high as 50 percent) and generating social and economic pressures that will threaten the very viability of many African states, in some cases begetting disintegration or implosion. The debris, without drastic action, will be the fodder upon which terrorists and transnational criminal elements will find refuge and sustenance. The pandemic—with surreptitious but undeniable force—is shaking some of the fault lines upon which tomorrow's wars will be fought.

Southern Africa is the canary for the rest of the world. By 2010, the National Intelligence Council predicts, China, India, Russia, Nigeria, and Ethiopia will have between 50 to 75 million infections, and possibly more (overtaking the 30 to 35 million projected in central and southern Africa).

By 2025, one expert estimates, AIDS will cripple China's, India's, and Russia's economies, such that they will only be able to produce flat to nominal annual economic growth. The aftershock will generate seismic reverberations throughout the global economy.

Already facing serious economic challenges and a chilling demographic crisis—Russia's population is expected to decline from 145 million by as many as 30 million in the next several decades—Russia faces the additional possibility of 8 million HIV infections in the next ten years. AIDS will imperil Russia's tenuous democratization, and will precipitate instability in a power already struggling to safeguard thousands of nuclear weapons and large quantities of nuclear materials. Poised to explode in India and China, the disease threatens to destabilize these other nuclear states as well, possibly contributing to internal, or even regional instability and conflict.

These "next wave" countries comprise roughly 40 percent of the world's population. The pandemic's near-term incursion heralds only the beginning. The toll taken thus far is merely a harbinger of what is still to come.

Throughout the rise of the AIDS pandemic, the United States has been the world's largest donor and its most vocal mouthpiece in the fight against the disease. No other country had experienced AIDS the way the United States had. More than any other wealthy nation, it bore the visceral scars of its very own AIDS epidemic. The experience placed it in a position to lead.

During the same period, the United States grew into a position of military, economic, and cultural power unrivaled in modern history. In 2003, the U.S. military budget would come to exceed military spending by the rest of the world combined. Its economy was by far the world's largest, comparable to the entire European Union. The breadth and influence of American culture and values, its "soft" power, was unmistakable. The combination placed the United States in a unique position of leadership.

America's peerless global reach meant that it would be particularly vulnerable to the economic and geopolitical instability the pandemic was poised to beget. It also meant that the U.S. response to the pandemic would have a profound bearing on the global response at large.

The "global community" is generally only as strong as the commitments of its nation-state members. Despite flourishes of leadership from others—such as the Scandinavian countries, too small to recalibrate the global response by themselves—U.S. policy consistently set the bar for the rest of the world. By and large, as went the U.S. response to global AIDS, so went the global response.

AIDS is a global catastrophe that requires an international response. It is critical to examine the national leadership of the most affected countries and the global community at large. They are part of the story, and indeed, they are part of this story. However, the primary focus here is the U.S. response: How has the mightiest, wealthiest, most advantaged country in the world responded to the defining humanitarian catastrophe of our time?

In a speech at the Kennedy Center in Washington, D.C., on June 11, 2003, Secretary of State Colin Powell shared the results of a recent analysis his staff had prepared. One could add up all the deaths in the twentieth century from weapons of mass destruction, Powell said, multiply that number by ten, and it still wouldn't equal the number of people that would die of AIDS in the next twelve months. Months earlier, a *Washington Post* editorial suggested that the pandemic was probably "the most underestimated enemy of all time."

Throughout the pandemic's twenty-year flight, the United States has shrunk from its strategic imperative and its moral obligation, failing at almost every turn to lead a comprehensive global response to the pandemic. The account herein tells an inglorious chapter in our glorious national history. Yet, the exploration that follows has been spurred by a profound faith in the singularly American capacity to harness its unique sense of mission to achieve a transcendent aim. It has been driven by a hope that history might evince the mistakes of the past, so they need not be the mistakes of the future.

The U.S. response is a very human story, and it is told here as such.

This is the story of the invisible people. It is the tragedy within the tragedy. It is about our refusal to see them.

A Feeble Beginning
(1983-1990)

ONE

A Contentious Start, Buck Passing

Sauntering through the halls of yet another international health conference on a soft summer day in June 1983 in Arlington, Virginia, Dr. Joe
McCormick wasn't entirely in his element. Forty years old, McCormick
had already become the head of the Special Pathogens Division at the
Centers for Disease Control, or CDC, the world's technical center of excellence for the surveillance of disease. McCormick's job was to hunt down
emerging and reemerging infectious diseases. That meant frequent trips to
formidably intemperate far-flung corners of the globe. McCormick would
identify the disease, take stock of the scale of infection, and, when possible,
take the steps to control the outbreak.

It was a life of science and adventure that, growing up on a farm in Indiana, was well beyond McCormick's wildest boyhood dreams. With his
slight country accent, intense eyes, and mischievous scowl, McCormick
appeared every bit the part. In a division of "virus hunters," McCormick had
earned himself special distinction—colleagues knew him as a "disease cowboy," the public health equivalent of a Delta Force captain.

Despite his preference for fieldwork, McCormick's presence at the conference was crucial. Over the past several years he had become one of the
world's leading experts on hemorrhagic fever, the topic at hand. Following
one of the sessions, McCormick struck up a conversation with Dr. Jan
Desmyter, a clinician from Belgium with whom McCormick had a casual
acquaintance.

A few minutes into a cordial side-conversation, Desmyter remarked, almost in passing, "You know, we've been treating a good number of people

who have come in from Zaire seeking treatment for what seems like that same disease that they've spotted in New York and Los Angeles." Still largely mysterious, the disease had only recently, just ten months earlier, been dubbed Acquired Immune Deficiency Syndrome, or AIDS.

As a young man fresh out of Southern Florida State College in the early 1960s, McCormick's church paid for him to spend a few years teaching science to youngsters in Zaire, formerly the Belgian Congo. He grew enamored with African culture and life, and the continent called McCormick back time and again in the decades to follow. Through it all, he had become intimately acquainted with Africa's vast equatorial plains and its dense northeastern jungles. He'd basked in the continent's natural splendor and he'd known its cruelty.

In 1976, he was summoned to Yambuku, Zaire, to investigate a virulent outbreak. Yambuku, McCormick would learn upon his arrival following a punishing trip from Kinshasa, the country's capital, was plunged into chaos and despair, struck with a viciously lethal virus that McCormick and his colleagues would later name after a nearby river: the Ebola.

He'd be called back to investigate yet another Ebola outbreak in 1979, this time in Africa's northeast region, in a similarly devastated town in the Sudan called Nzara. McCormick arrived in the Sudan with only one other colleague, lab technician Roy Baron, in tow. In short order, the two were directed to a makeshift hospital that seemed to McCormick more like a dank hut, in a nearby town called Yambio. The disease, transmitted through blood, is highly contagious and almost 100 percent lethal; there was no vaccine and no treatment. Wearing full body protective suits and peering through respirator face masks, the two looked out at a macabre spectacle of more than twenty patients writhing in agony. McCormick worked through most of the first night in unbearable humidity taking blood samples and conducting tests that would reveal the extent of the outbreak.

Two nights into the investigation, he tended to an elderly lady whose fever had spiked to dizzying heights. Seemingly delirious, she had recently suffered a seizure. She seemed to McCormick a textbook case. Wearing latex gloves, he inserted a needle into her frail arm and pulled back the syringe to draw out her blood. To McCormick's shock, she gave a powerful lurch. Stunned, it took him a few moments to realize that upon pulling back, he had stuck himself with the blood-filled syringe. His glove was ruptured. There was blood, and it was McCormick's. He had punctured himself.

A wave of nausea struck. He didn't panic, though. There was one possible measure he could take, even if it was a long shot. For years there had been some mumblings in scientific circles that transfusions of convalescent blood (blood from those who had recovered from Ebola) might help stem infection. McCormick had come to the Sudan armed with a few bags of the blood, extracted from these rare cases from Zaire, just in case.

That night, Baron gave McCormick a transfusion. They washed down the anxiety with more than half a bottle of whiskey. McCormick, sure that he was already dying, got back to work the following morning.

He soldiered on, conducting his investigation of the outbreak in the days that followed. A few days later, the woman's blood sample came back yellow—she tested negative. He could breathe again. He felt, he would later tell friends and colleagues, as if he had been given his life back—as if he'd won the lottery.

In the years to follow, McCormick would move from disease to disease, always chasing the next great outbreak. Usually, he would go to the outbreak. On this summer day in 1983, it had come to McCormick. As the Belgian doctor's offhand comment sank in, McCormick felt a familiar rush.

"How many patients do you have?" he asked Desmyter.

"About thirty," he remembered his colleague answering.

McCormick's deductive train of logic began generating steam. There was no way, he knew, that even 1 percent of the Zairean population could possibly afford the travel expenses to make it from Zaire to Belgium. If Desmyter was right, there weren't thirty cases in Zaire. There were thousands.

"All kinds of lightbulbs began flashing above my head," recalled McCormick, thunderstruck by the realization: AIDS was global.

Like most of his colleagues at CDC, McCormick had been intrigued by the new illness ever since June 5, 1981, when the CDC Weekly Morbidity and Mortality Report chronicled strange cases of cancer, primarily in younger to middle-aged homosexual men in New York City and Los Angeles. Little of the science behind the disease was known. What was known was that all of the patients' immune systems seemed to have deteriorated to the point of dysfunction. Tests revealed that at their death, patients had a shockingly low store of what are medically described as T-cells, or thymus-derived cells. These microscopic cells function as the intelligence agent of the body's immune system, identifying invading pathogens and signaling the rest of the immune system to respond. Without these cells, patients became helplessly vulnerable to opportunistic infection or disease.

Through 1981 and '82, the ranks of the disease's victims in the United States swelled to the hundreds and pushed close to one thousand. Doctors could do almost nothing except watch as their patients drifted to their demise. Scientists were unable to identify the cause of the disease, its origins, how to test for it, how many people were infected, or how (with verifiable proof) it was transmitted. They knew only that it was lethal, and there was no cure.

Speculation far outpaced prudence, and as a consequence fateful mistakes were made early on. Because most of those early cases in the United States involved homosexual men, the disease had originally been designated in both health and media circles as gay-related immunodeficiency disease, or GRID. By 1982, as the health and scientific community struggled to achieve a more comprehensive and precise understanding of the disease and its dimensions, it was becoming clear that it was not simply a gay disease, or, as some called it, a "gay plague." Incidence had sprung up among intravenous drug users. By year's end a seven-year-old boy and an infant, both hemophiliacs, were also infected. In New York, Dr. Frederick Siegal reported that Mount Sinai's first "GRID" patient was a woman of Dominican descent. To health and science journalist Laurie Garrett, it seemed evident that "she, clearly, was not a gay man." Dozens of cases would spring up in New York and Miami in the summer of 1982, among both men and women of Haitian descent, all of whom seemed heterosexual and non-intravenous drug users.

While the questions far outnumbered the answers, the experts at CDC knew this new disease would not remain consigned to one subpopulation. It was transmissible via blood transfusion, and the evidence strongly suggested that it was transmissible via heterosexual contact.

In response to this evidence, the CDC, in August 1982, quietly dropped the "GRID" designation, replacing it with "AIDS." While the gay label would fall, the misperception and stigma in which it was conceived would linger—a distorted prism through which wide swaths of Americans would perceive the disease through its flight.

In February 1983, the CDC reported the 1,000th case of AIDS in the United States. The disease was clearly on an alarming upward trajectory.

Scientific uncertainty was tacitly abetting its rise. The thirst for findings and answers among the science and health community was acute.

Officials at the CDC and elsewhere in the scientific and health community had their hands full grappling for resources, and laboring to produce scientific insight. As a consequence, no one in the U.S. science or public health establishment had given substantive thought to the global dimension of this emergent and virulent disease.

Joe McCormick would change that in the summer of 1983.

Upon arriving back at CDC headquarters in Atlanta, Georgia, following the health conference, the first thing McCormick did was to seek out Dr. Jim Curran. Curran, then thirty-eight years old, was a staid, mild-mannered, though politically savvy Ivy League CDC veteran of more than ten years. He was a family man, with a wife and two kids. Nothing in Curran's accomplished career at the CDC could have prepared him for the mantle he assumed as head of the Center's AIDS Task Force. He would find himself in the eye of some of the fiercest scientific and political battles ever attending any matter of health, science, or disease in U.S. history. Already a party to some of those maelstroms by the summer of 1983, Curran was desperate for hard data that might yield answers to the plethora of questions that still abounded.

McCormick relayed the chance encounter with Desmyter in Arlington. He told Curran that he wanted to lead a CDC-sponsored investigation into the heart of Zaire to test his hypothesis, and, if he was correct, to explore the dimensions of the disease in Africa.

Curran consented immediately. If McCormick found AIDS in Africa, and it had been there for some time, he would be able to unearth answers that had so far eluded Curran and his team: the disease's origins, its incubation period, and most importantly its definitive mode(s) of transmissibility. Curran assured McCormick he would have the financial and technical support needed to conduct the six-week investigation in Kinshasa.

While McCormick was eager to shed light on those big questions, and help Curran advance his agenda, there was much more to it. If his intuition was on target, there were thousands, quite possibly tens or hundreds of thousands, of AIDS victims in Africa. African leaders had to know about it. The world had to know about it.

McCormick enlisted Sheila Mitchell, an experienced virologist well schooled in administering and assessing blood samples, to join him. Shortly before leaving, he got a call from John Bennett, the head of the epidemiology program at the CDC, asking him to link up with other interested parties. Among those with whom McCormick would soon join forces was Dr. Peter Piot, who was leading a Belgian team with the same agenda. Then in his mid-thirties, Piot had already earned an international reputation as something of a prodigy, making his mark on the same Ebola investigation that had brought McCormick to Zaire in 1976. McCormick knew, respected, and was fond of his younger, passionate colleague. Piot, it turned out, like Desmyter, had seen African AIDS cases in Belgium, and he had made the connection, perhaps even before McCormick.

The American-Belgian team arrived in Kinshasa in mid-September. On each of McCormick's sojourns in Zaire's capital, it seemed there was always a fresh crisis of some sort brewing. This time there had just been a massive devaluation of the Zairean currency. McCormick, Piot, and his colleagues felt like "mafiosi" as they strolled out of their hotels with suitcases full of money on their way to a Greek restaurant to go over the team's strategy the night of their arrival.

The next day McCormick met with Zaire's health minister, Dr. Tshibasu, a tall man with graying hair who cut an elegant and somewhat reserved figure. McCormick's reception was cordial, but stern. Tshibasu asserted that existing health issues—including malaria, malnutrition, diarrhea, tuberculosis, sleeping sickness, and measles—were already overwhelming the national health system. He would be happy to cooperate, but he warned in polished French, "Don't count on finding much interest or support from us for the problem you are interested in. . . . We can't even cope with the ordinary problems I just told you about."

With Tshibasu's consent, the team was afforded comprehensive access to Mama Yemo Hospital, named after the mother of Zaire's former dictatorial leader Mobutu Sese Seko, in Kinshasa. One of the nation's largest health facilities, Mama Yemo was a vast structure with high, rusting tin roofs and dark cement floors stained, McCormick would write, with "countless miseries." Each ward was able to house about thirty beds. Most of the mattresses were stuffed with cotton and grass, and many wards didn't have mattresses at all. There were few bathrooms, and they rarely functioned. Fitful moans and wails punctured the heavy African air that wafted through Mama Yemo, echoing throughout the hospital's halls.

On their first day at Mama Yemo, the team moved through the hospital's wards examining patients. It would be weeks before Sheila Mitchell could provide technical confirmation that the patients were infected with

AIDS. But to McCormick, Mitchell's tests were almost academic. He could tell that AIDS had struck Kinshasa with impunity. He strode through the wards and counted dozens of women, their hair fallen out, unable to move, emaciated to fifty or sixty pounds, their faces "sallow and eyes sunken, lips studded with raw sores, tongues encrusted with yeast infection . . . livid, bulging blotches of Kaposi's sarcoma," a cancer of the blood vessels of the skin common in AIDS patients.

Among the sea of dying patients McCormick met during the investigation, none remains more transfixed in his memory than Yema, a twenty-one-year-old woman brought to Mama Yemo by her mother. Years before, Yema's family had moved from Zaire's rural hillside to La Cité, a sprawling and densely populated slum in the middle of Kinshasa packed with countless houses made of wood, tin, cement, mud, and cardboard, hoping to save some money to move on. With Yema's father gone for long stretches looking for work, the family was left behind to contend with want and hunger.

After the family had exhausted all of its options, Yema joined the thousands of other femmes libres in La Cité, exchanging sex for money, goods, or gifts. Her work provided food for her family, but by the time she was twenty Yema had already had two abortions. She had also contracted the virus that would later be dubbed HIV.

At first she had sick spells. Later the severe coughing and chills became incapacitating. Eventually, Yema could not rise from bed. She was a young woman, barely an adult, but physically unable to stand. Her mother had tried to care for her, she explained to the workers at Mama Yemo. But there was nothing more she could do, she cried, and so she brought her daughter to the hospital—to die.

The hardened "disease cowboy" had to fight back tears "of anger and frustration" on more than one occasion. He had never seen anything as devastating, and there was absolutely nothing he could do about it. He clung to the one pillar of hope that would sustain and drive him: "if we could understand the processes we were observing, someone, somewhere, might find some solution."

Slowly, the data began coming in from Mitchell's blood tests, validating McCormick's worst fears. Mitchell's work provided McCormick with the proof he knew he would need to buttress his case back in Atlanta. It was a job well done. The immediate sense of satisfaction, though, gave way to a staggering personal remembrance: 1979 in Nzara, Sudan.

Of course, in that act of desperation back in 1979, McCormick had had his friend Roy Baron give him a transfusion with blood from Ebola survivors. The episode, he had presumed, was history, a tale to tell over whiskey on a ski trip or in the field with colleagues. But AIDS was flourishing in Africa. In trying to save himself from Ebola, had McCormick infected himself with AIDS? He had a familiar sinking feeling.

He had Mitchell test his blood. When the results came back negative, McCormick felt like he had won the lottery, twice.

With Mitchell's blood test results, there was no denying that AIDS had already become rampant in Kinshasa. But it wasn't just the disease's prevalence that struck the group. They noticed a roughly one-to-one prevalence ratio between males and females; that is, as many females were infected as males. Transmission, it appeared, had been occurring almost entirely through heterosexual contact. All of the surveillance work, interviews, and other epidemiology confirmed the fact. To the team it seemed irrefutable.

Immediately, the team moved to draft and publish the results of their findings, with Piot as the drafter and McCormick the senior author. Eager to share their groundbreaking findings with the international health community, they submitted the paper to *The New England Journal of Medicine*. The journal's peer review panel, however, rejected it. Another dozen or so journals similarly refused to publish the team's findings, all incredulous that the disease was heterosexual. To the team's outrage, the paper went unpublished for almost an entire year before it was finally included in *The Lancet* in July 1984.

Such a scenario was emblematic of the misperception that framed the international scientific community's discourse on the epidemic through the mid-1980s. Only months before McCormick and his team set out for Kinshasa, in April 1983, John Maddox, the editor of England's prestigious journal *Nature*, drafted an editorial entitled, "No Need to Panic About AIDS." He cautioned the scientific community not to exaggerate what seemed to Maddox a "perhaps non-existing condition," and chided the "pathetic promiscuity of homosexuals." Even prominent men of science were wont to reach hasty, stigma-laden conclusions. In those early years the facts were all too often subsumed in cursory judgments and ill-conceived contention.

The reception by the scientific community was as painful as it was perplexing to McCormick. His findings were not merely data points on a scientific paper, but images forever etched in his memory of human suffering, of young women emaciated to skin and bones, left alone to their demise. He was outraged, but compelled to press on.

Upon arriving home in Atlanta in early November, he sought out his old mentor, Dr. Bill Foege, the legendary, soft-spoken, but quietly forceful director of the CDC. Many years earlier, McCormick had done his residency under Foege. As director, Foege held a post that was scientific, but also political. McCormick admired Foege, estimating that few at his senior level were able to navigate between the two demands with greater dexterity and integrity.

Foege's directorship was coming to an end, though. Fortuitously, his replacement, a Reagan appointee named Dr. James Mason, was at CDC headquarters the day McCormick approached Foege with his findings. Foege perused McCormick's results. He was deeply alarmed. The team had demonstrated that AIDS had secured an ominous foothold in Africa. Most notable of the findings was that the disease was transmitted almost entirely through heterosexual contact in Africa. It had obvious ramifications for the burgeoning U.S. epidemic. It also meant that AIDS wasn't an issue for subpopulations in Africa—the entire population was vulnerable. The worst-case scenario was imponderable. McCormick and his colleagues, it seemed, had discovered a pandemic in its nascence.

At CDC, things began to move with a sense of gravity and urgency. Foege convened an extended group of senior officials including Mason and Curran in his spacious office at CDC headquarters. They dialed the number for Dr. Edward Brandt, the assistant secretary of the Department of Health and Human Services, or HHS. With Brandt on the speakerphone, Foege turned the call over to his junior colleague. McCormick carefully spelled out the details of the investigative effort, the sort of research that had been done, the data, and the team's conclusions.

It took several minutes for McCormick to complete his presentation. He had woven, he estimated, an airtight yarn. The denouement arrived when McCormick declared: AIDS is rampant in Africa and it is heterosexual.

The group in Atlanta sat eagerly anticipating an answer. On the other end of the phone: a long silence.

Finally, Brandt spoke up. "I don't believe it," McCormick remembered him saying. "You must have got it all wrong. . . . There must be another explanation for your findings." He asked if McCormick had considered other vectors, such as mosquitoes. In other words, could mosquitoes be transmitting the disease, as with malaria?

"Mosquitoes," McCormick later wrote, "were obviously easier for him to talk about than sex." The scientists in Atlanta were aghast.

No one on the Atlanta end of the call knew much about Brandt. They knew only that, like Mason, he was a Reagan appointee. It was an administration that campaigned on a conservative platform. And while Foege and others knew that Reagan's health and science officials had politically conservative backgrounds, they were unsure just how far and how deeply those conservative tentacles extended.

AIDS had become a political hot potato, and the Reagan administration's strategy, to the extent there was one at all, was to avoid it. The subpopulations suffering in the United States were not part of Reagan's constituency. AIDS was sexuality and death: not the stuff that politicians are wont to gravitate toward. If the disease was truly heterosexual, then it was a bigger problem (at least politically) than the administration had estimated. They would have to address it, and they didn't want to do that unless they had to.

Understanding the stakes, McCormick continued to plead his case to Brandt. "I don't think the evidence supports that, sir. So far we've found very little disease in children. And children get just as many mosquito bites as adults—probably more," McCormick explained. "What we saw with the disease were definite chains of infection . . . clustering around sexual contact."

Brandt could not argue with the data, but, according to McCormick, he seemed "hell-bent" on settling on another theory to explain the disease's stronghold in Africa. The discussion went on for twenty minutes. Brandt proved immovable.

Foege hung up the phone. Dumbfounded, the group stared at each other, as if looking for confirmation that what had transpired had really gone on. It was, for McCormick, the grossest instance of politics over science and truth he had encountered in his career.

No one in Foege's office in Atlanta would yet know that in fact approximately forty thousand lives had already been lost, and 1 million infections had accrued around the globe.

With Foege's blessings, and McCormick's drive and gumption, leadership at the CDC persevered, intent on continuing the international effort that had been started. They were professionals. They were, perhaps, too professional.

With budget slashing the order of the day, all areas of the federal health effort were under siege, and the CDC was no exception. Foege calculated that he would be better off moving things around and making do with existing resources, rather than taking on a controversial and still largely unknown disease, and perhaps risking further cuts and wrath from the executive branch.

As public health officials went, Foege was a deft political operative. But he was able to measure himself against a very low bar in that regard. America's leading scientific and health officials were trained in science, medicine, and public health and were among the foremost technical experts in those fields in the world. Those who rose to positions of stature and power in public health and science, though, were generally ill schooled at the sort of political advocacy necessary to secure the resources and political capital they needed to effectively do their job.

The episode in the fall of 1983 was a classic instance. Foege and his entire team did the best they could within the system, but no one sought to jolt the system. No one cultivated relationships with the media or used it to scream about the team's findings or the significance of the disease's stronghold in Africa, the disturbing global dimension that had just been discovered. They did not forcefully lobby the administration or seek to galvanize domestic political constituencies to the issue.

Of course they were facing a panoply of problems and constraints: their budget was under siege, they did not have their own administration's support or leadership, they were struggling to amass resources for the wide range of prevalent U.S. domestic health problems, including the domestic AIDS epidemic brewing in the United States, and relatively little was known about the international dimension at the time.

McCormick would later assert that "by steadfastly refusing to acknowledge the true dimensions of the AIDS crisis, the Reagan administration made itself an ally of the virus." Brandt's negligence struck an ominous note at a seminal juncture.

It was a cause, in 1983, in search of a political champion.

On the memorably inauspicious morning of April 23, 1984, HHS Secretary Margaret Heckler stood at the podium at the department's headquarters in Washington, D.C., with Dr. Robert Gallo in tow, wearing a wide and sprightly smile. Gallo, the director of the eminent National Cancer Institute and one of the world's foremost experts on retroviruses, had earned his spot in the limelight next to Heckler, she announced, because he had officially "discovered" the virus that causes AIDS. It would be dubbed, shortly thereafter, the human immunodeficiency virus, or HIV.

Heckler's unbridled enthusiasm seemed to give the announcement great occasion, as did her buoyant pronouncements. "Today's discovery," she proclaimed, "represents the triumph of science over a dreadful disease." She suggested that the discovery would pave the way for a vaccine that would be ready for testing within two years.

Wild miscalculations would continue to abound through the year that followed.

In the summer of 1984, the McCormick/Piot article would be released in *The Lancet*. In addition, a handful of prominent epidemiologists had been drawn to the global dimension of the disease. One of them was Dr. Robert Biggar, who published a set of very bold estimates in *The Lancet* in that same year. Many more would follow, including Gallo himself.

The World Health Organization, or WHO, on the other hand, had extricated itself from global AIDS. An internal 1983 WHO memorandum stated that AIDS "is being well taken care of by some of the richest countries in the world where there is the manpower and the know-how and where most of the patients are to be found." It was of course, a grossly mistaken presumption on all accounts. WHO would have been a logical clearinghouse for the science—estimates of incidence and features of the disease, for example. Without WHO's participation, disparate sets of teams set out, intent on capturing data on the global dimension. The results would be divergent, leading to contention and chaos.

In April 1985, the CDC organized what would become the first International AIDS Conference, to be held in Atlanta, Georgia. It would attract approximately two thousand scientists, public health officials, and journalists, brought together with the aim of sharing knowledge, and reaching common ground and consensus.

Peter Piot had been working on a CDC-sponsored AIDS longitudinal study that McCormick had helped to set up in Kinshasa. Studying the disease in Africa, Piot had developed a keen sense for the urgency of the problem brewing. He was ecstatic about the opportunity in Atlanta. Piot had even encouraged several of his African colleagues to make the long journey. He believed that the experience would be of value in their work, and that their perspective would enrich the proceedings.

As the scientists took to the stage to present their findings, Piot watched, befuddled. Some of the world's most prominent scientists were presenting estimates of incidence of HIV in Africa that were absolutely stratospheric, off the charts. Some estimates purported that in certain regions of Uganda, children tested 66 percent positive for the virus; others suggested that 88 percent of the female prostitutes in Rwanda carried the virus. Robert Biggar of the U.S. National Cancer Institute estimated that between 1982 and 1984, roughly half of the Kenyan population had been infected with the disease.

Piot had hoped that the international scientific community would acknowledge the severity and magnitude of the epidemic. He had been living in Africa for a year and he knew from firsthand experience, however, that the numbers presented here were gross overestimations. Confounded and despondent, Piot kept a close eye on his African colleagues. Their goodwill and support was the bedrock upon which his presence was made possible in Zaire.

When Harvard scientist Max Essex averred that the origins of the disease could be traced back to monkeys in central Africa, Piot's trepidation grew. Sure enough, a group of journalists found their way to Piot's African colleagues and asked them, "Is it true? Do Africans have sex with monkeys?" The African scientists were aghast.

Hours later, sitting alone in a stairwell, Piot was utterly dejected. "This is a disaster," he said to himself.

Shortly after the conference it would be verified that almost all of the estimates proffered were wildly erroneous. The blood tests used—still terribly unrefined and clearly inadequate—yielded positive results for traces of malaria and other unrelated pathogens. All of these cases were captured in the results, inflating the AIDS estimates. Almost all of the African populations tested had, at some time, been exposed to malaria in varying capacities. It was a wonder, then, journalist Laurie Garrett wrote, that the estimates did not report even higher levels of incidence.

The immediate reaction was panic—it seemed all of a sudden that the continent was about to erupt in a terrible conflagration. While the inaccuracy of the estimates would be redressed in short order, the social and political fallout of the conference would generate debilitating consequences that would reverberate for years to come. The inflated estimates would breed skepticism among U.S. policy makers, the public health establishment, the media, and the public.

On the African side, political leaders, ever sensitive, particularly in light of the imperial legacy and the stereotypes they knew to abound in the

West, grew incensed at the false estimates. "African AIDS reports are a new form of hate campaign," Kenyan President Daniel arap Moi fumed. Already grappling with crises like drought, famine, civil war, poverty, and a panoply of existing health issues, African leaders were furious about western scientists grandstanding and painting a near apocalyptic depiction of Africa. The inflated estimates would plant seeds of skepticism that would help breed denial among the continent's leaders for the next decade and a half. African denial would, in turn, serve as a crutch for U.S. inaction.

When the estimates were later brought down to single-digit incidence rates, the immediate reaction was one of relief—"It's not as bad as we thought." With that sentiment as an undercurrent, what little attention Africa had garnered was seamlessly redirected within America's borders, where incidence was escalating precipitously.

———•—•———

While no one could claim a commanding grip on the magnitude of the pandemic, by 1986 certain progress had been made. The misestimates proffered in Atlanta had been debunked and more reasonable and accurate ones offered in their place. The research effort that McCormick had worked to establish in Kinshasa, Zaire, had been up and running since the middle of 1984. Called Project SIDA (the French acronym for AIDS), it was yielding a great deal of useful data. Finally, WHO had taken up the issue and established the Special Program on AIDS, or SPA. Its leader, Dr. Jonathan Mann, would in time become a pioneer and a legend. Already by 1986, he was a credible and forceful advocate for the world's response to the pandemic.

Despite the Reagan administration's continued refusal to address the disease, Congress was able to ensure that funds for the domestic epidemic were scaled up. Priority number one was vaccine development. A vaccine would, of course, have positive ramifications for the global dimension of the disease, but the politics and constituencies driving the effort were almost entirely domestic-centric. The global dimension was not considered at all, and had received entirely no funding or political leadership.

That would change in 1986. A small handful of figures in the Congress were starting to take notice. Primarily through the efforts of Pat Leahy, the towering, gray-haired senator from Vermont and a staunch internationalist whose politics leant to the left, Congress was able to appropriate an inaugural sum for global AIDS.

By the end of that year a quarter of a million people had died of AIDS worldwide. Almost 4 million had been infected with HIV. The total U.S. appropriation for global AIDS in 1986: $2 million.

Leahy and other early champions, including Representative David Obey from Wisconsin, knew that it was a woefully inadequate amount. But the White House was entirely disinterested, if not averse, to the effort, and it was notoriously difficult to create any new line item on the budget, particularly in the foreign assistance bucket. It did not help that this was taking place against the backdrop of the gaping deficits being generated under Reagan's aggressive supply-side economic plan. It was, they hoped, a start. And a most needed one at that.

But where would it go?

Now that Congress had appropriated the money, what branch of the government, what department or agency, would tackle global AIDS? There was no one obvious candidate.

In time, AIDS would begin to eviscerate national economies. At the outset, however, the Treasury Department, the area of the U.S. government empowered to oversee matters of international finance and economic development, was not interested. Treasury had its hands full managing what were becoming unprecedented budget deficits. In the Reagan era, framed by the Cold War, "globalization" had yet to catch on. The world was still divided into two camps, and the idea that the world's economic well-being was interwoven among all the world's nations was weak in currency. Officials weren't accustomed to thinking in terms of "nontraditional" economic issues like health or the environment.

At the Department of Defense, Reagan's hawks had their hands full defeating the "evil empire." Managing the U.S.-Soviet great power rivalry and the NATO alliance, building up the U.S. missile arsenal, developing Star Wars and deploying U.S. intermediate range ballistic missiles in the European theater kept Defense busy through the mid-1980s. In a prescient 1980 article in Foreign Affairs, entitled "Redefining Security," Richard Ullman argued that the strictly politico-military conception of "security" ignored other pressing "nontraditional" security issues. In time, forward thinkers would emerge willing to push Defense to revisit Ullman's call for a "redefinition" to include threats such as global AIDS. In the 1980s, though, the idea was ahead of its time.

As the diplomatic arm of the U.S. government, the State Department was able to highlight and prioritize emergent international crises and champion resource allocation for them. It was able to press foreign leaders to engage matters of import to the U.S. foreign policy agenda. Yet few at State, even through the late 1980s, demonstrated serious interest in upgrading U.S. policy to tackle the burgeoning pandemic. A handful of ambassadors voiced concern through the State hierarchy on several occasions. But they were more the exception than the rule. At a critical point in the Cold War and on the eve of a "New World Order," U.S. diplomatic capacity was stretched and focused elsewhere.

In the late 1980s, the Soviet Union, East Germany, and their satellite "minions" launched a propaganda campaign in Africa, claiming that the CIA had created the disease to kill black Africans. Leaders at State's Africa Bureau were shaken by cables that seemed to forewarn of "apocalypse," but they spent more time and energy digesting the reports and debunking the Soviet-led propaganda campaign than pressing for U.S. involvement or spurring African leaders to lead. State wasn't opposed to U.S. engagement, one bureaucratic operative explained, "it was more benign neglect."

The Department of Health and Human Services, or HHS, seemed to many the logical place to house the U.S. response. HHS, though, would join the leading U.S. departments in passing the proverbial buck on global AIDS.

Among the most stung, HHS found itself waylaid by the Reagan budget cuts. Assuming office, Reagan proclaimed, "Government doesn't solve problems, it subsidizes them." Adhering to his mantra, Reagan eviscerated the funds available to the department responsible for the health of the American people. From 1981 to 1983 Reagan slashed the HHS budget by approximately 25 percent. Amid the siege, HHS was doing all it could to fight America's biggest killers, heart disease and cancer. The domestic AIDS epidemic was thrown into the mix at a time that was less than propitious. The Department was overwhelmed.

Importantly, HHS's official mandate extends only so far as matters of "domestic" health. Paul DeLay, a longtime U.S. health official, later to become a leader in the U.S. response, remarked: "HHS was seen as not only not having the mandate, but not really understanding what was involved. . . . They didn't have the experience [necessary to tackle the problem]. How many people," DeLay asked, "at HHS have passports? How many had been to Africa?"

There was an arm of HHS, though, that was brimming with rough and tumble "virus hunters" who had spent more than their fair share of time in

Africa and other international locales. The CDC is the United States's center of technical excellence for disease surveillance. "Bug busters" like Joe McCormick had been all over the earth, searching for and combating emerging and reemerging infectious viruses. They knew how to identify them, how to conduct surveillance, and, when possible, how to control the outbreaks.

But CDC, like HHS and all the other aforementioned departments, had no international mandate per se. Dr. Kenneth Shine, former president of the Institute of Medicine, explained, "CDC has no international surveillance responsibility. The CDC operates under the assumption that if an outbreak of something occurs they will be called in to investigate." But international surveillance, let alone intervention, strictly speaking, was not a mandatory responsibility.

The calculus to fly McCormick and his colleagues halfway around the world and sponsor their investigations was generally driven by U.S. national interests. If there was an outbreak, even in a faraway locale, it behooved the U.S. scientific community to know about it so that they would be well schooled in the threat and thus able to protect the U.S. population at home and abroad. Funds were tight and humanitarian efforts were a luxury, not the norm. Congressional oversight generally saw to that. American taxpayers, after all, were funding CDC's activities.

"In the beginning," Dr. Helene Gayle, an African-American woman who would later oversee the CDC's global HIV/AIDS effort, explained, "because CDC primarily has a domestic mandate, a lot of what drove the ability to work in international settings was the fact that there were lessons to be learned from the international setting that could be used for domestic populations." The CDC would launch surveillance efforts in Zaire, and later Côte d'Ivoire and Azerbaijan. The CDC's surveillance work would yield insights that would benefit developing nations as they fought the pandemic in their own backyards. But the impetus driving the CDC's engagement had its origins in a domestic mandate and U.S. concerns.

There was a sense, anyhow, that the CDC was equipped to conduct surveillance and do research, but that was where their competency ended. What was needed abroad, global AIDS advocates argued, was intervention.

The CDC may not have been "set up" to lead interventions, but they had done it in the past, and they had done it with astounding success.

Counters Dr. Jeffrey Harris, a CDC official at the time, they "did it on smallpox, did it on diarrhea and immunization. They had done a good job."

AIDS demanded a more ambitious intervention, though, and resources were scant. Initiating an intervention effort would have been, or at least was perceived as being, extramandatory. CDC figures like Helene Gayle would expend a good deal of energy through the late 1980s and 1990s trying to expand CDC's efforts. But until the late 1990s, global AIDS was viewed as only one emergent health issue among a vast panoply of diseases and sicknesses already claiming millions of lives a year.

Early on, CDC's leadership could muster neither the foresight nor the political will or ingenuity to marshal the resources and political support to broaden its range of involvement. A decade and a half later, the CDC, like its parent department, HHS, would join the State Department in a loud chorus pleading for resources to expand its efforts in fighting the pandemic. At the moment, though, when their engagement might have done the most to preempt the pandemic's global explosion, all of these centers of government were willing simply to pass the buck. And the buck—all 2 million of them—would stop, it turned out, at the United States Agency for International Development, or USAID.

USAID was created by the Kennedy administration in November 1961 to provide developmental assistance to countries in need. Like the Peace Corps, it was an outgrowth of the "New Frontier" ethos of international service. The agency was quickly consumed, though, by the geopolitical context into which it was born. All major U.S. international initiatives during the Cold War were to a great extent either a function of, or greatly influenced by, the overarching U.S. foreign policy imperative of the epoch: containment of the Soviet Union.

USAID, though perhaps born of a noble impulse, would prove pervious to that phenomenon. USAID's grant making and developmental assistance functions became yet another weapon in the U.S. arsenal to fight the Soviet Union. Grants and assistance were doled out not on the basis of need, but to countries friendly to the United States. Assistance was used as leverage both to keep countries in the U.S. camp as well as to woo countries away from the Soviet bloc.

Confusing the agency's mission further, it would come to award hundreds of millions of dollars in contracts to U.S. companies or nongovernmental organizations (NGOs). As such, a veritable cottage industry grew around the agency, competing for money and becoming a political lobby in the beltway.

Financed with billions of dollars a year, and with missions and deeply dedicated foreign officers, the agency was able to do significant good all over the developing world. By the mid-1980s, however, the agency's clarity of mandate, its operational efficiency, its credibility, and its sense of purpose were all foundering.

A decade earlier, in the 1970s, health was added to its long and extremely diverse list of priorities including, but not limited to, agriculture, famine, democracy promotion, family planning, and education. By the mid-1980s, USAID's leadership began attempting to upgrade the agency's health effort. Dr. Kenneth Bart, a prominent CDC official, was brought on to head the agency's Health Office. Funds were scant though, and were disbursed based primarily on geopolitical considerations. What little remained was meted out to the multitudinous array of offices and divisions at the agency. The funds available to Bart and his Office of Health were mostly earmarked for child-related programs. The agency's polio immunization effort and its support of the development for a malaria vaccine were among their most prominent efforts for a long time. Child-centric health issues, which circumvented issues of sex or dubious behavior, were viewed by most at the agency as a safe sell, a particularly important consideration in the conservative Reagan years.

As a consequence of all these factors, in tackling the world's major health problems and crises, Bart and his Office of Health were able to pack only a very meek punch. And though HIV/AIDS had been an emerging global crisis for several years, "we weren't rehearsed on infectious disease," let alone HIV/AIDS, Paul DeLay said of USAID's health effort.

If, as the Chinese philosopher Sun-Tsu suggested, every battle is won or lost before it is even fought, then the U.S. response to the pandemic would be framed from the get-go to fight a losing battle. Enlisting USAID to tackle the pandemic was, in the words of a former National Security Council director, "like asking the JV team to come and play the Giants."

The decision of just what to do with those inaugural $2 million would fall, along with the very mantle of commandeering the U.S. response to the burgeoning pandemic, into the lap of a neophyte entirely green to the world of Washington bureaucracy and politics, a thirty-year-old fresh-faced doctor hired to work on diarrheal disease with no experience in AIDS.

The Prism of the U.S. Experience, Absence of Leadership

Without that weekly trip to the capital, Jeffrey Harris would have gone stir-crazy. Stationed throughout 1984 in the "Middle of Nowhere," Bangladesh, with his young wife, Judy, herself an accomplished, up-and-coming doctor, Harris was working on cholera vaccine trials for the CDC. A pediatrician's son, at age three Harris had boldly proclaimed to his extended family in Dallas, Texas, that he, too, was going to be a doctor. Something of a prodigy, Harris entered the University of Texas Medical School at eighteen years of age and graduated at twenty-two. A thirst for adventure and a strong sense of moral purpose—Christianity had played a big role in his upbringing—brought him to the CDC's Epidemiology Intelligence Service, or EIS, where he envisioned an "exotic" and adventure-filled life of helping people in need.

Harris's romantic vision ebbed, in short order, into the spartan grind of his new daily reality. In a rural outpost, hours from Dhaka, the country's capital, Harris made do in a small cinder block house with a concrete floor. His quarters were envied among those in the community, though, for having a toilet, a rare luxury.

Because there was a well-established field station focusing on diarrheal disease, Bangladesh had attracted a stream of young CDC officials. Few, however, took the time to learn the language, immerse themselves in Bangladeshi culture, and cultivate meaningful relationships with locals. Jeff and Judy were determined to forge a different path. Upon their arrival, they lodged at a local monastery for six weeks, and immersed themselves in Banghali, taking lessons for ten hours a day. Eventually they became proficient. Gregarious and kind, they became popular in their new community.

There was little activity around their small hamlet, though, and so they made it a habit to venture into Dhaka almost every weekend, hazarding the two-and-a-half-hour journey in order to preserve their sanity. After a ferry ride, Jeff and Judy would hop into a shuttle, a rugged white Toyota van, well suited to tackle the inclement weather and muddy, bumpy, inchoate roads they traversed on their way.

The journeys gave Harris time to read. With a curious intellect, he was determined to stay abreast of the latest developments in science and public health. One summer morning, on Harris's weekly trip into the capital, he stumbled upon an article in *The Lancet* submitted by Dr. Robert Biggar. The later-notorious article had posited wildly exaggerated estimates of AIDS incidence in Africa.

Years earlier, in 1981, Harris had read that first CDC report chronicling the first AIDS cases in the United States. Harris remembered his reaction: "I turned to the intern and said, 'This is going to be a big deal.' It was interesting that [even] as a non-epidemiologist, I picked up on this."

Now, halfway across the world, Biggar's article made a whopping impression on Harris. Though eager to follow the evolution of the epidemic, Harris was on the fast track at the CDC, and content to stay in Bangladesh to continue his work. But by March 1986, Harris's tour of duty ended. After a few years in the field, he and Judy were eager to get back to the States, where a prestigious fellowship awaited Judy at Johns Hopkins, and comfortable beds and functioning bathrooms promised a welcome change.

The CDC had awarded Harris a grant that would fund his master's in public health. Upon arriving back home Harris learned that his grant had been rescinded, a casualty of budget cuts. He still could have had his pick of research fellowships, but he didn't want to be in a laboratory. He wanted something a little more program-oriented, something a little more tangible.

The CDC old-boy network kicked into gear to take care of one of the center's up-and-coming stars. A senior colleague mentioned that an old-time CDC veteran, Dr. Kenneth Bart, had recently become the head of the Health Office at USAID. Harris had heard Bart deliver a lecture on measles a few years earlier in Seattle. He had been impressed by Bart's bearing, his passion, and the force of his personality. He conveyed a strong sense of mission and purpose unencumbered, it seemed, by self-doubt.

In need of a job that would challenge and advance him, Harris sought out his older colleague at USAID. He was invited to come in for a meeting at the agency's headquarters, then in Rosslyn, Virginia, on Wilson Boulevard in a tall building with ugly green glass. Sitting across from Bart, in his relatively spacious seventh-floor office, in short order Harris won Bart's favor. By meeting's end, Bart had offered Harris a post at the agency, as head of the diarrheal disease program, Harris's specialty.

"By the way," Harris remembered Bart asking, "have you read anything about this HIV/AIDS stuff?"

"Oh, yeah," Harris said, "I've been reading Biggar's stuff on Africa."

"Well, we want you to do that one day a week. We want you to coordinate our AIDS program one day a week. It's twenty percent time and we think after six months it will go away. . . . Trust me," Bart assured him, "we're sure this will blow over."

Harris had been on the job for only days in early September 1986 when the end of the government's fiscal year was approaching. It was a time for bureaucrats to make sure that they had used every last coin in their coffer. With some loose change available in Harris's budget, he scurried to put together a tour of the African continent for the middle of the month.

Meeting with African health officials and touring hospitals all over sub-Saharan Africa, it became clear to Harris that contrary to Bart's assurance, AIDS wasn't going away. In fact, it was just beginning.

When he arrived back in Baltimore that fall, he told Judy, "This job is going to kill me, but it's going to be the best job I've ever had."

Jeffrey Harris, at thirty years of age, was appointed head of the incipient division of HIV/AIDS at USAID. It was to become the locus of the U.S. government's response to the burgeoning pandemic. It was a division of one, just Harris.

Harris found he had little company as he fixed his sights beyond America's borders. The rest of the country, when it thought about AIDS, by and large found itself consumed with the epidemic exploding at home. From the outset, the U.S. response to *global* AIDS would be conceptualized and perceived through the distinct prism of the U.S. experience.

When the neighborhood is on fire, the question goes, do you tend to your neighbor's house first, or your own? "We are fighting a war here," declared Emilio Carrillo, a New York City hospital official. It was a war that public health officials and concerned policy makers would continue to lose throughout the 1980s.

Throughout the decade, the epidemic proliferated all over the United States, leaving a searing trail of death in its wake. On July 8, 1982, the CDC reported 452 diagnosed cases of AIDS, and 177 AIDS deaths. By decade's end there were almost 115,000 diagnosed cases, and more than 70,000 deaths. By the end of 1995, roughly 500,000 diagnosed cases had accrued, and more than 300,000 Americans had died of AIDS.

The public policy around the domestic epidemic became a political firestorm. Policy makers championing increased resources met strong resistance from the White House and conservative figures in Congress. The media had much to write about and report on with the science, the policy, and the cultural dimensions of the domestic crisis. AIDS activists groups, such as the AIDS Coalition to Unleash Power, or ACT UP, the high-profile and flamboyant group founded in February 1987, generated controversy and attention. They had grass roots, though, and spoke out almost exclusively for local constituencies.

The United States was waging a war, and to those fighting it, the battle lines seemed to be firmly entrenched within U.S. territory. "How can anyone think globally, when the United States is burning?" most who were involved in the issue in the 1980s asked.

In 1987, the fire metaphor turned literal, when a group of miscreant arsonists torched the home of an Arcadia, Florida, family with three HIV-positive hemophiliac sons. It was only one of a wave of hate-based or violent acts perpetrated in the mid- to late 1980s. The family was able to escape, but the nation was unable to escape the smoke-filled cloud of stigma attached to the disease.

It was not a new phenomenon for U.S. society. Harvard University public health expert Allan Brandt wrote in his authoritative work *No Magic Bullet:* "Since the late nineteenth century, venereal disease has been used as a symbol for a society characterized by a corrupt sexuality. In particular," he wrote, gonorrhea, syphilis, and other venereal diseases all "came to be seen as an affliction of those who willfully violated the moral code, a punishment for sexual irresponsibility."

AIDS, even more so than its predecessors, seemed to strike those engaging in American society's least tolerated, most hot-button activities: promiscuous homosexual sex, prostitution, IV drug use. Perceptions of the modes of the disease's transmissibility met a collective pathology of great anxiety and unease because so little was verifiably known about the disease. It was a recipe for hysteria and hate.

Levels of stigma in the United States ranged from passive to virulent. Seventy-five percent of respondents to a *New York Times*/CBS poll in 1988 said they had "no sympathy for homosexuals suffering from AIDS." Nineteen percent of those polled said that they had no sympathy for any AIDS patients at all, even transfusion recipients and infants.

With America burning, and the disease shrouded in a smoky haze of misperception and anxiety, Americans, by and large, were either fighting for scarce resources to put out the inferno, or sticking their heads in the sand, preferring not to think about an uncomfortable stigma-laden disease. There was no groundswell, no impetus, from American society at large to address the global dimension of the catastrophe percolating. To engage the pandemic in its nascence, then, would have taken foresight, will, and political courage—the stuff of leadership—from the country's highest political echelon. None was forthcoming.

Ronald Reagan would preside over the "discovery" of the disease and its flight into a full-blown pandemic. Through his presidency, he would barely mention the term "AIDS."

At a Pediatric AIDS Foundation dinner in January 1990, a star-studded audience listened as a public statement submitted by former President Ronald Reagan was delivered at the gala. "We can all learn and grow in our lives," the statement began, "and I've learned that all kinds of people can get AIDS, even children." It was a mea culpa directed toward the AIDS community. As apologies go, however, it was a decidedly obtuse and tepid one.

There is no evidence to suggest that the fortieth president of the United States, the former B-movie star turned world leader, dubbed the "great communicator," who brought a stunningly simple ideology to world affairs and the role of government in American life, ever really understood that a seismic pandemic was generating steam on his watch.

"It's a virus like measles? But it doesn't go away?" Reagan asked his doctor in 1985. "Maybe the Lord brought down this plague," he wondered aloud in the spring of 1987.

Two years after Reagan's assistant director at HHS, Edward Brandt, rebuffed Joe McCormick, the disease cowboy received an invitation to a tented gala benefit by the Potomac River in Washington, D.C., thrown by Elizabeth Taylor and funded by a wealthy Japanese businessman. The historic summer evening in 1985 would later come to be known as the infamous "Meeting on the Potomac." It was there that Ronald Reagan, four years after the CDC introduced the disease to the public health and science community, acknowledged publicly for the first time the existence of AIDS.

The benefit was an ostentatious affair. McCormick was bemused to be included in the potpourri of guests—numbering roughly four hundred—including movie stars, industrial titans, lobbyists, journalists, and scientific luminaries. Having spent a good portion of the two previous years setting up a research effort in Kinshasa, and deeply frustrated at the dearth of leadership and support from the administration, McCormick was skeptical about what the unusual evening might bring.

Taking everything in, he noticed a familiar tall bearded figure enter the tent and felt a jolt at the thunderous applause directed toward the man. Surgeon General C. Everett Koop was a conservative and a well-known opponent of abortion, but he was also a staunch and anomalous champion of AIDS engagement and education within the administration. The gala was thrown to honor Koop's leadership on AIDS education.

The president was tightly managed by a small cadre of hard-line conservatives, including senior domestic policy advisors Gary Bauer and Patrick Buchanan. Reagan's handlers had systematically stymied Koop's efforts to publicly address the disease.

The administration's core constituency of Christian conservatives, including a myriad of notable figures, spoke out vociferously, and on occasion venomously, against government involvement in AIDS. Perhaps most famously, the Rev. Jerry Falwell proclaimed in a 1983 television sermon: "AIDS is God's punishment. . . . The scripture is clear," Falwell preached. "We do reap it in our flesh when we violate the laws of God." Reagan aide Patrick Buchanan joined Falwell, pronouncing: "The poor homosexuals—they have declared war upon Nature, and now Nature is exacting awful retribution." Ronald Godwin, director of the Moral Majority, averred: "What I see is a commitment to spend our tax dollars on research to allow these diseased homosexuals to go back to their perverted practices without any standards of accountability." Imposing a vituperative, ill-informed brand of moralism on policy, these conservative leaders were making it clear to the administration that there would be a political price to pay for engaging AIDS.

It was a message that had been heard at 1600 Pennsylvania Avenue, and managed by Bauer, Buchanan, and other operatives. On the few occasions he was able to circumvent the cordon, Koop found the president very inquisitive and eager to learn and to do more. The surgeon general remembered that the president's handlers advised against engagement, however. AIDS was affecting marginalized subpopulations, and they told the president it was a "lose, lose" issue.

Reagan would not utter a word on the matter, even as it became a hotbed political and cultural item in the national discourse, until the summer night he took to the podium by the Potomac. As he stood to address the crowd, he received only a lukewarm reception. In fact, there were a few boos and hisses from various pockets of the intimate crowd. It was an enormous rarity that Reagan would be exposed to such a reaction, let alone at a luxurious gala.

His remarks in honor of the surgeon general were warm, brief, and extremely vague. He acknowledged the existence of the disease and told his audience that AIDS was a public health problem. He did not speak to his administration's policy, and did not allude to the global dimension.

Two years later, on April 2, 1987, with nary a mention made in the interim, Reagan again took to a podium, this time at the College of Physicians in Philadelphia, to deliver his first "major speech" on the epidemic. He surprised critics, calling the disease "public enemy number one." By then the epidemic's scope and lethality could no longer be ignored. Unwilling to engage the notion of an administration policy, or to tackle issues like education and "safe sex," Reagan called for abstinence.

One month later, on May 4, 1987, during an issues lunch in the Cabinet Room, the subject of AIDS came up again. The president mused, "I saw a TV show on AIDS in Africa the other day—they spread it there like the common cold." No one responded and the discussion turned to a memo submitted by a Reagan aide proposing the sequestration of AIDS patients in the U.S.

C. Everett Koop believed that Reagan's handlers were the crux of the problem. Koop felt that to Bauer, Buchanan, and others, global AIDS "was something over there." According to Koop the sentiment was: If we're not going to worry about it in this country, why should we worry about a bunch of black people over there who have the same thing.

By 1987, Reagan had appointed a Presidential Advisory Council on AIDS. It proved an empty political gesture, though, as the administration repeatedly bypassed the council's recommendations for an upgraded U.S.

response. In one of its later reports, the council pointed the administration to the global dimension of the disease, and suggested that early engagement would be critical. Despite the warnings from experts at WHO, testimony from his own agency, USAID, and his own presidential council, the global dimension never registered on the administration's agenda throughout Reagan's tenure.

In early June 1987, sitting vice president and presidential candidate George Herbert Walker Bush arrived at the Hilton Hotel in Washington, D.C., to participate in the Third Annual International AIDS Conference. The number of those participating had swelled from around two thousand in Atlanta two years earlier to more than ten thousand scientists, public health officials, policy makers, and journalists.

Bush was unlike his predecessor in many respects. He was an internationalist, who had served as U.S. ambassador to China and the United Nations and had been the director of the CIA. Though most of the power base in the Republican party expected Bush to provide them with a third Reagan term, Bush was his own man, and somewhat more centrist than his wildly popular predecessor.

In short, Bush seemed an outstanding candidate to grasp the gravity of the emerging global catastrophe, and make AIDS a global priority. His participation at the International AIDS Conference was an excellent opportunity to emerge as an international leader on the issue. It was not to be.

When Bush approached the podium to address the crowd, throngs turned their back to him in protest of the administration's negligence. Activists from ACT UP held aloft protest signs. Hundreds of scientists, in an impromptu demonstration of solidarity and exasperation, joined those in protest.

In the presidential campaign of the following year, Pat Robertson brought the issue to the fore, forcing Republican candidates to choose sides. Scalded by the inauspicious introduction in Washington that prior summer, and intent on maintaining his standing with the conservative power base in the party, Bush veered away. On global AIDS, at least, he would never come back.

The internationalist president could not, in his wildest dreams, have conceived of a more dynamic international political landscape against which to assume the presidency. The Berlin Wall would fall soon after his inauguration, a prominent domino auguring the ripple effect that would culminate, on Bush's watch, in the peaceable dissolution of the Soviet Union and the end of the Cold War. It was a world transformed, and it was Bush's. Later he would preside as commander in chief over the biggest U.S. military mobilization since Vietnam in the Persian Gulf War.

It was an epoch for the history books, and Bush jumped in eager to realize his vision of a peaceful, prosperous, democratic "New World Order." There was much to be done in managing the transition from old threats, though scant time, or perhaps inclination, to consider emergent ones.

In July 1990, in Bush's second summer in office, the National Intelligence Council, or NIC, essentially the think tank arm of the CIA, exploring "new" post–Cold War threats, released a report that managed to slip under the radar screen of almost every decision maker in the U.S. federal government. Entitled "The Global AIDS Disaster," the report estimated that the pandemic would yield up to 45 million infections by 2000. There were not that many combatants killed in WWI, WWII, Korea, and Vietnam combined, wrote journalist Bart Gellman. (The report would underestimate the actual tally of cumulative global infections. By the end of 2000 there were close to 55 million.) The reaction, according to the principal author Kenneth Brown, was "indifference."

The NIC report would never get to the president's desk. The issue never registered as a priority for the Bush I administration.

The administration did, however, have a flagship policy on international AIDS. Rather than tackling the catastrophe, though, it stipulated that all foreigners with HIV or AIDS were to be kept out of the United States. It was a policy born in part from irrational fears about the modes of transmission, and in part from a grave concern that an influx of HIV-positive visitors or immigrants would put a tremendous burden on the U.S. national health system at a time when it was encountering gaping budget cuts and attempting to cope with the disease at home.

The policy summoned domestic activists to begin to look beyond America's borders, heralding in some respects the birth of the domestic community's global consciousness. When HIV-positive foreigners were precluded from entering the United States to attend the 1990 International AIDS Conference in San Francisco, many foreign scientists and public health officials boycotted. There was a strong, though still a fringe, movement among U.S. activists to boycott the conference as well, in deference to their foreign counterparts. In 1992 the pressure from all quarters escalated, and after much deliberation the conference was moved from Boston to Amsterdam. It would never return to the United States.

Then an assistant secretary of state, Princeton Lyman, a seasoned diplomat at the State Department and soon to become the U.S. ambassador to South Africa, explained the U.S. response to global AIDS through the Bush years: "There wasn't a lot of attention [paid]. It wasn't a big issue in those days." There were a lot of resources and attention devoted to the domestic dimension, but the linchpin of U.S. global AIDS policy through the Bush I years was the "policy of keeping people out—keep it away from us. So, there was very little U.S. money going into it."

Though by marginal increments, the little that was appropriated did increase during Bush's tenure from the $2 million allotment made available in 1986 to a baseline annual commitment of around $120 million for 1993. The increases happened not because of, but rather in spite of the Bush administration, which never demonstrated meaningful support.

The leadership came from an emerging cohort of congressional figures, led by a fiery, liberal representative from the state of Washington. With a barrel chest, a sturdy frame, and a thick head of white hair, Jim McDermott looked the part of the populist-legislator unafraid to speak his mind. Appearances, in this case at least, did not deceive. McDermott was a doctor, a physician-come-legislator, in the small but notable tradition of American politicians dating back to Dr. Benjamin Rush, a prominent founding father and later congressman from Pennsylvania. Upon his arrival in the Congress in 1989, McDermott had little company as he began shouting about the emergence of a dire global humanitarian catastrophe.

During the mid-1980s, before running for his seat in the House, McDermott had served as a regional medical officer for sub-Saharan Africa with the U.S. State Department. Stationed in Zaire, he was responsible for all of the embassies south of the equator, from Gabon to Somalia to South Africa. The itinerant doctor had a long-standing passion for travel as well as for the developing world, and so it was a position that he relished.

Traveling from embassy to embassy all over the subcontinent, McDermott was roaming the epicenter of the looming global catastrophe. Through the late 1980s and early 1990s, South Africa had reported only several hundred infections to WHO. A colleague of McDermott's at the State Department knew that the official estimates belied a much greater base of infection. McDermott remembered his colleague fuming, "Because of the sanctions [then still in effect because of apartheid] we're not doing anything. We're committing genocide in South Africa."

When McDermott arrived in Washington to assume his seat in Congress, he wasted no time. The first-term representative brazenly approached then Speaker of the House Tom Foley and made a passionate case for U.S. congressional involvement. Foley became an early convert, providing McDermott essentially with a blank check to "go and figure it out."

He pored through reports released by USAID and WHO, and began to appreciate that beyond Africa, the pandemic had gained menacing footholds in Latin America, Asia, and elsewhere. By the late 1980s, it was clear that AIDS really was global. And by the end of the decade more than 9 million people across the globe had been infected with HIV, and almost 1 million had already died of AIDS.

Over the next two years, with Foley's blank check in his back pocket, McDermott spent a good portion of his time traveling to try to get a handle on the pandemic. In addition to Africa, he traveled to India, Thailand, the Philippines, Honduras, Jamaica, and Brazil. The trips confirmed his worst fears. The lethal duo of AIDS and denial were rampant everywhere McDermott toured.

On a trip to India, he asked senior officials from India's national health ministry to show him Bombay's red-light district, where hundreds of sex workers line the streets looking for johns. It had been established that AIDS had emerged in India by the mid- to late 1980s, if not earlier. Attempting to engage his Indian inerlocuters, McDermott was met with ardent denial. Seeing the strips, teeming with prostitutes, truckers, and others, McDermott foresaw a horrific explosion in India. His hosts showed little concern.

In Thailand, internationally known for its thriving sex trade, in 1989 the rate of infection among prostitutes in Chiang Mai was roughly .04%. That rate of infection increased over the next twenty months to 70 percent. As in India, the Thai government avoided acknowledging the presence of the disease for years, in part out of national pride, in part out of discomfort in dealing with sex, and in part due to a lack of resources that mobilizing against it would require.

Stigma was taken to an entirely new level abroad. Throughout Asia, HIV-positive patients were often subject to quarantine, imprisonment, or even death. Thai policemen told journalist Laurie Garrett that Burmese officials, for example, had injected cyanide into women they had found to be

HIV-positive and set their bodies afloat in a stream, as a warning that they would not tolerate the disease's presence.

This sort of cruelty, McDermott knew, would only further stigmatize the disease, precluding open discussion, breeding misperception, and driving those infected further underground or to the margins of society, where they would no doubt continue to participate in the sort of activities that spread the disease. It seemed a disastrous runaway train. To McDermott, though, there seemed an evident and critical role for the United States to play in combating it.

Back in Washington, McDermott, with Foley's blessing, started the congressional Global HIV/AIDS Caucus to drum up awareness and resources among colleagues. McDermott would host conferences, bringing in experts to brief congressmen and senators. It was rare that he was able to get more than five to attend any one session. If he was lucky, senators or congressmen would send senior staff to attend in their stead. "No one wanted to go, they all thought it was a good idea, but they weren't particularly interested," he said.

A small band would get on board though. Key supporters included Senator Pat Leahy, Congresswoman Nancy Pelosi, Congressman David Obey, and a handful of others. These early congressional champions pushed—against the wishes of the White House—for increased funding year in and year out, accounting for the steady, though marginal, increases.

McDermott tried to engage the administration in his effort, but found no interest at the White House. "There was very little understanding in the administration about this issue. I don't remember anybody coming to me from the administration to ask for my help or to talk about what we could do."

Political will and support were scant. Despite his best efforts, McDermott found himself exasperated at his colleagues' lack of interest. "What difference does it make if there are half a million people infected in India, for most people. It doesn't affect their district. They don't see it as an impact on their economy, or really anything."

It was clear to the doctor-legislator that the disease would become a destructive force to national economies, and eventually even to the global economy. He shuddered at the social devastation and the human toll the disease would extract.

If he was screaming at the wind, it wasn't like McDermott to stop. He would just have to keep screaming and wait for an opening.

———•◆•———

At five o'clock on a September morning in 1986, Jeffrey Harris rolled out of bed to get ready for his first day of work at USAID. Living then in temporary housing in Baltimore, with Judy settled at Johns Hopkins, Harris knew he'd have to get used to the early rise. For the next three and a half years, he would make that same commute from Baltimore to Rosslyn, Virginia, catching a 6:15 A.M. train to start his workday by 8:00 A.M. But he was full of youthful vigor, and eager to tackle the unique opportunity he would have at USAID.

His office, he found, was a tiny ten-by-twelve-foot box on the seventh floor of that glass structure in Rosslyn. He would come to know it well, working eighty- or ninety-hour weeks for stretches at a time.

Shunting aside his diarrheal disease portfolio to focus exclusively on global AIDS shortly after his arrival, Harris felt like the new kid on the first day of school, without a friend. The operatives to whom Harris would report were extremely skeptical about the disease and USAID's role in combating it. Anne Van Dusen, an experienced senior operative at the agency who oversaw the Office of Health recalled an "acute skepticism" in the early days. There was a host of other health issues, and the budget was already stretched. With little experience in infectious disease and little knowledge about the disease itself, the agency's leadership conferred little favor or attention on the issue early on.

Dr. Kenneth Bart, the head of the Office of Health, estimated that he spent roughly one-twenty-fifth of his total time on global AIDS. "That's probably not a bad estimate during those early days," he explained. "I don't think there was nearly the appreciation that we have in hindsight of the importance of what was being done at that time."

Disengaged and entirely unequipped to tackle the disease, the agency's leadership decided to pass along almost all of the $2 million to the new global AIDS program at WHO. They felt that what was needed was an international coordinating capacity, and with little to offer, and little enthusiasm about engineering an effort, they passed the funds to the fledgling WHO effort. At USAID, "there was," Anne Van Dusen remembered, "a let's wait and see attitude."

Determined to build up his own division, engage the problem, and make his personal mark at the agency, Jeffrey Harris began to dig into the issue and conceive of ways that USAID might actually grow into the role it professed to wear—global leader. Because the effort was entirely new, Harris was thrown in headfirst. Bart said that his introduction was "sort of like medicine—watch one, do one, teach one." Like everything he had done before, Harris proved a quick study in the erstwhile foreign domain of Washington bureaucracy. "Jeff was one of the finest health officers I've ever run into," lauded Brad Langmade, the agency's deputy administrator and second senior ranking official.

The first thing Harris, like every other bureaucratic operative, learned was that he would need money. Resources were very tight, though. The agency comprises regional bureaus that focus on geographic areas and technical bureaus that focus on specific issues or fields, such as health.

From time to time the agency was able to muster significant resources for an emergent issue, but they were usually for imminent "emergencies" like a widespread famine or drought or humanitarian relief due to a war or conflict. Otherwise, officials were wont to guard their purse strings and positions with an almost primal intensity.

Having trouble organizing a reallocation of funds, Harris sought to align himself with one of USAID's biggest bureaus, Family Planning. Harris felt his division could leverage the bureau's resources and range of technical expertise in sexual behavior to his division's benefit.

But this was the Reagan era, and Family Planning had fallen into the vise of what would later become dubbed the "Mexico City Policy." The policy dictated that no U.S. foreign assistance dollars would go to groups with any involvement in performing abortions. It became a polarizing policy, and Family Planning found itself struggling to meet its targeted goals.

Highly wary about affiliating itself with activities that might court additional controversy or scrutiny, Family Planning rebuffed Harris's attempts to leverage potential financial and technical synergies. Harris praised the senior officials who oversaw Family Planning for being generous with their time and encouragement. But that was where their support ended. Harris explained: "They thought we're going to put two political tar babies in the same box—this isn't good." And they were diligent in segregating the two efforts, leaving Harris orphaned.

"Under their wing, we could have handled about $500 million a year with their tutelage and blessing." But it wasn't offered, which Harris considered a tragic opportunity lost: "I think we could have done great things."

While Harris's division did not get access to the resources or expertise from Family Planning that it sorely needed, it would come to adopt the same fear of reproach from the White House and conservatives in Congress, and, in time, come to assume a similarly clandestine modus operandi. When Harris and colleagues should have been screaming about the impending pandemic to anyone and everyone who would listen, instead they did all they could to keep a low profile, hoping not to disturb the apple cart. "We were always ambivalent about media attention. We weren't sure we wanted it," Harris said. "We were in a Republican administration. We had focused early on sexual transmission. We had watched what happened to Family Planning. . . . Let's not kid ourselves," he continued, "we were a very big supplier of condoms and that's not a fact that we wanted out there." The division supported, for example, gay not-for-profits in Latin America that, said Harris, "would have curled conservatives' hair. . . . That was something we didn't want to read about in *The Washington Post*."

The predicament created a bizarre dynamic: a division within an agency under the aegis of the executive branch, working for the president, was in actuality enacting an agenda that they deemed in precise contradistinction of the wishes of that administration. All along, they couldn't pursue their real agenda in earnest because they feared getting chopped off at the head.

Interestingly enough, the administration would bring almost no direct pressure to bear on the division's activities. They amounted to a minuscule effort dealing with an issue not on the administration's radar screen. "I certainly felt that I was free to do almost anything I wanted to do," remembered Brad Langmade, who oversaw Harris's efforts. "I was not getting serious pressure." If Harris was hearing from the White House at all, it was to change the word "prostitute" to "commercial sex worker" in the division's literature: conservatives deemed the former inappropriate language to be included in program descriptions that were receiving funding from the U.S. federal government.

Harris recalled a report proffered by Partner Maulding, a legend, "a grand old man," at the agency. The study found that the *fear* of censorship turned out to be a much bigger factor than censorship itself, "in other words *self-censorship* was the bigger problem" for bureaucrats. "I think," Harris said, "to some extent we did that to ourselves."

Against the backdrop of a myopic administration, gaping budget deficits, and an emerging, still unclear, threat, Harris and his colleagues—those empowered to lead the U.S. response—would have faced a decidedly uphill battle in seeking to recalibrate the U.S. response in those early days.

But it was a fight that should have been waged, Harris now senses, and it never was.

He would meet with Peter McPherson, a staid academic born and raised on his family's farm in Michigan, who as USAID administrator ran the agency. The two developed a strong rapport that was unusual for an administrator and a relative underling. McPherson would read Harris's memos. Sitting in his boss's spacious office, filled with heavy, dark furniture and government paraphernalia, Harris would paint a picture of the devastation poised to beset the African continent.

Having McPherson's ear was a key advantage. But Harris wasn't thinking big. "In the McPherson time $100 million would have been our wildest dream." He would never even ask for that amount.

When McPherson retired in 1987, Harris's division lost a champion. His successor was Allan Woods, a successful lawyer who seemed sympathetic but tragically died of colon cancer only months after assuming his post. The seat of leadership at USAID then remained vacant for roughly a year, before Ronald Roskins, a conservative university president from the Midwest, was named to fill it. Subordinates had a hard time making out precisely what Roskins's agenda was. He seemed disengaged. One senior USAID official thought that Secretary of State James Baker simply "wanted someone who would stay out of his way." Roskins seemed to do as much, never demonstrating any particular interest in global AIDS. Through Harris's tenure, leadership at the agency was fitful and uninspiring.

There were other obstacles within USAID itself. Harris felt impeded by the agency's lack of "capacity" to distribute additional funds. The division developed an "outsourcing model" whereby it would award contracts— which focused primarily on prevention (disease surveillance, provision of technical expertise, communications campaigns, behavioral modification such as condom distribution)—to American nongovernmental organizations, or NGOs, primarily family planning or population groups. There weren't many NGOs available with this brand of expertise, and there was a limit to what they could accomplish. Furthermore, there was a lack of certitude about how exactly to tackle the global dimension. The disease was still young, and little was known.

Many of these problems would have been remedied by leveraging the resources, expertise, infrastructure, and capacity of other larger U.S. Departments like State, HHS, and CDC, or even by providing greater support to multilateral initiatives like the program at WHO or leveraging the UN's various agencies. But, once USAID had the "mandate" and, more important, the money, it clung to it, adhering to priority number one in bureaucratic politics: turf rules.

With the sense that only nominal resources would be made available, Harris, Bart, Van Dusen, Langmade, and others chose instead to disburse their funds to a wide swath of recipient nations. By the early 1990s they had doled out funds to more than seventy countries. It would have been a remarkable accomplishment had they not been such meager slices: several hundred thousand dollars here, a million or two there. These small chunks of change were hardly moving the meter abroad, and the division's efforts through the early to mid-1990s have since been written off as "experimental." A landmark August 1993 USAID report assessing the first six years of the agency's response concluded that "available resources were spread too thin, and that fragmentation and duplication" were abundant and crippling.

All of these impediments assailed USAID's ability to function as an effective leader, to marshal an effectual U.S. response. But, there was something even more fundamental missing: a strategy. Brad Langmade conceded: "To be perfectly honest we didn't spend a hell of a lot of time on that question—because the resources needed were always so gigantically larger than the resources that were going to be available." Harris, Langmade, and others anticipated that obstacles would have been insurmountable, and the amount of resources unattainable. Foreseeing a political dead end, they didn't dare to formulate a strategy to combat the pandemic. And so, without finite goals, a timetable, and a schedule for the resources required to get there, the USAID effort was consigned to aimlessness. Bureaucrats at the agency were serving process and procedure, not the solution, and certainly not the suffering.

In Jeffrey Harris's long and distinguished career, there would never be another time comparable to his tenure at USAID. He brought vigor and intellectual acumen to the post. In turn, he won the universal admiration of his colleagues. On a daunting track of steep hurdles, he ran a better race than anyone might have expected from a thirty-year-old neophyte with no experience in the matter at hand. He built a division of one with $2 million into a division of almost twenty with a budget of roughly $120 million in less than six years, and he was a consistent and credible voice within the federal government trumpeting the issue. Harris took pride in those accomplishments.

Still, the effort he led was a pittance measured against the magnitude of the threat and the resources needed. Beset by the stasis inherent in the agency, he sometimes felt like he was running on a treadmill. The hours, the commute, the sense of moral obligation all took a tremendous toll on Harris. The job hadn't killed him, as he had once quipped to Judy that it would, but it had left him thoroughly exhausted.

He spent more than a quarter of his time—at spells as much as one third—abroad, traveling to oversee the agency's effort. Toward the end of his tenure, in November 1990, Harris found himself immersed in preparations for an upcoming trip to Africa. The excursion had attracted interest and participation from an impressive cross section of senior operatives from State, HHS, CDC, USAID, and elsewhere. They would investigate the toll of the disease and check on the agency's work on the ground. Harris was looking forward to the chance to preach the gospel to a wide and important audience.

With plans for the trip still in process, Harris left the States for a quick jaunt to attend an AIDS conference in Switzerland. Late one evening, he picked up the phone in his hotel room in Geneva to shocking news. It was Judy. Six weeks before their tenth wedding anniversary, in the prime of her life, she had been diagnosed with ovarian cancer.

The diagnosis shook Harris deeply. Still, he seemed set on going on the Africa trip. The choice between being there for Judy and fulfilling what had become something like a moral crusade constituted a wrenching dilemma. After much deliberation, he opted to stay with Judy. Later, doctors would tell them that Judy had, in fact, received a misdiagnosis, and the original prognosis had been much overstated.

The time with Judy had given Harris pause for thought. He noted that the division could actually run without him and estimated that a replacement could do a fine job. He felt that against great obstacles, he had accomplished much during his tenure, and that he needed a change. He would spend another year at the agency completing work in process and making sure that new projects were up and running. Then on February 16, 1992, at the age of thirty-six, he tendered his resignation, ending an era in the U.S. response.

He would never have another experience like it. "I really did have the sense of history being made," he recalled, "that we were dealing with something cataclysmic and we were in the center of it."

THREE

—⚏—

A Maverick Goes to Geneva, Turf Wars

On October 22, 1985, a steady stream of rain pelted the high tin roof of an airy lecture hall made of cement blocks in Bangui, the capital of the Central African Republic. Inside, Faqry Assad, the head of communicable diseases at WHO, a portly five-foot-six-inch Egyptian in his early sixties, sat eagerly awaiting the presentation that was, in large part, the reason he had made the journey.

For months, through the summer and into the fall of 1985, Assad, famed for his boisterous, bellowing laugh, had been fielding phone calls from his old friend and colleague Joe McCormick, with whom he'd worked on those Ebola investigations in the mid- and late 1970s, helping to control the outbreaks. McCormick was hammering away at Assad, making the case that there was something new looming on the continent. It was ill understood, and the international science and public health response was tangled in confusion and discord. McCormick argued that the world needed a global vehicle to examine and combat the new disease—a clearinghouse for scientific and epidemiological exchange, a center of technical expertise and, perhaps, advocacy. McCormick was hoping that Assad might agree that WHO was the place to house the effort.

The two had long since established a friendship and working relationship forged on endearment and mutual respect. Assad heeded McCormick's alarm call, and asked McCormick if he would like to run the new program. Still engrossed in his work on other diseases and affairs, McCormick declined.

He convinced Assad, though, to agree to come to Bangui later that

October. When you get to Bangui, McCormick assured him, "you're going to meet someone who would be an excellent candidate to run the program."

A little less than two years earlier, McCormick had placed a call to New Mexico, where Jonathan Mann, a CDC veteran then thirty-seven years old, was serving as the state epidemiologist. Mann had a lanky frame and a penchant for European suits, almost always worn with his trademark bow tie. A voracious reader with an engaging personality, Mann had an urbane air about him.

McCormick did not know him well, but had heard him present at a handful of conferences and was impressed each time by Mann's intellectual acuity and his magnetic presence. He had heard through the grapevine that Mann was restless in New Mexico and looking for a new challenge.

Mann picked up the phone in New Mexico in January 1984 to hear McCormick's voice. McCormick asked Mann if he would be interested in an opportunity to run the first longitudinal study of AIDS in Africa. It would be a chance to examine the pandemic in its nascence, to glean early scientific insights, to spearhead international surveillance, and to get a grasp on the dimensions of the pandemic brewing.

Mann had never been to Africa, and it wasn't even on his list of possibilities, he explained to McCormick. He had many questions: What would life be like for his wife, Mary Paul, his daughters? What would happen to their schooling—they were approaching college age? McCormick's years of experience in Africa made him a good man to answer Mann's queries. Eager to get Mann on board, and the effort under way, he persisted in selling the opportunity.

A week later McCormick got a call from Mann: "When do we leave for Kinshasa?" he asked.

That winter and spring McCormick joined Mann out in Kinshasa, showing him the lay of the land, making key introductions, and helping him put in place the infrastructure for the program. The two spent full days in a backroom of the American Embassy, where McCormick tutored Mann on a cutting-edge computer technology called word processing as well as the CDC's latest data entry programs. They developed a mutual admiration that would serve as the foundation of a lifelong friendship.

Leadership was a role that suited Mann well. He assumed the reins of Project SIDA (the French acronym for AIDS) by the late spring of 1985, and instituted what would become the largest, most productive international surveillance effort on AIDS in the world. Perhaps more than any other vehicle, its findings would alert the world to the disease's international dimension.

By the time Mann took to the podium on that rainy day in Bangui to make his presentation to an international audience of Americans, Africans, and Europeans, he was one of the world's foremost experts on the pandemic. His command of the material, his clear grasp of the extent of the pandemic, and the eloquence of his presentation made an indelible impression on Assad.

Assad made a beeline for McCormick immediately following the presentation. "There's no question," he exclaimed, "this is the guy I want."

The Egyptian introduced himself to Mann and asked him if he would like to come to WHO to start the Special Program on AIDS, or SPA. Mann grasped that it was a unique opportunity, and jumped at it. Over the next six months he began traveling back and forth from Kinshasa to WHO headquarters in Geneva.

In the SPA, the pandemic would finally command a global stage, and in Mann, its finest player.

On his first day, Mann arrived at WHO headquarters, a modern glass structure set against the backdrop of the Alps, in Geneva, in late 1986 to a tiny sparse office, a part-time secretary, a minuscule budget, and no full-time staff. The road ahead appeared daunting.

Mann's efforts, it was agreed at the outset, would have to be extrabudgetary, meaning that little to no funds would come out of WHO's budget. Mann would have to do his own fund-raising. AIDS was not a priority for the agency.

Having recently eradicated smallpox, WHO was coming off of a relatively successful epoch. Its agenda, however, was fixed primarily on "basic" health care issues: immunization, water supply, and the prevention of certain existing communicable diseases. The donor countries in the World Health Assembly, or WHA, the agency's governing authority, were either rich countries who had the resources to tackle AIDS on their own, or poor countries still focused on other pressing health threats.

Faced with resistance from the agency's existing programs, and without support from its governing authority, Mann needed a champion. In characteristically brazen fashion, he went straight to the top, appealing to the agency's director general, or DG, the well-respected, experienced Dutch

official, Halfdan Mahler. At first, Mahler seemed impervious to Mann's entreaties.

Two factors would turn him around, though, in 1986.

The first was the unusual case of Uganda. The country's leader, Yoweri
Museveni, had only recently seized the reins of political authority via military coup in January 1986. Having replaced the notorious despot Milton
Obote, Museveni's regime was green and not yet entirely stable when he
started to receive deeply disturbing reports from senior military officials.
Fidel Castro, it seemed, citing incidence of a mysterious, debilitating, and
seemingly infectious disease, was returning Ugandan soldiers from Cuba,
where for years they had gone to be trained.

The reports jolted Museveni, still enormously reliant on the strength
and stability of his military. It was the bulwark of his fledgling regime.

Unlike almost all of his political contemporaries around the continent,
Museveni did not indulge in denial. Losing little time, he launched an
ambitious multisectoral—government, industry, religion, and civil society—
effort aimed at combating the disease. Early acknowledgment and leadership would, over the following decade, make Uganda the archetypal success
story. Museveni's early and comprehensive response helped curb the pandemic.

At the outset, the Ugandan strategy sought to engage the international
community. When Uganda's minister of health placed a call to Mahler to
plead for resources and attention, the DG took notice.

No factor, though, was more central to Mahler's awakening than
Jonathan Mann's advocacy. "That's what Mahler told me," explained
Daniel Tarantola, an amiable Frenchman and a veteran of the UN system
who would later become Mann's most senior and trusted deputy. Tarantola
remembered Mahler telling him, "Yes, the countries were important, but
Jonathan was an even more important factor. He was able to show me what
the problem was."

Mann combined a peerless intimacy with the disease and all its facets
with his natural powers of persuasion, and pounded on Mahler's door relentlessly in the first few months after his arrival in Geneva. He was so
convincing, in fact, that by August 1986, Mahler had done nothing short
of a 180-degree turn on the issue. The former skeptic proclaimed: "We
stand nakedly in front of a pandemic as mortal as any pandemic there has
ever been. In the same spirit that WHO addressed smallpox eradication,"
he pledged, "WHO will dedicate its energy, commitment, and creativity to

the even more urgent, difficult, and complex task of global AIDS prevention."

Armed with Mahler's support, Mann set out to devise a strategy to combat the pandemic. For months, Mann hunkered down in his tiny office, and almost single-handedly, in only minor consultation with colleagues from USAID and CDC, began to draft a seminal document entitled "Global Strategy for the Prevention and Control of AIDS." Dated 1986, and adopted by the WHA in 1987, it was the blueprint for SPA's strategy.

The approach to battling the scourge worldwide was innovative and audacious. Comprising a three-pronged plan of attack, the plan was remarkably prescient.

Prong one: surveillance. "Only if you have the proper information," world-renowned German epidemiologist Bernhard Schwartlander later noted, "can you take the proper action." Poring over existing data to arrive at their best estimate, Mann and Tarantola were stymied. There could be anywhere from 100,000 to tens of millions of HIV-positive cases in Africa in 1987, they estimated.

The uncertainty about the magnitude of the disease bespoke a crippling deficiency in the global health surveillance system. In response to this shortcoming, Mann would later write: "AIDS is trying to teach us a lesson. . . . A worldwide 'early-warning system' is needed to detect quickly the eruption of new diseases or the unusual spread of old diseases. Without such a system we are essentially defenseless, relying on good luck to protect us."

Without a proper international network, WHO customarily relied on reports from national health ministries to construct its estimates. AIDS presented a stark dilemma, though. The countries most acutely affected were also those that lacked surveillance capacity, the same countries most encamped in denial.

Mann and his colleagues could scarcely rely on these national estimates. In response, they focused on building in-country capacity, providing nations with as many tools as they could muster and as much expertise as they could impart. They also launched an independent effort, deploying experts to conduct tests and collect data. They recruited some of the world's most renowned epidemiologists to oversee data collection and modeling at the program's Geneva headquarters.

Under the stewardship of a leading American epidemiologist, Jim Chin, by the late 1980s the program was able to proffer some of the world's first credible regional and global estimates. In 1989, Chin projected that there were 8 to 10 million infections worldwide. The numbers were startling and attracted their fair share of skeptics. Dismissed and even disparaged, they would later prove far short of actuality.

Prong two: prevention. The linchpin of the prevention strategy called for SPA to support the installation and promotion of national AIDS programs, or NAPs, in affected countries. The idea was to make inroads with national leadership and prompt them to create their own national effort to combat the disease.

Mann deputized Tarantola to run this corridor of the strategy. "My job," he explained, "was to go to countries and to convince politicians and public health officials that rather than neglecting HIV or responding in a haphazard manner, what was needed was public recognition that there was a risk of HIV present in the country and that prevention was feasible." It was no mean undertaking. Many leaders didn't want to acknowledge the disease for fear that it may divert foreign investment, or cripple the local tourism industry. If their militaries were infected, they didn't want their adversaries to know about it. Some leaders' denial was even more visceral: they were worried that they themselves might be infected and couldn't come to terms with it.

SPA responded to national leaders' recalcitrance in three ways. First, its leaders became tireless advocates, traveling the globe several times over, meeting with national leaders, shouting to the press or anyone who would listen, trumpeting the necessity for creating NAPs. Second, they dangled the carrot of financial assistance. The resource-stretched developing nations would receive resources if they exhibited a willingness to pursue NAPs. Finally, SPA demonstrated that it could achieve demonstrable progress immediately. Drawing on their own funds, if need be, they were able to install short-term programs, usually six to twelve months in duration, with which countries could take initial measures to address the disease. They would then move to incorporate a medium-term program—usually with a four-to-six-year time horizon—with which the country would be encouraged to pursue meaningful structural change to mobilize society to curb the disease.

The rate of progress was blistering. After only a year and a half, one hundred countries had adopted NAPs. "There was a certain chain reaction that was quite significant," Tarantola remembered. "Countries were in-

creasingly feeling comfortable talking about HIV. That was important."
More than acknowledging the disease, though, countries were taking steps
to institute structural changes to combat it.

Finally, prong three: place the disease in a larger context than just
health. To address the root causes of its proliferation, the global response
would have to engage issues such as human rights and, later, social equality
and development. The idea that a disease needed to be conceptualized
within a broader milieu was nothing short of revolutionary.

Mann had gleaned a key insight into the disease: the vicious cycle of
marginalization. The disease tended to affect segments of society already
on the margins: those engaging in promiscuous, extramarital sex, prostitutes, homosexuals, drug users. Mann found a fitting French phrase to describe these peoples: "les exclus."

The tendency in most corners of the developing world was to punish
those who became infected. Mandatory testing, quarantine, imprisonment,
and even torture or death were deemed viable solutions in many parts of
the world. But rather than curb the disease, these policies helped it to
flourish. Those potentially infected wouldn't get tested. Rather, they would
end up further underground, closer to the margins of society, still engaging
in the same behavior. These policies amplified the degree of stigma attached to the disease, precluding societies from engaging in an open, con-
structive discourse.

Mann was troubled that these misguided policies were based on misconceptions about the modes of transmission as well as base prejudice. Far
from helping societies, they would only degrade and debilitate those already suffering enormously.

"His vision," Tarantola said, "and one of the things for which he is given
credit and for which he should be given credit, was that very early on he
recognized that if there was to be a response to HIV in the United States
or anywhere else in the world that it had to be based on respect for human
beings and protection of their privacy and human rights."

Peter Piot, who had continued to work in Kinshasa on AIDS, and would
later become a global leader on the issue, believed Mann's contribution cannot be understated. "I'm not convinced that if someone other than Jonathan
had been the first director of the [SPA], the whole response to the epidemic
would have been different. For example," Piot explained, "we [might] have
gotten into a repressive approach, perhaps using quarantine. Because let's
not forget that in the early days there were many calls for that."

Trumpeting human rights not only prevented an untold quantity of infections, but also provided elemental human dignity to millions of lives across the globe.

By the late 1980s, Mann was fleshing out the paradigm even further, contending that underdevelopment and social inequality helped to abet the disease's proliferation. Where societies lacked resources to build a health infrastructure, to educate and communicate with the populace, where mores precluded women's sexual empowerment, the disease would flourish. If the world was serious about stopping the scourge, it would have to think more broadly.

Meeting stiff resistance at almost every turn, Mann would keep pushing, never flagging, to meet the enormity of the catastrophe with a commensurate conceptual framework with which to fight it. In the "Global Strategy" Mann had constructed a comprehensive and visionary blueprint to combat the pandemic across the globe. To execute the strategy, Mann would bring on, during 1986 and 1987, an experienced and dedicated cadre of deputies who shared his sense of urgency.

By 1987, it was a strategy rearing to be implemented, but still in desperate need of financing. All of Mann's plans would be for naught without funds, and in the early days the program's coffers were all but empty. Mann took to the air, traveling the globe, spreading the gospel to everyone and anyone—nation-states, not-for-profits, wealthy individuals—who he was able to get to sit still long enough to listen. The Scandinavians—famed for leading the world in international assistance as a percent of their GDP—signed on early. Beguiled by Mann's power of persuasion, a wealthy Swiss countess sold many of her family's treasured paintings to help give SPA a start. Above all, Mann had high hopes for his own country, the United States.

It began as a seamless relationship. When Mann looked to the United States to open its pockets, he was pointed to USAID and the Office of Health. Dr. Kenneth Bart, then running the office, was pleased to hear from Mann, an old classmate from the CDC's elite EIS unit. Their encounter around the middle of 1986 was, for both, propitious. Mann was in need of money. Bart and his colleagues were sitting on a $2 million allocation that they needed to spend.

Easily enough, USAID passed along its inaugural $2 million to SPA and Mann. And just like that the United States became the largest single donor to SPA—and as such the leading nation in the global response—contributing close to 40 percent of SPA's 1986 fund-raising total.

Mann sensed that for the United States, it was the tip of the iceberg. He had connections, the country had deep pockets, and he knew that there were people in Congress who cared about the issue. Congress became Mann's stomping ground. He came back time and again over his first two years, testifying about the pandemic brewing, how a commitment up front might avert mass catastrophe down the road.

At first, Bart, Harris, and others at USAID couldn't have been more thrilled about Mann's advocacy. They were doing their best to keep a low profile, because they didn't want to chance White House interference in their programs. But it was still very much in their interest for Congress, the media, and others to hear and to think about the pandemic. Mann was doing USAID's advocacy work for them.

Harris recalled, "WHO had been beating the drum more loudly and more effectively than any of us combined. . . . Jon Mann was a very charismatic guy." USAID would benefit, and in turn, become SPA's largest donor.

By the time SPA was renamed the Global Program on AIDS, or GPA, in 1988, U.S. support was helping to fuel the program's meteoric rise.

At the end of 1986 Mann had only a $5 million budget and a handful of staff. In 1987, SPA's budget jumped to $30 million, and then to $50 million in 1988, due to Mann's tireless advocacy. By 1989, GPA would have a budget of $90 million. Staff now numbered roughly four hundred people.

Along the way, Mann broke precedents and tore down barriers. On October 26, 1987, Mann became the first WHO functionary to address the General Assembly of the United Nations. His appeal led the UN, for the first time in its history, to pass a resolution on a specific disease. The next year, in 1988, with WHO's backing and the labors of his colleagues and extended network, Mann successfully convened the largest gathering of health ministers ever assembled—117 in total—for a conference on AIDS in London. The U.S.'s senior most health official opted not to attend, sending his deputy instead.

As a speaker, Mann was electric. At the London conference, Mann exhorted his audience: "Our opportunity is truly historic. . . . We live in a world threatened by unlimited destructive force, yet we share a vision of creative potential—personal, national, and international. The dream is not new—but the circumstances and opportunity are for our time alone.

The global AIDS problem speaks eloquently of the need for communication, for sharing of information and experience, and for mutual support. AIDS shows us, once again, that silence, exclusion, and isolation—of individuals, groups, of nations—creates danger for us all."

He was able to shine the spotlight on the catastrophe as well as the deficiency of the global response, yet frame the predicament as an opportunity, a chance to realize transcendent human aspirations. He would showcase AIDS to strike a more fundamental human chord, and it would play with wild appeal. A hit with international audiences, Mann earned similar acclaim from his own staff.

He brought flair and personality. Quirky, he was fastidious about keeping his office immaculate. He began his day with two briefcases—one for documents he was already carrying, the other for anything new he would pick up that day. Constantly in between television interviews, it was not uncommon for colleagues to see Mann at formal meetings or conferences wearing makeup and perhaps even a bib to shield his dress shirt.

A leader by example, Mann approached his work with a missionary's zeal. His self-imposed work schedule was unrelenting. He allowed himself only five or six hours a night of sleep. Traveling almost constantly, he would work on flights.

It was clear from the outset that Mann would employ a bold and innovative vision for his program. Rigidity, red tape, and business as usual would have to be bucked. The crisis required a commensurate response, and without hesitation, Mann proceeded to craft a different sort of enterprise.

Mann grew the staff at a rate that far outpaced other programs. He brought on a young, passionate, international group, many of whom had backgrounds in law, development, or the humanities, giving the staff a decidedly unique flavor.

The pace of work was fanatical. On weekend mornings, swaths of GPA staff could be seen making their way into WHO headquarters for a long weekend of work. Mann could often be found in the lobby, shaking hands, ushering his staff in, showing his appreciation for their dedication. On Friday nights, Mann and his senior colleagues began a tradition of having wine parties for the staff. It was a chance to build camaraderie, take stock of a hard week's work, and let off some steam.

Bonded and propelled by a shared sense of mission and culture, the program, by 1988, was proving stunningly effective. By the end of the year, in fact, GPA was working with over 80 percent of the countries on earth. The program had pledged financial support to over 130 nation-states. Data collection and surveillance were improving radically. The program organized regular regional conferences that, over time, helped sprout an international collaborative network.

In short, GPA was making countries acknowledge the disease, but much more than that, it was making them devise and pursue strategies to combat it. It was providing them with technical guidance and expertise as well as resources. It was serving as the international clearinghouse for scientific insight and surveillance intelligence.

The program was an international hit, and its leader, the global voice for the pandemic. "The global AIDS effort," in those early days, remembered Brad Langmade, "was Jonathan Mann."

GPA had, in less than two years, built nothing short of a global platform with which to launch a truly comprehensive effort to battle the pandemic. Then cracks started to appear in the foundation.

Compelled to respond to the crisis but with only little time and scant resources, GPA was cutting corners. The international donor community would not be forgiving.

GPA was doing a poor job of managing donor expectations. In a rush to attract funds and attention for the pandemic the program was rightly trumpeting an "emergency response." Whereas other emergencies like earthquakes, or even most disease outbreaks, explode and then dissipate, AIDS was clearly a long-term crisis. Expecting fast results, many donors felt that GPA had not sufficiently managed their expectations for what would be a long and painful effort. The perception damaged the program's credibility.

Donors also alleged that GPA did not sufficiently account for its flow of funds. Only half of the NAPs that the program supported could account for their funds. Similarly, donors like the United States who sought verifiable, even quantifiable, results—in other words, proof of a return on their investment—were disappointed.

The program further came under fire for pursuing a top-down, "boilerplate model" in installing the NAPs. "The fact that programs developed with countries were often based on a blueprint, [that] they sometimes lacked a sensitivity to country specificities," was, Daniel Tarantola conceded, "a shortcoming."

Mann and the program's leadership generally recognized the problems and the need to address them. GPA had achieved so much in so little time with so few resources, and against such a catastrophic threat, that the program's leadership assumed that the donor community would afford them the time to iron out these creases.

The blemishes surfaced, though, at a time that was less than propitious. The Cold War was dissipating and anti-UN sentiment was high. The geopolitical imperative for foreign assistance had waned. Beset by "donor fatigue," donors were looking for excuses to clamp down on foreign commitments. Donors began to narrow in on the program's "deficiencies." The specter of all of these other issues certainly left GPA's leadership wondering if the pressure from donors was serving the global response or, perhaps, unrelated national interests.

Nowhere was this phenomenon more evident than in the fissures developing in the relationship between USAID and GPA.

In 1986, the dynamic was simple enough. USAID had funds and didn't know what to do with them. GPA didn't and did. By 1987, though, under Jeffrey Harris's leadership, the Division of Global HIV/AIDS was growing at USAID. The U.S. funding pie was still terribly paltry, and now there were two vehicles, both growing and both in demand of funds.

Mann was convinced that the dollars would be best spent at GPA. Testifying before Congress, he practically said as much. He would not only advocate for increased U.S. spending on global AIDS, he would press to earmark those funds directly for GPA, as opposed to USAID. "There was tension," Harris remembered, "because Jon—honestly, if Jon would have had his way—I don't know what he would have wanted—but he certainly would have had most of the resources come to him."

But in Rosslyn, Virginia, under Harris's leadership USAID was also growing. U.S. NGOs, like Family Health International and Population Services International, originally with no experience in AIDS, popped out of the woodwork and began lobbying Congress and the agency for funds. With the U.S. organizations buzzing around in the Beltway, insisting that American taxpayer money should be spent, after all, on American organizations, USAID grew increasingly parsimonious with their contributions to GPA.

Mann's star and his aggressive tactics began to draw the ire of some at USAID. In turn, Mann was frustrated at USAID's inefficiency and its apparent insistence that SPA's budget be capped, in effect handcuffing his efforts.

"There was a lack of clarity occasionally," Daniel Tarantola remembered, "as to who was leading the global response to AIDS. Was it GPA or USAID? Who was part of whose initiative?"

Cooperation continued to wane through the late 1980s, as both efforts grew increasingly competitive over a small pie of resources. The tenor of the relationship grew increasingly contentious in Washington, and it filtered across the globe into efforts in the field, where duplication and discord were the net result.

Stark tension, and even at times animosity, between GPA and USAID thus ushered in a critical theme in the history of the U.S. response to the pandemic: should the United States respond bilaterally, that is through U.S. mechanisms directly, or multilaterally, that is by pooling U.S. resources and expertise with other nations and actors, and attacking the pandemic with an aggregated, global effort?

With earnest hindsight, Dr. Kenneth Bart assessed the position from the bilateral camp: "There's also the chauvinism of an organization that wants and needs to maintain its own integrity. So shouldn't we keep the money for ourselves and give it to our own missions?" Increasingly through the late 1980s, the bilateral camp would find itself winning the battle, even as it was losing the war.

Through the turmoil and vicissitudes, Mann could always count on support from his boss, Halfdan Mahler. His door was always open and the two would meet regularly. Mahler would confer privilege and priority on Mann's program, providing Mann with a free rein to tackle the scourge that Mahler himself had elevated, in a few short months, from the bottom of his agenda to the very top. But Mahler's long and successful tenure was coming to a close. 1988 was an election year at WHO, ushering in an era of new leadership, a new director general at the agency.

Their introduction could not have been less auspicious.

It was the sort of occasion Mann relished. WHO's Western Pacific region was holding its first conference on HIV/AIDS in Australia. It was still early in Mann's tenure, but it was a chance to enfranchise a new cohort of scientists and public health officials, a chance to alert the media and the populace in a new region to the global crisis. It was, for Mann, yet another chance to save lives.

As the area's regional director, Hiroshi Nakajima, the Japanese bureaucrat who favored traditional WHO protocol, arrived from regional head-

quarters in Manila to preside over the conference. Nakajima, whose background was in pharmacology, generally preferred the scientific or medical
approach to public health. He knew little about AIDS, spoke very little
English, and was terribly uncomfortable at the conference.

Mann, on the other hand, was entirely in his element. He savored the
glare of the media spotlight. He had an ambitious strategy to share. The
conference, in short order, became the Jonathan Mann show.

Mann, in a breach of protocol, had not officially requested Nakajima's
permission to attend the conference. Watching from the sidelines as Mann
usurped the spotlight in Australia, Hiroshi Nakajima felt slighted. It was an
incident that he would not forget.

Over the next year or two, Mahler noticed donors becoming increasingly critical and parsimonious. Mann and many others, who admired
Mahler enormously, hoped that he would run again for another term, or at
least agree to a short-term extension, so that an exhaustive search could
yield a worthy successor. Mahler was fed up, though, and after a long and
productive tenure, ready to leave.

At the same time, many on the American political scene resented the
UN, and the disproportionate share of the burden they felt they had been
saddled with. There was a strong push to coerce other nations to increase
their dues payments. This discussion, of course, was taking place against
the backdrop of a relative decline in U.S. economic wealth vis-à-vis Japan.
Key diplomats advanced the argument that, given its wealth, Japan was
free riding. After some diplomatic jostling, Japan consented to pay a higher
share of the burden. But the Asian powerhouse also insisted on quid pro
quo. Japan would increase its dues, but in return it wanted greater represen-
tation at the UN's senior level.

When elections approached in 1988, then, Japan made it known to all
that it was expecting some good news. Two new directorships, Japanese officials learned to their delight, would be awarded to the Japanese. One was
the DG spot at WHO.

The dynamics behind the selection were hardly a secret. "Nakajima
wasn't picked as Nakajima," explained Sally Grooms Cowal, a seasoned
U.S. diplomat who spent much of her career in the UN system, "but as the
Japanese candidate for the WHO."

Shortly after Nakajima's election, the WHA, WHO's governing body,
had to render another decision. The Palestinian Liberation Organization,
or PLO, had applied for membership to WHO. It was a stunt the PLO had

pulled before, using the WHA gathering—the first in the season of gather-
ings among UN agencies—to gauge the international community's support
for their inclusion. Predictably, the United States objected. According to a
delegate to the WHA, Nakajima went to work as a "floor manager," bro-
kering alliances to ensure that the WHA would deny the PLO membership. In return, Nakajima demanded free reign from leading donors to
manage WHO's global AIDS effort, which by then had begun to overshadow much of the rest of the agency.

Huddled in a corner at a cocktail reception the night after the "bargain"
was struck, both Mann and Tarantola were wrought with anxiety. They
feared the worst, "that the days of the program," in Tarantola's words, were
"counted." Nakajima would be able to reshuffle and reorganize the program
the way he wanted, clip its wings in terms of fund-raising and profile, stran-
gle its convening power, and decentralize authority to the regional offices.

As Mann and Tarantola brainstormed, with the sound of cocktail banter
in a myriad of foreign tongues simmering in the background, they noticed
Nakajima making his way over to them. He was usually serious and his
countenance was generally fixed. On this evening, though, he seemed in
decidedly good spirits as he approached the pair. He looked at his new colleagues with a "sarcastic smile" and said in perfect English: "Now I can
begin the surgery."

During the next two years, many of Mann's greatest fears were realized.

Nakajima was formal and rigid, a technocrat's technocrat—everything
that Mann disdained. His background was in science and medicine. He
knew little about, and was averse to consider involvement in, public health
interventions. For Nakajima, sex, drug use, and the other activities that
spread the disease were taboo and he was deeply uncomfortable addressing
them.

Laurie Garrett remembered interviewing Nakajima when TB was
sweeping through South Asia. "He was a drug company nut . . . I remember
my jaw dropping when I interviewed him once." When she asked how he
planned to deal with the epidemic, he replied, "I think in short order that
drug companies will be able to invent a new drug, and in the meantime
we'll just have to muddle through." She was livid: "He didn't know anything about infectious diseases. He had no concept of contagion at all."

On another occasion, journalist Bart Gellman reported, Nakajima was overheard telling a wealthy WHO donor: "Ah, don't talk to me about AIDS; I have malaria which is a much bigger killer of people, on my hands."

The new DG implemented an even more rigid, stratified culture at WHO headquarters. Over the course of Nakajima's tenure, donors would become at first dissatisfied, and then indignant at Nakajima's ineffectual brand of management. At a time when the United States and other donors were particularly averse to big UN bureaucracy, Nakajima was trying to build himself a small empire in Geneva.

Senior staff grew, in the early stages of his tenure, from 66 to 107. Staff salaries consumed 76 percent of WHO's budget, and less than one third of WHO's staff was in the field. Anil Soni observed, "only nine nations were scheduled to have more money spent on WHO country programs than WHO would spend on paper, pens, and pencils."

Eventually, Nakajima would confirm others' gravest apprehensions as well. Dan Spiegel served in the Clinton administration as ambassador to the UN in Geneva. At first, Spiegel remembered, the goal was to foster a positive, workable relationship with Nakajima. That course, however, soon proved untenable. "It was patently obvious to us that everything he did from appointments to budgetary priorities, that he did [these things] to gain favor with various countries and groups. Ultimately, he was a full-time campaigner for himself. . . . It was clear that the organization was totally mobilized for him, not for global health." For almost the entire decade, WHO was a discredited and hapless actor on the world stage.

Life changed for Jonathan Mann and GPA following Nakajima's inauguration. Mann went from having weekly or biweekly meetings with the DG to rarely meeting at all. Nakajima reined in Mann's contact with the media. All of Mann's public statements would have to go through Nakajima's media director. Mann now needed documented permission from Nakajima's office prior to all of his travel engagements and in order to convene or even participate in special events.

Wherever and whenever he could, Mann ignored or circumvented the red tape put up by Nakajima.

Some point out that Mann was a party to the acrimony developing as well. "Jon put Nakajima in a very difficult position for an international civil servant from a place like Japan," Ken Bernard, a U.S. emissary to WHO, explained. "You can't, if you're working for someone, publicly disobey them. If you're the head of a big UN agency and it looks like the people who work for you are not doing what you ask them to do, it's untenable."

Many felt that Mann was egotistical, that he simply couldn't bear the constraints of authority. Ambassador Sally Grooms Cowal explained, "Jonathan Mann didn't come to WHO and sit there and run a nice little bureaucratic program, he began to build it as a power center . . . he increasingly became a threat to Nakajima and he deliberately provoked Nakajima."

Tarantola conceded that Mann and GPA could have done a better job with "internal PR," and that they were not always as sensitive as they might have been to procedure and process. Perhaps a little more time spent greasing the wheels, and a little less time spent bulldozing might have paid dividends. But it wasn't Mann's way.

In their meteoric rise, Mann and associates were collecting enemies and they didn't pay it serious thought. In fact, it helped stoke the fire and codify their self-selected image as renegades fighting the good fight against all odds and foes.

Many suggest that Nakajima was not necessarily the culprit he was made out to be. Many, even perhaps Tarantola, believe Mann could have done much to bridge their differences. But each incident, each provocation added to the other, and the two obstinate, self-assured men would never reach out to the other.

By March 1990, Mann was approaching his breaking point.

A conference was to be held in Copenhagen early that month, and the Eastern European countries comprising the former Soviet bloc would be attending. Although it was known that HIV existed in these societies, they had largely failed theretofore to acknowledge the disease. For Mann, the conference was going to be a wonderful opportunity to engage this part of the world and their health officials in the global fight. He was also keen to learn more about their health systems at large. Not much had been shared during the Cold War. He hoped to use the opportunity to enfranchise Eastern Europe in his crusade.

On the eve of the conference Mann sat in his office alone, fuming. The authorization he needed from the DG's office to attend the conference remained unsigned. He would have to miss the conference entirely.

The following day, Tarantola found Mann, still furious, sitting at his desk in his office at WHO headquarters. He motioned Tarantola over and pointed to his letter of resignation.

His colleagues were up in arms. First, they argued with him to stay. "There was no going further though," Tarantola remembered well. "He had already signed his letter of resignation and so we knew that this was it." Tarantola said of his longtime colleague and friend: "Jonathan was never a person who could work within an institution having a boss telling him what to do. Jonathan was just not like that." And so it was. Fanatically loyal, Mann's senior colleagues offered to tender their resignations as a sign of solidarity. Mann insisted that they stay. They were needed to continue the work.

Mann submitted the letter, a scathing denunciation of WHO's senior leadership and Nakajima, to Le Monde, the popular French newspaper. It made a splash in the international media.

Mann's dedicated staff was crushed. Supporters would describe the time to follow as "soul destroying. All those years lost!" A female GPA staffer bemoaned, "It was like a slow torture."

During the eight years to follow, the world's response to global AIDS would founder. In that time 32.9 million people worldwide would become infected with HIV, and almost 10 million would die of AIDS.

On a melancholic day, the 11th of March 1990, Jonathan Mann shut his office door at WHO headquarters in Geneva for the last time. He was wrought with piebald emotions: furious, despondent, nostalgic, and deeply grateful to staff for their labors, dedication, and affection.

As Mann made his way down the long corridor past his program's offices, at eleven o'clock that morning, swarms of GPA staff members and admirers from other programs wishing to pay their respects lined the walls, forming a walkway of honor to escort Mann out. It was totally impromptu. "We had never seen anything like that at WHO for anybody before," Tarantola recalled.

Mann was shaken. At first the crowd stood still and somber. As he moved forward, people began clapping, then hollering until the crowd, roughly two hundred strong, broke into wild roars and cheers.

Unable to find his tongue to address his colleagues and admirers, tears streamed down Mann's face as he ambled into the crisp Geneva morning.

Quiescence
(1990–1996)

—ᴍ—

Voices in the Wilderness, Race and Space

On November 11, 1989, the Berlin Wall came tumbling down, giving way to a sea change in the international political landscape. Change was in the air, and Africa was no exception. Only three months later, at 3:30 P.M. on February 11, 1990, the famed political dissident Nelson Mandela embarked on the last leg of his "Long Walk to Freedom." Mandela had spent twenty-seven years, or roughly ten thousand days, imprisoned on the infamous Robin Island.

South Africa's Nationalist president F. W. DeKlerk had informed Mandela of his long anticipated release roughly forty hours earlier. It was to be the opening salvo in the South African government's dismantling of apartheid, the country's half-century-long system of racial separation. Mandela's release evoked wild celebration. The promise of what was to come stirred the national spirit. For tens of millions of black South Africans it meant political freedom, social equality, and human dignity—the realization of a dream long struggled for.

For Princeton Lyman, it meant the opportunity of a lifetime.

In 1992, the fifty-seven-year-old U.S. diplomat, a gentleman-statesman staid in dress and manner, was nearing the apogee of a remarkable career in the U.S. Foreign Service. The son of Lithuanian immigrants who ran a grocery in a low-income, predominantly African-American area of San Francisco, Lyman spent his boyhood in a home brimming with books, mostly old-world literature. He developed a love of learning, listening, and a keen fascination with the vastness of the world that lay beyond his immediate reality. As an undergraduate at Berkeley Lyman delved into political theory and sensed that service through diplomacy might be his calling.

In his thirties, Lyman was working as an official at USAID when a mentor pointed the newly minted Harvard Ph.D. toward Africa, a continent for which he would develop an abiding passion. Later he moved to the State Department and became the deputy assistant secretary for African Affairs. In the 1980s, he received an ambassador posting to Nigeria. Then he came back to Washington to serve as assistant secretary of state for Refugee Programs.

Seasoned and in the prime of his career, in 1992 Lyman was named the U.S. ambassador to South Africa. At the time, the vast majority of the country's population was intoxicated by the promise of a new, free South Africa. Several leading experts, however, were not as optimistic. The transition would be an enormous challenge laying bare long-held animosities and tribal divisions. The experts worried that the country might degenerate into chaos and/or conflict. The country's trajectory going forward would have enormous impact on the rest of southern Africa and the continent at large.

Around the time of Lyman's confirmation in 1992, a new organization had emerged in South Africa. The National AIDS Committee of South Africa, or NACOSA, sought to bring together governmental and nongovernmental organizations to enhance dialogue and promote action on the issue. When Lyman learned that Nelson Mandela had opened the new committee's proceedings and had pledged his full support, the new ambassador was pleased. Mandela's national and international prestige was at a stratospheric level, even then, two years before he assumed the presidency.

Global AIDS had come on Lyman's radar screen early on. At a cocktail party in Washington in the mid-1970s, Lyman bumped into a social acquaintance, a doctor from Boston who mentioned to Lyman that he had noticed abnormal reports of clusters of strange cancer cases in Zaire. The doctor asked Lyman for funds to investigate. Then in the Office of Development Resources at USAID, Lyman was focused on investments in long-term development. Back then health was considered a social good, not an investment. Lyman didn't have the resources and had to turn him down. More than a decade later, Lyman ran into the same doctor. "I was on to something, wasn't I?" he said to Lyman, who agreed that it was possible that a rare historical window had been missed.

By 1985, Lyman had moved to the State Department. Project SIDA was well under way in Kinshasa, and a senior colleague and good friend of Lyman's, Frank Wisner, was hearing reports from a family friend, a doctor at Harvard, about the disease's foothold on the African continent. Wisner broached the issue with Lyman: "This AIDS problem is really serious," he said. "We've really got to do something."

"Frank, you're absolutely right," Lyman responded sincerely. But there were other issues that seemed more pressing at the time, and there didn't seem to be much interest at the African bureau. Nothing happened.

Eventually Lyman would have another chance in South Africa. As he immersed himself in the affairs of the country, he began to hear more and more from both American and South African diplomats and public health officials about AIDS. In 1990, less than 1 percent of pregnant women throughout the country tested positive for HIV. By 1994 the number had soared to almost 8 percent. In Africa, antenatal HIV prevalence is one of the best benchmarks by which to gauge prevalence of HIV in the adult population at large. The figures suggested that national infections were escalating at a staggering rate.

Up to 1994 the United States had done little about it. The CDC had deployed a full-time expert and USAID funding had reached approximately $3.5 million a year. It was "a paltry sum," Lyman wrote later. If the trend line continued, the CDC expert estimated back in 1994, there would be more than 5 million people infected with AIDS by 2000 in South Africa alone. "Alas, he was too close to the truth," Lyman would write in 2002.

The numbers shook Lyman. It was an alarming prognosis for a country already beset by a daunting litany of political, economic, social, and health issues. After decades of hardships, degradation, and toil, South Africa's black majority was finally on the verge of securing political freedom. But if these numbers were right they were also hurtling toward a terrible precipice.

"We were so focused on the transition and avoiding civil war and getting through the election and the new government. That was our overwhelming priority," Lyman recalled. U.S. foreign policy was transfixed on the historic opportunity. Policy makers were determined not to veer off point. "I can't say [AIDS] stood out among all the other issues in that transition period," Lyman said.

There was also a strong sense that it was not the right juncture to focus on AIDS. Prior to elections, the white-governed Nationalist regime remained in power, and firmly in command of the nation's public health system. During apartheid, injustice and neglect had created an irreparable breach of trust between the white government and the country's blacks.

Lyman and other colleagues felt that pushing the government to move on AIDS prior to a successful transition would have been for naught. The people would never trust the government, and they would not respond to any of their initiatives. It made more sense to weather the transition, and then to move on the issue following the election to be held in May 1994.

When Mandela eventually came to power following the election and appointed Dr. Nkozasana Zuma, an outspoken woman who had directed a USAID-funded HIV/AIDS NGO, as his administration's minister of health, Lyman was hopeful. Right away, she moved to generate an open public discourse on AIDS. Aiming for national attention, she put together *Serafina II*, a high-profile musical production replete with HIV/AIDS awareness themes.

The flagship effort quickly backfired. Many deemed the program unseemly or puerile. The issue became controversial and politically polarized.

Lyman watched aggrieved through the mid-1990s, as South Africa systematically failed to address the impending catastrophe, and was shocked as Mandela said nary a word about the crisis during the rest of his presidency.

For his part, Lyman did attempt to make inroads on the issue. He ensured that crime and AIDS were the only "non-political" items on the U.S. agenda through the transition period. But the issue would languish at the bottom of that agenda. The disease was an emergent, long-term threat always looming on the horizon, subjugated to political or economic matters deemed more high profile and more imminent. The United States would provide tens of millions of dollars in financial aid and untold quantities of human capital to facilitate South Africa's peaceful political transition. It would set up several binational committees with South Africa during that time to address the issues deemed most urgent to ensure the country's stability and well-being through the transition. There would be committees on trade, business, education, and other sectors, but not on health.

By the time Lyman left the country in 1996, the transition had gone better than most anyone might have expected. The country's major public and private institutions had survived a peaceful, orderly election very much intact. South Africa had emerged a vibrant, functioning emblem of multiracial African democracy.

Lyman had indeed been a "Partner to History." But the State Department had sat on the sidelines as the AIDS pandemic burgeoned wildly in South Africa. Experts had told senior officials of the impending catastrophe. Measured against more high-profile, imminent issues, however, State would afford scant time, will, or resources to engage the threat.

"We did not have the handle we thought we had on this issue," Lyman wrote later, "and the results are grievous."

The U.S. approach to the AIDS crisis in South Africa would be a microcosm of the response at large throughout the 1990s. After a tempestuous beginning wrought with contention, misperception, and turf wars, the U.S. response faded into a dim period of quiescence. Stephen Morrison, a U.S. State Department official for much of the 1990s, recalled, "The figures were taking off, yet the response remained relatively static." There were, in Morrison's words, "lone, loud" voices scattered throughout the wilderness of the U.S. government. Yet those voices were disparate and dissonant. They would be drowned out by a powerful wave of contextual currents that worked against U.S. engagement in the issue.

Through the 1990s, the U.S. response languished in a larger complex of U.S. neglect of Africa. It was a complex fueled and perpetuated by U.S. perceptions—or more accurately, misperceptions—about Africa, a deleterious brand of passive racism, geopolitical change and strategic considerations, and an attendant U.S. "fatigue" with both foreign aid and AIDS.

———◆———

By the early 1990s, it was clear to anyone who had bothered to look that AIDS was a crisis of global proportions. As early as 1982 American doctors had diagnosed cases in Haitian immigrants, establishing the disease's presence in the Caribbean. A decade later the pandemic was exploding in corridors of Latin America, most acutely in Brazil. AIDS was also taking a vicious toll in Asia, where Thailand was emerging as that continent's most high-profile hotbed.

Still, as the decade closed and a new millennium dawned, approximately 85 percent of all AIDS deaths had occurred in sub-Saharan Africa. More than 70 percent of those living with HIV/AIDS and 95 percent of AIDS orphans lived in the subcontinent. Through the 1990s, if global AIDS had a face, it was an African one. The distinction would have an enormous bearing on the U.S. response.

As the Cold War thawed, scholars and pundits seemed ebullient about the future prospects of democracy and free-market capitalism, the antecedents, it was assumed, to peace and prosperity. The United States had emerged wildly victorious with unrivaled military and economic power. Waves of democratization and free market reform throughout Eastern Europe, South America, and Africa reinforced the scope, intensity, and influence of U.S. ideology. At times, promise seemed boundless and the zeitgeist of the moment might best be described as "triumphalist."

It was a phenomenon that did not sit well with at least one thinker. Robert Kaplan, a leading realist thinker-pundit-author, set about to disembarrass the United States of its foolish optimism. The world was a messy place, and the United States ought to think twice before committing itself to foreign adventures—military, economic, or humanitarian.

In *The Coming Anarchy*, first published in article form in February 1994, Kaplan's Africa was a macabre spectacle, an anarchic, miasmic postmodern wasteland coming apart at the hinges. He wrote of "the withering away of central governments, the rise of tribal and regional domains, the unchecked spread of disease, the growing pervasiveness of war." He described Conakry, the capital of Guinea, for example, as "one never-ending Shantytown: a nightmarish Dickensian spectacle to which Dickens himself would never have given credence." The piece was clearly posited as a tonic for U.S. ebullience, and it was sobering stuff to be sure.

Kaplan's portrayal would not give much consideration to the democratization, the economic progress, and the potential inherent in the continent. It seemed to evince an implicit admonition: Americans beware. Involvement seemed likely to exact a price in blood and treasure.

Kaplan's work enjoyed much attention among policy makers and elites. President Clinton read it and passed the article around to senior administration officials. To many, the message had a stark resonance.

Jack Chow, the U.S. ambassador for Global AIDS during the Bush II administration, a youthful-looking Asian doctor turned diplomat from California, described the mind-set: "It's Africa," he explained, "it's the victim of 1980s widespread famine, civil war, and the Somalia incursion." He spoke of "the ongoing television pictures of disaster after disaster after disaster." To many Americans, each crisis seemed part of one long, uninterrupted narrative of death and suffering in a faraway land. Pounded with negative images, the result seemed only inevitable: "People's minds just click off. And then you have AIDS and people just think, oh, it's just another disaster."

At a foreign policy conference in Washington, D.C., in the fall of 2002, Ambassador Stephen Lewis, UN Secretary General Kofi Annan's special envoy for Global HIV/AIDS, addressed an international crowd of diplomats and public health officials. Renowned for his passionate oratory, the former Canadian member of parliament pondered aloud: "I do not understand the complex of reasons that allow millions and millions of people to die needlessly under the glare of the world's spotlight. How is this possible?" He confessed: "I don't want to face the answer: subterranean racism that resists the continent of Africa."

The historical record is highly unlikely to reveal any instances of policy makers opposing engagement in the issue because black Africans were dying. Rather, there was simply less of an impetus to move policy because it was black Africans who were dying. This alternate brand of *passive* racism undergirded U.S. inaction through the pandemic's flight in the 1990s and beyond.

When, in the late 1980s, the National Intelligence Council debated whether or not to invest even nominal resources in investigating the pandemic and its repercussions, viewpoints were scattered. Bart Gellman explained that some were of the view that "it will be good for Africa because Africa is overpopulated anyway." AIDS deaths among senior military officers, others suggested, might "boost morale" in the military if they appeared likely to result in increased opportunities for advancement. Along those same lines Gellman cited a 1992 World Bank study, which said: "If the only effect of the AIDS epidemic were to reduce the population growth rate, it would increase the growth rate per capita income in any plausible economic model."

In neither case was there anything overtly racist. Nevertheless, one finds it hard to imagine the intelligence or financial institutions speaking of demographic or economic gain in the event that an insidious disease were poised to kill 20 to 30 percent of the population in North America or Western Europe.

Activist Jamie Love proffered "a 30 million white person test," in which he suggested, "we'd move kind of like it was an emergency." Peter Piot, the director of UNAIDS exclaimed, "If this would happen in the Balkans, or in

Eastern Europe, or in Mexico, with white people, the reaction would have been different."

There are strategic—military and economic—and cultural reasons why the U.S. response might have been different had the disease taken a comparable toll on another continent. But even noted policy makers got the sense that race played a powerful, though amorphous role. In the early 1990s, Russia reported its first cases of HIV. In 1994, with 163 official cases reported, former AIDS Czar Patsy Fleming remembered a rare moment of hope: "At the beginning of the epidemic in the former Soviet Union countries, I thought, well, maybe now they'll pay attention to it, these are white people."

It's not that U.S. policy makers, the media, or the public at large wished death upon black Africans, argued Mark Schneider, a former Peace Corps director and USAID deputy, it was that it simply "made it easier to look away."

Paul Zeitz was never very good at looking away. As a teenager growing up in Philadelphia in the 1970s, Zeitz attended Hebrew School every afternoon. One of his teachers was an elderly lady, a Holocaust survivor who had lost most of her family in the genocide. Often, she would grab a box of Kleenex and assemble the class in a circle and tell them the story of her life, exhorting them, "Never forget. Never again." Zeitz couldn't understand how such a thing could have happened.

As a medical student in Philadelphia in the mid-1980s, Zeitz found that his interests differed from his classmates'. On rounds, they were interested in treating the patient. Zeitz wanted to know why the patient's illness couldn't have been prevented. At a conference in Russia during his second year of medical school, Zeitz listened to a presentation about children's health. He learned that millions and millions of children were dying annually of preventable diseases. He had found his calling.

After finishing his master's in public health at Johns Hopkins and a stint doing epidemiology at the CDC in Atlanta, Zeitz joined USAID in Washington, where he worked through the early 1990s. Working on an inaugural health strategy for Zambia, an impoverished country in the central part of Southern Africa, Zeitz was riding the metro to work one morning in 1994 and reading a newspaper article about the genocide unfolding in Rwanda. Reading the wrenching account, Zeitz gleaned a painful insight. "I am the reason this genocide is happening," he thought to himself. "I'm riding the metro to work like it's any other day and I'm not doing a thing about it."

Zeitz was determined to follow through on the Zambian project, and he resolved to go to Africa. In the fall of 1996 he was appointed senior technical advisor both to the Zambian government and the USAID Mission in Zambia. Zeitz found the transition difficult. He had uprooted his wife and three young children, moving them to a foreign continent. The U.S. government had paid for a spacious white house in Lusaka with sprawling grounds, enough to accommodate a cultivated garden, a fruit grove, and a swimming pool. Hiring a nanny, a cook, and other help, Zeitz found himself living a "neo-colonial" life.

Still, it was difficult to settle in. Spending most of his waking hours at the office working on strategic issues, and increasingly gravitating toward the emerging Zambian orphan crisis, Zeitz had little time for socializing. He was happy, then, to make a new friend. Also in his mid-thirties and with young children, Justin was a member of Zambia's central board of health. In charge of developing communication strategies for HIV/AIDS and child survival programs, he was one of Zeitz's main contacts.

A sharp dresser with a magnetic personality, Justin was welcoming and extended himself to Zeitz immediately. He shared his American colleague's passion for children's health. He helped orient Zeitz in his new milieu. He also had an exceptional sense of humor. At Zeitz's home after hours, during working lunches, or in car rides to and from meetings, he kept his colleague in good humor.

In Washington, Zeitz had studied and analyzed the brewing Zambian AIDS crisis. Now, he was living in it. Early on, his family had become close to the children's nanny; close enough for her to reveal that three of her siblings had died of AIDS, a bold admission given that the disease carried enormous stigma, and most refused to acknowledge it. It was clear to Zeitz that the intermittent ailments that beset his secretary, a warm single mother with a four-year-old child, were striking her because of a deteriorated immune system. She clearly had AIDS, but she would never admit it to Zeitz, a trained physician who could have helped.

The disease was everywhere. It was striking nannies and secretaries, but civil leaders were not immune. Soon after his arrival, Zeitz discovered that the woman who led the nation's nutrition effort, a strong leader with an irreplaceable depth of experience, had died of AIDS. Staggered, Zeitz felt compelled to get a handle on the magnitude of the disease. He shunted aside other commitments and focused on putting together a set of national projections. By the middle of 1997, the results were becoming clear. There was a 20 percent adult national prevalence rate; the rate was one in three in urban areas and 14 percent in rural areas. Far from cresting, the epidemic was still gaining steam, and Zeitz predicted that the crisis would not peak until 2005.

Back at his USAID mission and on the telephone with Washington, Zeitz was pleading for funds and resources. In 1996, Zambia received $2,268,645 from the United States to tackle AIDS. His entreaties were for naught though. Funding would barely move through the end of the decade.

Though death was all around him, Zeitz had not yet been to an African funeral. Late in 1997, he would go to his first. Weeks before, Justin had fallen ill, and as in so many African AIDS cases devoid of proper drug therapy or care, death came quickly. Zeitz had lost a dear friend, and the country had lost a leading official in its effort to battle the disease.

The sun was pounding down on a sweltering Zambian morning as Zeitz set out to pay his final respects. Smothered in a meandering line of hundreds of mourners, Zeitz waited his turn to take his moment at the casket, which rested in a concrete-block building a few hundred feet from the gravesite. Normally, Zeitz found the Zambian people mild-mannered and reticent. As Zeitz passed by the casket to say good-bye to his friend, he could hear the wails of hundreds of mourners piercing the air.

The women were dressed in traditional garb and most of the men in suits in the procession escorting the coffin to its final resting place. Zeitz could see at least three other burials happening within a few dozen yards. The separate groups of mourners seemed to meld into one. Once Justin's coffin had been manually lowered, Zeitz took his turn throwing a fistful of dirt down the grave onto the coffin. The wailing continued. He looked at Justin's kids, the same ages as his own. They seemed lost. The experience, he recalled, "shook my soul."

With the images of the funeral still fresh in his mind, Zeitz went back to his work. Leaving the University Teaching Hospital one morning on a route he'd taken dozens of times before, Zeitz couldn't believe what he was seeing. Incredulous, he had to pull his red Jeep over and into the shade. Parked at the side of the road was a white minivan belonging to a Christian youth aid program. Alongside it were a bunch of young kids. They were selling coffins.

Zeitz was starting to believe that the system was failing. He was getting radicalized.

———•◆•———

For all its attendant costs and anxiety, the Cold War had had the effect of imposing a finite order on global politics. The U.S.–Soviet rivalry neatly divided the world into a bipolar power structure, in which the two superpowers jostled restlessly for prestige and influence. A gain for one would be a loss for the other. The underlying dynamic meant that almost no corner of the globe could be left unattended. In the Cold War, then, Africa mattered.

As the iron curtain lifted, ushering in the new post–Cold War era, Africa seemed to lose its geostrategic relevance. It was deemed a poor continent in which the United States had no major economic partners. It represented a small export market. There were no major military flashpoints that threatened to spill over into other regions. There were no nuclear weapons on the continent. No Southern African country presented a particular military threat—to U.S. interests, at any rate. There was no major domestic political constituency driving U.S. engagement in the continent.

All the factors that drive the strategic calculus seemed to rate low when it came to Africa. According to Chester Crocker, the senior African policy maker in the Reagan administration: "The end of the cold war produced a strategic disengagement" from the continent.

The calculation would overlook several critical inputs. A wave of economic growth would ripple through the continent over the course of the 1990s. Fourteen of the continent's countries would grow by more than 4 percent per year. Three or four would be among the fastest growing economies in the world. Africa was rich in resources and minerals, such as iron ore and manganese, that were vital to U.S. industrial and military interests. The United States imported roughly 15 percent of its oil from the continent.

Still, Africa seemed a region of strategic irrelevance, the perfect place from which to pare down commitments to secure a "peace dividend" for an increasingly insular American public.

Wasting little time, the United States moved to scale back accordingly. First, it would steadily slash its diplomatic presence on the continent. Roughly sixty officer positions were eliminated at the State Department's Africa Bureau, which also lost a deputy assistant secretary of state position.

Stephen Morrison was a senior official in the U.S. State Department
Policy Planning Staff, concentrating on Africa, for most of the 1990s. "We
were shutting down missions. We were shutting down intelligence stations.
We were shutting down things all over the place. . . . We dropped our
coverage in Africa dramatically." As a result, "Large stretches of the continent—particularly areas suffering acute conflict—[were] no longer regularly covered by on-site diplomatic personnel." Through the 1990s the
continent was, in fact, as one *New York Times* journalist opined, "the neglected stepchild of American diplomacy."

Concomitantly, U.S. foreign aid, at large, decreased substantially over
the course of the decade. Measured against the growth in the U.S. economy during the same period, U.S. foreign assistance to Africa, specifically,
fell off precipitously.

Jack Chow, former U.S. ambassador for Global AIDS, noted: "there is
this baseline antipathy towards foreign aid as a whole." The reasons for
that "antipathy" begin with a powerful misconception harbored by most
Americans. When Americans are asked to estimate what percent of the
U.S. budget goes to foreign assistance, one poll showed, the median guess is
15 percent. When asked if they think that number is appropriate, most answer that it seems too high. In actuality, though, through the 1990s, U.S.
foreign assistance totaled approximately 0.1 percent of the national
budget—1/150th of the median American's estimate. Most of that aid was
apportioned to Israel, Egypt, and Colombia—allocations clearly driven
more by strategic considerations than a needs-based calculation.

U.S. insularity, the demand for a post–Cold War "peace dividend," and
U.S. misconceptions about foreign aid at large were all factors in generating declines in U.S. foreign assistance. And they would find a voice, and a
powerful one at that, in an elderly conservative senator from North Carolina named Jesse Helms.

After a long career in Congress, Helms became chairman of the Senate
Foreign Relations Committee when the Republicans took control of Congress in 1994. Though Helms denounced adversaries who called him an
isolationist, he made it clear that U.S. foreign commitments ought to be
scaled down, and focused only on those threats he deemed "vital" to U.S.
national security interests.

U.S. foreign assistance became Helms's battering ram. It seemed to the
old-line conservative the epitome of liberal profligacy. He proclaimed that
foreign assistance was tantamount to throwing money down a "rat hole."

Helms argued that foreign assistance merely siphoned funds from U.S. taxpayers to inept despots or corrupt regimes who would not use funds efficiently or judiciously. The money rarely went to those in need, he maintained, and when it did, it helped make recipients dependent on American aid, perpetuating a negative cycle that stood against the interests of all involved.

Against the backdrop of gaping budget deficits and a strong movement in the mid-1990s to balance the budget, Helms's view held sway over most of the Republican-controlled Congress. Helms would spend much time trying to abolish USAID, or move it under the aegis of the State Department, so that at least its activities might yield strategic benefits.

Paul DeLay, who would run the Division of Global HIV/AIDS at USAID in the late 1990s, remembered, "Helms was a constant thorn in our side." He was constantly looking to cut funding at the agency. DeLay recalled a certain NGO in Senegal, one of the hundreds of groups the division supported on the continent. On one occasion Helms got wind, according to DeLay, that the NGO had some vague links to "voodoo"—not, in DeLay's view, a particularly troubling irregularity. Helms used the tidbit to cut back funding and hold the division in a vise.

The senator was a constant source of frustration to Congressional champions like Jim McDermott. "Once the Senate goes over to the Republicans [in 1994], you had a guy who was homophobic as the chairman of the Foreign Relations Committee, and who was certainly AIDS phobic. . . . That was a dark period," he averred. "Some of the inaction has to be tied to the fact that Jesse was wielding a pretty strong hand."

Those averse to foreign aid commitments, as well as the much larger group who was merely disinterested, had found a powerful paladin in Helms. The senator would unflinchingly employ his clout to quash the effort. He furnished a cogent argument to rationalize the position. It exempted disinterested policy makers from asking some of the harder questions, from digging deeper.

Foreign assistance levels were slashed accordingly. At the crest of the Cold War era, U.S. aid to Africa had reached roughly $800 million per annum. Aid levels would consistently taper down over the course of the 1990s, and by 1996, U.S. developmental assistance to Africa had dropped to around $600 million.

For Chow, U.S. disinterest in global AIDS began with the "baseline antipathy," and "then you have global AIDS, or AIDS in Africa, and then they lump it in to foreign aid." In other words, "foreign aid has negative connotations and they extrapolate that onto global AIDS overseas."

Since the early 1980s, AIDS had taken its toll on American society. It had taken hundreds of thousands of American lives, cost billions of dollars in resources, and it had been a point of intense political division. It had also forced the American public to talk about sex, drug use, and other taboo subjects in an unprecedented fashion. These were all uncomfortable matters.

By the mid-1990s, the rate of domestic incidence had begun to wane. There was a sense that the fires were now under control; that AIDS on the domestic front was going away. Most Americans were more than happy to consider the issue history.

AIDS fatigue was evident throughout the decade. Policy makers, the media, and the American public alike were disinclined, by and large, to confront the murmurings about an impending global catastrophe. Having retired from USAID in 1992, Jeffrey Harris would watch from the sidelines as American policy remained static through the next seven years. His explanation: "I think it's . . . that they were just tired of hearing about it."

———•◆•———

Donna Shalala first encountered AIDS in the early 1980s when she was president of Hunter College in New York City. A petite, fiery woman with short black hair, she was hardly afraid to challenge the system. When college employees began to come down with AIDS in 1982 and '83, Shalala circumvented the rules, ensuring that they would receive benefits.

As Bill Clinton's secretary of Health and Human Services, or HHS, Shalala was the nation's seniormost health official for most of the 1990s. During her tenure, Clinton broke with his Republican predecessors, and openly and forcefully declared the domestic AIDS epidemic a national crisis of the highest order. During his first campaign, he pledged to marshal resources and leadership to combat the epidemic.

Clinton's campaign promises were music to Shalala's ears. There was no health threat of greater import to the new Cabinet official. Upon assuming her post, Shalala declared that AIDS was her number one disease priority.

During her tenure she spearheaded a comprehensive national effort to combat the disease. She was able to secure billions from Congress for biomedical research, patient care, and a far-reaching prevention campaign, including the first nationally televised commercials. The prevention campaign helped decrease infection levels. In addition, during Clinton's tenure, effective life-extending antiretroviral, or ARV, drug treatment was "discovered" and made accessible, decreasing AIDS deaths markedly.

Despite her accomplishments, she would fail to keep the president from making an eleventh-hour turnabout on needle exchange programs, as he reneged on the campaign promise in late April 1998. It was a blemish on an otherwise remarkable record on the domestic front.

Shalala knew from the outset that there was a front beyond America's shores as well. But when she arrived in Washington early in 1993, she was also confronted with a series of steep obstacles. Her department's budget had been pummeled by budget cuts at the hands of a twelve-year Republican reign. There was a steep economic recession, and she was working for a president who would become intent on balancing the budget. Fiscal and political constraints would make it difficult for her to secure funding increases and throw her political weight behind more than only a handful of issues.

"We never saw AIDS as just a domestic issue," Shalala said of her department's perspective under her tenure. "It was very clear to me that there was an international crisis of unbelievable proportions." However, "all the pressure on us was on the domestic side."

Yet, Shalala would do more than any other Cabinet official during Clinton's first six years in office to elevate global AIDS on the U.S. agenda. Every high-profile speech she gave on AIDS had an international dimension. Every time she met with a foreign leader, she would include AIDS on her agenda. She was particularly vehement in her advocacy with India, China, Russia, and South Africa. To varying degrees, she said, "All of them were in denial."

In the summer of 1994, Shalala attended a notable international event on AIDS dubbed the Paris Summit. In a telling sign of the administration's position early on, there was a good deal of high-level rancor concerning whether or not the event was even worthy of the "Summit" designation. Some senior officials did not think the subject of the meeting was worthy of conferring the import that the word seemed to connote.

The Summit's primary by-product was the passage of GIPA, or Greater Involvement of People with AIDS, an agreement that aimed to enfranchise HIV/AIDS patients themselves in the formulation of government policy. A landmark achievement, in many ways it paved the way for the strong role that the AIDS community would play in policy making in the future. The Summit also helped draw attention to the pandemic. However, it would not substantially move U.S. policy with respect to leadership or funding, which remained stagnant at $120 million per annum.

The Paris Summit motivated Shalala to probe ways in which she might move U.S. policy. The funding picture in Congress was bleak. With Jesse Helms chairing the Foreign Relations Committee, Shalala said, "it was very difficult to get health money through on the international side." USAID's prospects appeared dim. Shalala sought, then, to exert influence on the issue through alternate channels.

To galvanize a global solution, Shalala began to appeal to the pertinent international organizations, attempting to upgrade their response. As long as Hiroshi Nakajima was at the helm of WHO, she believed, that agency's response would be feckless. So she began to set the diplomatic wheels in motion to ensure that Nakajima would not run for reelection in 1998. She was a leading voice in creating UNAIDS, the vehicle that would rise out of the rubble of the GPA. She would also enlist Jim Wolfensohn at the World Bank, a longtime friend and colleague, to focus on the issue. Wolfensohn did in fact become a convert, raising AIDS on the World Bank agenda and speaking widely and forcefully about the issue.

On two or three notable occasions, Shalala appealed directly to President Clinton on global AIDS. Despite the president's apparent interest, there would be no direct follow-up. Shalala did not exert considerable effort or expend much political capital to ensure that there would be.

Through the late 1990s, Donna Shalala could justifiably call herself the Cabinet's most consistent and ardent policy champion on global AIDS. It was a meek distinction, though. Ultimately, for Shalala global AIDS was a subaltern agenda item: "You can't look at this issue and think that we did enough. Not 10 percent of what we should have done."

Much of HHS's global AIDS effort came out of the CDC. Under the leadership of Helene Gayle—an African-American woman with a medical degree from the University of Pennsylvania and an MPH from Johns Hopkins—the Center's international HIV/AIDS effort had indeed expanded its programs over the course of the decade. The CDC had sizable surveillance projects in Kinshasa (Zaire), Thailand, Côte d'Ivoire, and Botswana. The CDC also had a presence in South Africa and India.

Gayle worked assiduously, given what resources were made available, to ensure that the CDC stayed on top of the issue. Slowly and methodically, she also sought to sow interest among her bosses at the centers, in the hopes that more resources would be made available, and perhaps that the CDC might expand its mandate on the issue. There was certainly much it could do given the centers' technical skills if the resources were provided.

Gayle had proven her mettle as a manager. In the tradition of leading public health officials, however, she had more trouble as a political advocate. Early on, Gayle was a junior official in a small area of the CDC afforded little priority or resources. Her official title changed no less than five times over the course of her tenure.

To the young public health official recalibrating the CDC's commitment seemed a daunting enterprise. With only a limited budget, the CDC had roughly eleven different centers. Each had its existing priorities, things like cancer, heart disease, and strokes. Gayle was hardly willing to suggest that resources be reapportioned away from the cancer and heart disease efforts—the two biggest killers of Americans—to focus on international HIV/AIDS. Instead, she took a moderate, incremental approach. "I can't say one day I walked into someone's office and I said, 'By gosh, I need money for international AIDS' and it happened. It's a long dance and it takes many years, based on many inputs and a whole range of people."

One of those key inputs was the U.S. Congress, who oversaw CDC's efforts and funding. Protocol, according to Gayle, precluded her from taking an aggressive tack with the Congress. "You don't press for more funding. You're not allowed to under the rules. When you work for the federal government you're not allowed to advocate for resources . . . there's a very well circumscribed way in which that was done. . . . Congress can ask questions, you can respond to the questions that Congress can ask you."

Under Gayle's stewardship, the CDC's surveillance efforts would grow over the course of the decade. The center would learn much that would later be of use about the disease and its international dimension. Nevertheless, these efforts were largely, if not primarily, rooted in an interest to exploit insights gained abroad to combat the disease at home. Moreover, the agency did not make prevention a priority until late in the decade. Despite Gayle's dedication and notable efforts, then, the CDC's effectiveness in combating global AIDS was nominal through the course of the decade.

Throughout the 1990s the global dimension would take a whopping backseat to the prodigious U.S. effort to combat the disease within its own borders. While there would be roughly 1 million Americans infected during the decade, the United States would come to spend more than $10 billion per year on the domestic epidemic. In that same period more than 40 million infections would accrue worldwide. The United States would spend little more than $100 million per year on the global dimension.

—∞—

No Advocacy from Above,
No Groundswell from Below

On June 7, 1993, Michael Merson strode to the podium at an expansive conference hall in downtown Berlin. Facing an audience of roughly 13,000 scientists, public health officials, activists, and journalists at the Ninth International Conference on AIDS, Merson began reading from a prepared text. He had been anticipating the day for months.

Merson, forty-eight, was a seasoned public health official with a raspy northeastern accent, neatly combed graying hair, and large round eyeglasses. Three years earlier he had replaced Jonathan Mann as the director of WHO's Global Program on AIDS, or GPA.

In most respects Merson was Mann's antipode. A blunt-spoken WHO veteran, he had been at the agency for twelve years upon assuming the reins at the GPA. He was a well-respected, fastidious operative, who was known to do things by the book. If Mann was a maverick, revered for his charisma and renowned for his vision, Merson was the archetypal WHO bureaucrat.

It so happened that in the spring of 1990, the WHO director general, Hiroshi Nakajima—who had been castigated by the international news media in the wake of Mann's departure—was in the market for the latter.

When Merson's phone rang that spring, he was surprised to hear a voice from Nakajima's office requesting a meeting. Merson, then running both the diarrheal disease control program and the respiratory infections program, did not know what to expect when he arrived to meet with Nakajima and some of his staff shortly thereafter. They told him that they wanted him to move programs, and become the acting director at GPA, until they could find a permanent replacement.

Merson was ambivalent. On the one hand, he was a consummate team player and GPA was the agency's biggest program. On the other, he was reluctant to leave his programs, and he hardly knew a thing about AIDS or GPA. "I had no direct involvement at all in AIDS. I won't say I knew nothing, but very little."

When he arrived at GPA, he found the residual trauma from the Nakajima/Mann war palpable. Staff was "very traumatized by his loss and I was aware of that. . . . For them he was a tremendous leader, a visionary. . . . It was painful for them." Many of Mann's loyal lieutenants were skeptical of Merson, whom they presumed to be a Nakajima puppet. None had grown closer to Mann than Daniel Tarantola, his trusted deputy and friend. The Frenchman had stayed behind at Mann's request, but in short order he grew disconsolate with the change in leadership.

As acting director, Merson was not interested in far-reaching change, or moving any needles. He marshaled most of his energies to focus on administrative and managerial affairs, with an emphasis on streamlining the program's operations.

Nakajima and his team seemed pleased with the change. Things were quiet at GPA. The program was staying out of the papers for the most part, running much more by the book, more in line with Nakajima's expectations of proper WHO protocol. Merson was offered the post on a permanent basis, and he accepted.

Not everyone was pleased. "To me it was a huge setback," Tarantola said. "Merson brought in bureaucracy that never existed. Mann was a visionary. Merson was a micromanager. Mann was daring. Merson was afraid. The program lost much of its efficiency and the enthusiasm vanished." Tarantola would resign in the next year. Much of Mann's staff would remain, and continue to work as hard as ever. Many would leave burned out and dejected. "It was tough," Merson remembered, "it was a very tough time."

Operationally, Merson adhered to Mann's overall vision for the program. GPA would still focus on surveillance, the national AIDS plans, or NAPs, and human rights. As Mann had, Merson would also divide his time between advocacy, fund-raising, and management.

In his first few years, Merson worked diligently to streamline GPA's operations and management, rectifying shortcomings for which the program had been criticized under Mann's tenure. "Under Merson more of the groundwork got laid, doing nuts and bolts," remembered Terje Anderson, a prominent AIDS advocate. "If you want to say 'professionalizing'—that's what characterized him." In his rush to ramp up the profile of his program and the pandemic and to gain footprints in as many nations as possible, Mann had moved furiously in those early years. Some of the "nuts and bolts" were overlooked. The rudiments were Mike Merson's specialty. He was a "technical" leader, in the words of Anil Soni, an international policy maker on the issue, and the program benefited.

Merson emerged as a credible global voice on the pandemic and the international response. He traveled extensively, delivering roughly 180 speeches during his five-year tenure. He reached a wide and prominent cast of national leaders and officials. Nils Daulaire, a senior health advisor at USAID for much of Merson's tenure, recalled: "Mike was a strong, capable, very energized leader."

The temptation to compare Merson with his predecessor, however, proved too strong for many to resist. Invariably, they found Merson wanting. "He wasn't the same guy who gave the keynote speeches and moved things," Terje Anderson explained. "Mann was clearly viewed as a more charismatic leader, a visionary. . . . I don't think Merson had that same kind of impact."

At Berlin, Merson aimed, in one dramatic turn, to raze all of the skepticism and to recalibrate the scope and intensity of the global response.

During his three years of tireless advocacy, Merson had grown indignant at the response he was getting from national leaders. They seemed steeped in denial, or even worse, apathy. Some would tell Merson, "It's not our problem. It won't happen to us." Merson believed that much of the denial stemmed from an undergirding view that there was nothing that they could do about the pandemic anyway. It was a lethal fallacy, and Merson didn't want to hear it anymore. Of his speech at Berlin he would say, "I wanted to say, 'Darn it, that's not true.' "

In the months leading up to the Berlin conference Merson had enlisted a sizable cohort of his staff to analyze, with the best and most timely data available, what it might cost the world to turn the tide on the global pandemic. He was determined to think big and to be bold. "I will attempt to show how we can get ahead of the pandemic," he pronounced in his opening remarks. Merson read from a seven-and-a-half-page prepared speech. He outlined the global dimensions of the pandemic, explaining that there were 14 million cumulative infections. In addition to Africa, the pandemic was burgeoning in South America, the Caribbean, and Eastern Europe, and its growth in South and Southeast Asia was "explosive." Merson highlighted the growth in incidence among women and children. In light of these alarming trends, he assailed the global response as "grossly inadequate. Even where budgets are growing," he asserted, "the increases are only incremental—at a time when we need a quantum leap in investment."

The capstone to the speech arrived when he exclaimed that the world could prevent 10 million, or 50 percent, of the predicted new worldwide HIV infections through 2000. "So many lives saved, so much suffering averted," Merson declared.

The WHO knew what was needed to launch a successful intervention effort. The plan would include: the promotion and distribution of condoms in the general population; treatment of conventional STDs because of their role in facilitating HIV transmission; AIDS information and education in schools and through the mass media; promotion of condom use by prostitutes and their clients; the maintenance of a safe blood supply; and needle exchange programs for drug users. They were measures that had already yielded proven results.

Of course, there was a slight catch. It was an ambitious plan, and it would cost money. The audience did not have to wait long before Merson got to the bottom line. The price tag would be between $1.5 and $2.9 billion per year, he explained. Merson called it $2.5 billion to be conservative. It was an outrageously low sum. It was barely enough to "buy one can of Coke for every person in the world," but it was enough to save 10 million lives.

In the most public forum he was afforded, the world's leading authority on the pandemic had laid it out for the international community: 10 million lives could be saved for only $250 per life per year. The ripple effect would mean that millions more would be saved, and tens of billions of dollars would be gained from economic productivity. It was an incomparable opportunity to do so much for so many for so little.

On that early June 1993 day in Berlin, Michael Merson had done something that few in an official capacity had dared: he outlined a strategic plan to combat the pandemic. There was a clear and ambitious goal, a list of the measures necessary to achieve it, and the price needed to finance it.

When Merson departed the plenary session for a press conference nearby, he was met with a flurry of questions. The story made several major newspapers including the *Los Angeles Times*, which featured an article entitled, "AIDS Cases Could Triple by 2000 . . . Speaker in Berlin Urges that $2.5 Billion More Be Spent Each Year to Fight Pandemic." The speech had made a stir and seemed to generate momentum. The moment would prove ephemeral though.

In the two years to follow, Merson continued to advocate for global AIDS awareness and resources, but he had left his boldness in Berlin. When it came to his interactions with U.S. leaders, he reverted to the same incremental advocacy that he had convincingly decried in his landmark address.

Following Mann's infamous departure from GPA, advocacy from above—i.e., the international level—was uninspiring and ineffectual. U.S. politicians and policy makers would have to be moved, it seemed, by a groundswell of political pressure from below.

———•———

"I don't know if they didn't believe me, or if they didn't want to believe me," Merson wondered later. By the late 1990s, Michael Merson was telling anyone who would listen that there were as many as 30 or 40 million people infected in the world. But, there was a critical caveat: "only a fraction were sick."

Former USAID senior advisor Nils Daulaire noted: "I think it's interesting that when you look at the time of infection to time of death with AIDS [it] averages eight to ten years. The fact is that [the global response] has consistently been that length of time behind the curve."

AIDS killed roughly 850,000 people worldwide in 1993, and annual deaths would increase to 1.3 million in 1995. It was a terrible toll, but it still fell short of perennial killers such as malaria and tuberculosis. It made the full dimensions of what was brewing "very hard for people to grasp," Merson insisted.

Congressman Jim McDermott remembered the sort of reactions he would hear from colleagues in the House: " 'We've got problems with things right here, right now,' a typical colleague might say. 'You're talking about things that are going to happen in ten years.' " The disease's inherent latency was, perhaps, its most lethal weapon. Nils Daulaire believed: "It is one of the subtle and pervasive effects of a virus that acts so slowly and insidiously as AIDS does, that it lulls us into inaction."

The disease's latency would help breed apathy and inaction, but it was also a great crutch, a rationalization to justify the more elemental problem—myopia and malaise. For most of the 1990s, they were also among the most prominent features of American culture.

During the decade, three forces underpinned the country's cultural condition in particular: a prolific economic expansion that generated unprecedented wealth, the dissipation of the Cold War and the emergence of American hegemony, and finally, technology's impact on how Americans experienced the world.

The prominent political scientist Tad Homer-Dixon likened the U.S. relationship to the world at large to a limousine cruising through the slums of the developing world. It was an apt metaphor, and its resonance would only escalate as the decade went on. Wealth didn't accumulate in the 1990s; it exploded.

From 1994 onward, America would find itself in the midst of an unprecedented economic expansion. The Dow Jones Industrial Average rose by 400 percent throughout the decade. The stock market would increase fivefold in value, from $3 trillion to $15 trillion. The expansion generated a concurrent surge in wealth. By 1997, almost 150,000 Americans were making a million dollars a year. By 1999, 6.5 million had assets of a million dollars or more. Had Microsoft been a country near its apex, it would have been the ninth largest economy in the world, just behind Spain.

"We were in a boom period," Congressman McDermott recalled. "Everyone's watching their 401K go out of sight." In noneconomic matters, "There was little attention paid to the rest of the world."

At times it seemed the United States didn't really have to. Through the rubble of the Cold War, America emerged as the world's greatest economic, military, and cultural power—a hyperpower, it was suggested. The new American world without apparent enemies or immediate threats helped breed complacency, which in turn, bred insularity. "Therein lies the great irony of the post–Cold War era," foreign policy scholar James Lindsay wrote in an article entitled "The New Apathy" in *Foreign Affairs*. "At the very moment the United States has more influence than ever on international affairs, Americans have lost much of their interest in the world around them." Henry Kissinger concurred: "Americans' interest in foreign policy is at an all-time low."

It was a decade in which some congressmen would boast that they did not even own a passport. Others bragged that they had not ever traveled out of the country, an apparent sign of patriotism.

The 1990s were, perhaps above all, a time of magnificent technological innovation. Though much of the technology had in fact been invented in earlier decades, it was becoming accessible in droves in the 1990s. Consumers were treated to a staggering proliferation in radio, cable and satellite television channels, Internet access, and a seemingly endless array of media and entertainment options.

Techno-optimists heralded a new world of boundless choice and convenience. In the process, they would evoke that most famous of American cultural critics, Henry David Thoreau, who cautioned America in an earlier age of innovation: "We do not ride upon the railroad, it rides upon us."

While some rode the technological wave, few could resist being dragged along by the current. Whether it was billboards, radio commercials, Internet banners, television programming, or consumer electronics, the sheer scope and intensity of stimuli was incredible and unavoidable. It had vertiginous and sometimes mind-numbing effects.

The American mind was hard-pressed to avoid becoming saturated with bright, flashy, fleeting images. In an article in *Harper's Magazine*, "The Numbing of the American Mind," cultural critic Thomas de Zengotita argued that the intensity and ubiquity of these technologies fashioned the American mind "clogged, anesthetized. Numb." Thus, when you "see your 974th picture of a weeping fireman . . . or when you hear statistics about AIDS in Africa . . . you can't help but become fundamentally indifferent because you are exposed to things like this all the time."

Amidst all the change and "progress," America found it hard to identify and coalesce around a unifying national purpose. Americans, particularly the emerging generation, were disengaged with foreign affairs and public affairs at large. A survey indicated that in 1965, 57.8 percent of college freshmen believed that "keeping up to date with political affairs" was either a very important or essential life goal. By 1999, according to the survey, that number had dwindled to 25.9 percent. Applications for entry into the U.S. Foreign Service declined markedly during the decade.

In Henry Kissinger's view: "In the globalized economic world, the post–Cold War generation looks to Wall Street or Silicon Valley in the same way their parents did to public service in Washington. This reflects the priority of being attached to economic over political activity."

In *The Best of Times*, journalist Haynes Johnson interviewed several seniors at Stanford University, presumably the elite, the best and most thoughtful of their generation. Echoing the sentiments of the rest of his classmates, one of the students lamented: "I wish we had something to fight for, something that brings you together . . . But for us, there's nothing to unite about."

Consumed with an explosion of wealth, encamped in "virtual" communities, awash in frivolous entertainment and a dizzying sea of technology, and smug in its seemingly impregnable might, it was an insular, frivolous and apathetic epoch for America at large.

Through the limousine's rose-tinted windows, it was hard to make out the millions dying of AIDS.

———•◆•———

Attending a conference in Harare, Zimbabwe, in December 1998, Eugene Rivers, forty-eight, an iconoclastic African-American minister from Boston with a stout frame and graying hair, ran into Kurt Shillinger, a reporter for *The Boston Globe*. Shillinger had come to know Rivers as a local celebrity. Born in a rough section of Philadelphia and abandoned by his father at an early age, Rivers was taken in by a street gang as a teenager. An inquisitive intellect and a series of chance encounters with unexpected mentors kept Rivers in school, where he would begin to excel.

Eventually, a Pentecostal minister took him in as a protégé, and Rivers fell in love with the church. Upon assuming his ministry in Dorchester, a predominantly African-American and Latino section of Boston with a high incidence of drug use and crime, Rivers found himself in a familiar milieu. His life experience was a testimonial that the community's problems were not insoluble. He planted his stake in Dorchester and with a messianic drive, a sharp tongue, and a hands-on and—if needed—combative approach, he began a life of tackling the community's social ills. His devotion and unconventional tactics won him international attention and even a *Newsweek* cover story as a renegade "street pastor."

A staple in the Boston community, Rivers was popular enough to help attract Shillinger to Harare, where the clergyman would be addressing the World Council of Churches on the role of the church in combating crime. Already acquainted, Shillinger and Rivers were engaged in a side conversation at the conference the day before Rivers was scheduled to deliver his address. As Rivers briefed the reporter from the *Globe* on the broad points of his upcoming speech, Shillinger interrupted, "Listen, do you know what's going on here with AIDS?"

"Yeah, it's bad here, I know," Rivers answered.

In the preceding years, Rivers had heard snippets about AIDS in Africa. He knew that it was an escalating problem. He had read the press coverage on the debate over pharmaceutical pricing and drug patents. But he hadn't noticed much discussion, or picked up on much press coverage about the magnitude of the crisis.

His reply was too quick for Shillinger. "No. You don't understand. There's someone you've got to meet."

Shillinger escorted Rivers to his car and drove him to a colonial-style building in downtown Harare, where the pair climbed the stairs to an office where a ceiling fan sliced through the stifling midday heat. Upon entering, Shillinger introduced Rivers to Michael Auret, an elderly white man and a devout Catholic theologian who had fought in Zimbabwe's armed struggle for independence.

Auret explained that Rivers could do much to help if he took up the issue and drummed up advocacy in the United States upon his return. Rivers liked Auret, and so he gave a direct reply, "Look, I'm busy doing other stuff and I don't want to be one of these people who ambulance chase."

Auret could see that Rivers wasn't getting it. He felt it imperative to muster support from fiery leaders in the States, and so he put it differently: "Seven out of ten high school seniors in Harare are infected," he said. "We are in the midst of an ecological crisis as a result of the deforestation due to coffin construction. If there's not a major mobilization, Africa will be reduced to beachfront property for Europeans."

Rivers sat shaken as Auret briefed him further. By the time he exited the downtown office he was in physical pain. That evening, Rivers redrafted his speech. The following day he delivered an impassioned address to the conference, stressing sexual responsibility and the plight of mothers and orphans.

By the time Rivers returned home to Boston later that month, he had come to think of the crisis as an African holocaust, and he was determined to jump into the advocacy arena from the other side of the Atlantic. He began looking into the response from the African-American community. He couldn't find anything. He had a few office administrators do a Lexis-Nexis search and then had them call around to leading national organizations. They couldn't come up with anything.

Rivers went to Shillinger at the *Globe* and then to Ben Bradlee Jr., one of the paper's senior editors, and asked who was leading the charge from the African-American community. No one, both said. Rivers was incredulous. There were 35 million African-Americans, and no one in black America was speaking out on the holocaust consuming Africa.

Rivers's contacts were right. Through the end of 1998, African-American leadership was mute on AIDS in Africa. Well-financed and wielding enormous political clout, the constituency's leading organizations, like the National Association for the Advancement of Colored People, the Urban League, and the Southern Christian Leadership Conference started by Martin Luther King Jr., did not address the issue. Later, leaders like Ron Dellums and Barbara Lee would emerge in Congress. However, the Congressional Black Caucus uttered nary a word about the crisis until 1999. Along with leading personalities like Andrew Young, Jesse Jackson, and Al Sharpton, also silent on the issue until very late in the 1990s, these organizations largely set the African-American political agenda.

Leaders like Julian Bond, chairman of the NAACP, who conceded, "For years the NAACP didn't do enough about AIDS," point to domestic challenges in the African-American community like crime, drugs, poverty, and incarceration. To be sure, the African-American domestic agenda was replete with pressing issues. The reasons for the community's abdication, however, run deeper.

From the outset, AIDS laid bare long existing tensions between the African-American community and the U.S. public health establishment. Particularly on matters of infectious disease, the relationship has been checkered with distrust and animosity. Through the twentieth century, both syphilis and gonorrhea would affect African-Americans at a disproportionate level to Americans at large. It helped breed accusations and fed prevailing racial stereotypes of the oversexualized African-American.

In the 1930s, scientists at Tuskegee University in Alabama enlisted over four hundred African-American males, all infected with syphilis, to participate in a long-term study on the effects of the disease. The scientists were particularly interested in the relationship between race and the disease. The subjects were awarded nominal compensation and benefits. The study spanned five decades, and in the 1970s, the country would learn that even as penicillin had become available, the scientists had withheld the curative drug from the test subjects. The patients would live their lives unaware of the treatment. Most would become intensely sick, or even die for having been deprived of the drug.

Tuskegee left most African-Americans indignant and spawned circumspection of the public health establishment. Laurie Garrett wrote: "The travesty of Tuskegee would continue to fester in both the public health and African-American communities, widening a credibility gap that was already vast. Eventually, all U.S. government public health pronouncements and programs would be viewed with hostility, even outright contempt, by African-Americans of all social classes."

The Tuskegee experience was not forgotten among most African-Americans when a new sexually transmitted disease began to surface in the United States in the early to mid-1980s. When the disease spread to African-Americans, many were hostile and accusatory. Doctor Kenneth Shine, former president of the Institute of Medicine, who was a physician at UCLA and tended to many of the first diagnosed AIDS cases in the United States, recalled that they felt victimized. Some African-Americans, he remembered, "charged that it was Jewish doctors in Chicago who injected the virus in blacks." One conspiracy theory held that the virus was actually created in a CIA germ warfare laboratory. According to one regional poll, 65 percent of African-American churchgoers either agreed with, or were unsure about the statement: "I believe AIDS is a form of genocide against the black race."

Smarting from historical experience, in which these diseases fueled racial stereotypes, and a history of being misled by the public health establishment, many in the African-American community were wary of engaging the disease at home or abroad.

Rivers acknowledged the historical wrongdoings, but he wasn't about to exonerate African-American leaders with excuses based on historical grievances. As incidence and death rates soared in Africa through the 1990s, Rivers sensed another factor at work in the African-American community: plain denial. Addressing the magnitude of the calamity presupposed acknowledgment of the sexual behavior driving it. Black promiscuity or sexual behavior was too sensitive and racially charged for African-American leaders to take on. Denial also stemmed in part from racial sensitivities: "There was almost a feeling that we're just the cosmic biological losers of the universe. Every time we turn around we have another problem." Rivers explained, "There was a sense that we can't handle another story about blacks as basket cases."

The United States comprises many racial, religious, or ethnic groups—Irish, Italians, Cubans, and Jews, for example—whose links to their home-land are strong. There have been notable efforts from African-American industry to make commercial inroads into Africa. During Africa's decolo-nization, pockets of support arose intermittently among African-American activists and political leaders. Many African-Americans engaged in anti-apartheid political activism in the 1970s and 1980s. There have certainly been ties. However, historically the African-American community has not looked to the mother continent with a similarly strong sense of diaspora.

Part of the reason must be rooted in slavery, which denied slaves their cultural and historical identity. As Rivers suggested, part of the reason also emanates from racial sensitivities that have led many African-Americans to decouple themselves from Africa. In the Oscar award–winning docu-mentary *When We Were Kings*, chronicling Muhammad Ali's "rumble in the jungle" with George Foreman, Spike Lee explained that for a long time, if an African-American called another African-American "African," it would be grounds for a fight. For many, "African" is tantamount to a pe-jorative. "You have a certain segment of black America," Rivers observed, "that is skittish around connecting with Africa. [They] say, 'we're Ameri-can blacks'—versus being black Americans—that don't feel any cultural or historical connection with Africa."

Inaction and quiescence among the African-American community through the 1990s would leave Rivers to ponder: "What verdict will our descendants render upon their ancestors who stood by silently as a genera-tion of African children were reduced to biological underclass by this sex-ual holocaust?"

Rivers's chilling question went unanswered, not only by the African-American community, but by every other domestic political constituency that had a stake in the issue.

By the early to mid-1990s, there had been a huge upsurge in political activism aimed at moving U.S. domestic AIDS policy. Megastars like Magic Johnson—who candidly disclosed his own infection in November 1991—Elizabeth Taylor, and Elton John galvanized Hollywood and called for greater resources. Increasingly well-funded organizations like the Pedi-atric AIDS Foundation broadened the scope of the AIDS community to include soccer moms and mainstream America. The deluge of attention and high-profile advocacy made it politically untenable for U.S. politicians to ignore the issue. Policy with respect to the domestic epidemic moved accordingly.

Through 1998, the domestic AIDS community would concern itself, with rare exceptions, only with the domestic dimension of the disease. The organizations that represent the AIDS community had grass roots. They arose in direct response to local needs. The disease continued to take a dire domestic toll through the latter part of the decade, and anything international was generally viewed as extramandatory, and off point. In addition, there was a grave misconception among domestic activists that increasing resources for global AIDS would take resources away from their domestic efforts. In fact, domestic funding came from HHS and NIH and international funding came from USAID. The pots were separate. But, for the most part, the domestic community did not dig deep enough or demonstrate enough interest to get beyond the misconception.

By the mid- to late 1990s, the domestic AIDS community had grown conditioned to railing against the government about injustices and shortchanges in funding. The government response was very poor from the get-go, and the activist community had to be relentless and aggressive. It bred inertia, a feeling that even a momentary lapse in focus might do the cause great harm.

The domestic AIDS community would gradually turn its gaze abroad in the waning years of the decade, but for most of the 1990s, it would exercise almost no political influence on the global dimension.

There were several well-established political organizations focusing on matters of global health in the Beltway. AIDS was, after all, a global health issue. For organizations like the National Council of International Health, however, global AIDS was a low priority until late in the 1990s. Through the decade, health threats like malaria, TB, diarrheal disease, and cholera remained priorities for these groups. Those were the issues that professionals at these organizations knew. They had done their graduate work on them. Perhaps they had worked at HHS, the CDC, or USAID in one of those areas. They had made it their life's work to make progress in combating these other killers.

The disease's latency also played a role. As did the perception that health interventions—despite Mann's and Merson's testimony—were too expensive, or still had unproven efficacy. There seemed to be many reasons why not to afford a politically dicey, emergent issue newfound priority on agendas that were already tight.

The developmental community did not grab the issue for many of the same reasons: a dearth of resources, professional inertia, and uncertainty about how, exactly, to tackle the problem. Perhaps most notably, the developmental agenda was enormous and diverse: malnutrition, education, agriculture, democracy promotion, human rights, population control, and market reform featured most prominently. With a long agenda, nominal resources, and against the backdrop of U.S. government and public disinterest in developmental aid, the developmental community was stretched as it was. Global AIDS wouldn't register on the community's agendas until late in the decade.

The domestic political constituencies that drive policy from below were silent, and policy makers were listening. Patsy Fleming, who served in the Clinton White House as AIDS czar during the early to mid-1990s, was among a very small group of White House officials interested in moving U.S. policy overseas. When she looked beyond 1600 Pennsylvania Avenue for support from constituencies who might have brought political pressure to bear, she found none. "The American people [were] not really saying we need the [pandemic] to be stopped. American people were . . . not very interested. Every president, every elected official, listens to what his or her constituents say when they make those decisions on policy. So, that's really an important reason why there was not more done."

———•◆•———

During his five-year tenure from 1990 to 1995, Michael Merson traveled from Geneva to the United States four to six times every year. The leading global voice on the pandemic and the global response, Merson was intent on waking the United States from its great slumber.

There was a tricky dynamic behind the challenge for Merson. The United States was the program's single largest donor. Therefore, he deemed it prudent to tread carefully with U.S. policy makers. U.S. commitment, however, was also a critical benchmark, and probably the key in moving the global response. Merson was straddling a fine line.

The archetypal risk-averse bureaucrat, he set his aim merely on maintaining his position on the tightrope, trying to win incremental support, unwilling to hazard the type of advocacy necessary to achieve a recalibration.

Merson would call on U.S. policy makers with the most reliable data and analysis then available. He told his interlocutors of the magnitude of the problem and how much of it might be averted for a relatively paltry commitment in resources and leadership. Policy makers responded, though, for the most part with only tepid interest or outright apathy.

"Prevention is silent, you don't see it. You can't see what you don't have," Merson explained. Engaging the disease offered policy makers little in the way of tangible accomplishment with which to extract political gain.

For some, the pandemic's explosion was simply overwhelming. Merson recalled: "People felt that they didn't want to hear it—it's too much to take, too much to believe." Only a handful of politicians seemed to have the forethought to think about the pandemic at all. The issue easily became subsumed under the exigencies of the hot-button political issues of the day.

While Merson had trouble obtaining policy makers' interest and support, there was a more fundamental problem. He didn't know precisely who he had to appeal to in the first place. It was entirely unclear to the global leader who or what was driving the U.S. response. It seemed to Merson that "the U.S. government was very fragmented. That was a huge problem."

On visits, Merson would shuttle from building to building and office to office, making sure he had touched all the right bases, rounding an unwieldy number of bases indeed.

First, there was USAID. It was clear to Merson that the agency played a critical role in funding allocation, which is to say that the agency was where the money was. There was a long list of people with whom Merson sought to maintain a dialogue at USAID. Many of its key officials would change throughout his tenure. After Jeffrey Harris vacated his position as head of the Division of Global HIV/AIDS at the agency, the post turned over several times during Merson's tenure. It was often unclear who exactly was running the show at USAID.

Of course, there was also HHS, which occupied the U.S. seat on WHO's governing board; as such, that department was a critical constituency. In the realm of health, there was also the CDC. The center's surveillance activities made it a player in the global response, and a requisite point of contact for Merson during his U.S. trips. Similarly, Merson would try to meet with officials at the NIH, who were leading the effort on the scientific, biomedical side.

The State Department was a critical stop. State exercised considerable influence, or had the potential at any rate to exercise political influence on funding and the U.S. political and diplomatic effort. At State, Merson would have to meet not only with officials at the International Organizations Bureau, but of course with a plethora of officials in the regional bureaus.

Whenever he could, Merson would jump at the chance to get an audience with Leon Fuerth, Vice President Gore's chief foreign policy advisor. Gore had always demonstrated an interest in "new" or nontraditional foreign policy issues like the environment or health. Merson would furnish Fuerth with statistics and updates and implore him to enlist the VP to champion the issue with Congress, the president, and other international leaders.

The most important players on Merson's "to see" list were in Congress, where he would lobby appropriators for funds. There were about a half dozen key figures including Obey, Pelosi, Leahy, and McDermott with whom Merson really sought to connect.

Merson's advocacy trips to the States were dizzying, invariably leaving him exhausted by the time he was scheduled to wrap things up in Washington and return to Geneva. "I had to do a lot of knocking on doors," Merson remembered.

It was clear that there was an enormous amount of fragmentation in the U.S. response. No one area of the government had a mandate to tackle the issue in a serious capacity. Merson recalled: "I would sometimes wind up telling one part of the U.S. government what the other part of the government was doing." Structural overlap and dissonance continued to shackle the U.S. response.

Michael Merson was a world-class public health official, an impeccable manager, and an exemplary bureaucratic operative. Regressing to incremental advocacy, though, he was not willing to champion his bold plan, to sound all the trumpets, or to exhaust all the means at his disposal to bring pressure to bear on the world's wealthiest national leaders.

Through most of Merson's tenure, U.S. global AIDS funding hovered between $100 and $125 million. At Berlin, Merson had publicly proclaimed support for a strategy requiring $2.5 billion per year from the global community. It would mean that the U.S. share (per its percent of global GDP) ought to be $600 to $750 million per year, roughly a five-to sixfold increase over its actual funding level.

Yet, Merson conceded, "My appeal to the U.S. was to maintain and if possible increase funding," and so funding languished at around one-fifth or one-sixth of the level Merson had trumpeted at Berlin.

Merson would stand in conference rooms or offices, flanked by an array of charts, graphs, and visual aids, and outline the trajectory of the disease and its toll on humanity. But when it came to advocacy, Merson's strategy was: "We're going in and saying, 'Look, you've got to maintain us, you can't cut us.'"

Fiscal matters were tight in Congress in those years. Merson's congressional liaison would tell him that funding increases were unlikely. The consummate professional, Merson would say, "I was always careful not to exaggerate the extent of the epidemic or what I thought resource needs were because I wanted to be credible in the political context."

Merson maintained his credibility, and his funding levels, sometimes even securing modest $5 to $10 million increases for GPA. But it was a far cry from the levels he had endorsed at Berlin.

"There are times I wish we would have been . . . a little more angry. . . . I have thought about that—maybe we didn't make enough noise and maybe we didn't scream loud enough," Merson said. The obstacles to recalibrating the world's response just seemed too impregnable. Merson still can't imagine any scenario in which funding could have even doubled during those years. U.S. policy makers—like their contemporaries internationally—seemed far too steeped in denial and indifference.

During Merson's international travels, he had a hard time keeping his mind off of developments back in Geneva. In May 1993, only one month before Merson delivered his noteworthy speech at Berlin, WHO's governing body had passed a resolution with enormous implications. The resolution called for a study on a modified, or potentially even a new UN-sponsored global vehicle to focus on global AIDS. It was a cannon shot across GPA's bow. It was the genesis of what would, on January 1, 1996, officially become UNAIDS.

Merson was streamlining and "professionalizing" the program's operations. GPA had a sound vision, devised under Mann, and a deep and dedicated international staff. The program had acquired an enormous girth of technical expertise and proprietary knowledge. But as time passed, Merson began to read the writing on the wall. He spent much time contemplating the direction of the global response at large. Was GPA still the right vehicle? By late in 1993, after the resolution had been passed, it seemed increasingly clear that the answer was "No."

In an exceptional turn, Merson departed from business as usual in the realm of international bureaucracy. "I worked hard to form it," Merson would say of UNAIDS, "I consider myself the reason it happened." From 1993 through his resignation in March 1995, Merson spent much of his time and energy devising the new agency and formulating how the transition might unfold.

After much painstaking deliberation, he decided that he would cede his own power center, his own seat of authority—in effect cannibalizing GPA—in the interest of the global response at large. It was a rare act of vision and bureaucratic selflessness.

The move would pay dividends. But those dividends would take years to be realized. If Mann's departure in 1990 hadn't fully done it, the resolution in May 1993 had effectively sounded the program's death knell, if not in day-to-day operations, then certainly in its capacity to lead the charge in a serious global response. GPA would unravel slowly through 1994 and '95 until the formal creation of UNAIDS. After that, it would take the upstart effort at least two years to find its footing. All of the bureaucratic noise meant that the world would be left without an effective, credible global vehicle, or global champion, if not from Mann's resignation in 1990, then certainly from 1993 to 1998.

Michael Merson did as best he could to captain a sinking ship. But the urgency of the moment called for something grander—a brand of leadership that could inspire, that could transform. Merson wasn't the right steward. On a frigid sunny day in Washington, D.C., in January 1993, it appeared as if another figure making his entrance on the world stage might be the right man to lead the charge in the global response. His name was William Jefferson Clinton.

—〰〰—

SIX

The Clinton Enigma,
Bunker and Hunker Down

E arly in 1991, Congressman Jim McDermott broke from his legislative duties to make his way to Tom Downey's office. Downey, a long-time Democratic representative from New York and a close friend of then Senator Al Gore, had called a few colleagues together to come and meet with a young presidential aspirant. With primary season months away, it was still early in the presidential cycle.

Reaping the fruits of a successful war in the Persian Gulf, the incumbent president's popular opinion ratings were still lofty. Downey's guest was the governor of a small Southern state who was still considered a little-known upstart on the national political stage. McDermott had heard some promising murmurings about him, though, and thought that the meeting might be worth his while.

McDermott found his new acquaintance disarmingly well informed and a keen listener. He was affable and had an exceptional presence. The maverick congressman used the occasion to discuss his pet issue, AIDS.

As governor of Arkansas and on the campaign trail, Bill Clinton had been open and aggressive about the issue. He had known people who had been infected with HIV, and had communed with affected families. Clinton's target constituency was also gravitating toward the issue, furious at ten years of Republican neglect. The issue was gaining some traction, and he would showcase it throughout the campaign.

McDermott liked what he was hearing. He tried to stress to candidate Clinton that AIDS was more than just a domestic issue. The disease was global. The United States needed to wake from its slumber and engage the brewing catastrophe, McDermott asserted. The new president, whoever he may be, had to demonstrate mettle and leadership on the issue.

Over the months that followed, McDermott watched from Washington as Bill Clinton waged an improbably brilliant presidential campaign. Bush's popularity had waned. The sheen of his foreign policy victories had worn. The country was mired in a nasty economic recession, and burdened with a crippling national debt. Voters started to see Bush as an out-of-touch patrician, a perfect foil for Clinton, who oozed empathy and seemed to embody a new generation's hopes, perspective, and promise.

The American electorate was also becoming increasingly insular. Economic troubles and day-to-day concerns were amplified. The world seemed at peace, and the time was ripe to focus on domestic affairs. The backdrop played neatly into Clinton's inherent strengths. He had spent little time abroad, most notably two years in Oxford, England, as a Rhodes scholar. He would leave Oxford without inhaling, he would later claim, and also without any degree or diploma. The prestigious Rhodes and a degree from Yale Law School, though, would serve him well during an impressive rise through state politics in Arkansas. Command of foreign affairs would do little to serve Clinton's political ascent, and he seemed to pay scant attention. He excelled at domestic affairs, his passion.

It turned out that the incumbent was strong on foreign policy and vulnerable on domestic affairs. Predictably, during the campaign, Clinton accentuated the latter, and avoided the former. Les Gelb, the prominent foreign policy expert, noticed something remarkable in Clinton's speech upon receiving his party's nomination at the Democratic National Convention in the summer of 1992. He wrote an article about it entitled, "A Mere 141 Words." Gelb had counted the total number of words Clinton devoted to foreign policy in a 4,200-word speech.

The foreign policy community was keenly aware that the tone of the campaign did not bode well for a strong and active U.S. foreign policy.

During the campaign, Clinton proved staggeringly adept at plugging into the public temperament. "It's the economy, stupid!" became the campaign's unofficial mantra. Clinton would tell voters that the country needed a president focused as much on the Middle West as the Middle East. He sold himself convincingly as the candidate who cared about the problems of Americans.

Of course, he couldn't duck foreign affairs entirely. The Clinton team scoured the foreign policy landscape for an issue on which Bush might appear vulnerable. They thought they had found one in Bosnia, where early reports had percolated from the State Department and the news media of mass murder, perhaps even ethnic cleansing. The Bush foreign policy team had been essentially inert on developments in the region.

It was a splendid chance for Clinton to differentiate himself. He could point out a Bush foreign policy weakness, and at the same time woo voters by appropriating the moral high ground, casting himself as the candidate who would champion the great cause of humanity. He proclaimed: "If the horrors of the Holocaust taught us anything, it is the high cost of remaining silent and paralyzed in the face of genocide."

When the electoral dust cleared, Bill Clinton had accomplished the unthinkable. The forty-six-year-old upstart from Arkansas had defeated a seasoned incumbent and had won the White House.

The AIDS community was ecstatic. After a decade of railing against what was perceived to be an immutable brick wall of Republican neglect, the community felt that its time had arrived. "Everyone was extremely hopeful," remembered activist Paul Boneberg, "the Clinton administration was perceived very positively."

Up on the Hill, Jim McDermott was similarly pleased. He had had some contact with Clinton in the year following their initial meeting. He would use every occasion to try and advance global AIDS. "I spent a lot of time. . . . So I started banging on him before he even got to the presidency," McDermott said.

Thinking ahead, McDermott knew that in a few months the president would be delivering his Inaugural Address. His speech would command the international spotlight, reaching all of the world's leaders and hundreds of millions of people around the globe. The address would be an opportunity to inspire and to commandeer. It would also help set the tone and agenda for the term to follow.

McDermott wrote to the president-elect to congratulate him. Directly and through back channels he also lobbied Clinton to include global AIDS in his Inaugural Address.

On January 21, 1993, the president-elect lifted his right hand from the Bible after finishing his oath of office, becoming the forty-second president of the United States. In his smart suit and light blue tie, the statuesque figure with a large florid face, a full jaw, and a thick head of graying hair stood in front of tens of thousands of onlookers stretched out across the Washington Mall. Against the magisterial backdrop of the Capitol building steps, Clinton began to deliver his long-anticipated Inaugural Address.

About two-thirds of the way through, he digressed briefly from a predominantly domestic-centric address. "To renew America," he exhorted the nation, "we must meet challenges abroad as well as at home. There is no longer division of what is foreign and what is domestic. The world economy, the world environment, the world AIDS crisis, the world arms race—they affect us all." He went on to declare: "We will not shrink from the challenges, nor fail to seize the opportunities, of this new world. . . . Together with our friends and allies, we will work to shape change, lest it engulf us."

The crowd applauded, offering perfunctory but convincing affirmation. The new president had placed global AIDS alongside the economy, the environment, and the arms race. The pronouncement seemed to augur a sea change in the priority the issue would be afforded going forward. Jim McDermott and Paul Boneberg were jubilant.

Upon assuming office, Clinton assembled an unremarkable foreign policy team. Warren Christopher and Les Aspin assumed the two most senior Cabinet posts, secretary of state and defense, respectively. They were qualified, but neither was a visionary, nor particularly commanding. Richard Holbrooke, a bold and seasoned foreign policy luminary, and Colin Powell, who remained chairman of the Joint Chiefs of Staff, were unarguably more talented, but were not summoned to top posts in part because they were headliners in an administration that sought to showcase domestic politics, and Clinton himself. Journalist Joe Klein opined that "the selection of a flaccid, almost purposefully obscure foreign policy team seemed further evidence of Clinton's relative lack of interest in the area."

David Gergen, a seasoned White House staffer, estimated that on average, a president spends about 60 percent of his time on foreign policy. Bush—in part due to personal proclivity as well as historical context—spent closer to 75 percent of his time on foreign policy. Clinton, in sharp contrast, spent closer to 25 percent of his time on foreign affairs throughout the first several years of his presidency.

The president's managerial style further impeded the effective conduct of foreign policy. His natural enthusiasm and empathy for a wide range of issues meant that aides and policy makers would continually flood in and out of meetings with Clinton thinking that they had made progress or even won the president's support on an issue. In the Clinton White House, policy makers would learn that "sympathy" or "agreement" did not necessarily translate into action.

It was against these currents that Clinton would pursue his (predominantly domestic) agenda during the first half of his first term.

True to his campaign pledge, Clinton turned to the task of economic reform immediately. He sought to implement fiscal discipline in order to stem the burdensome deficit and pull the United States out of recession. It was priority number one.

Even as Clinton's economic team labored behind closed doors to tighten the fiscal ledger, the flagship issue of Clinton's first term became health care reform. He enlisted his wife, Hillary, to join Ira Magaziner, a former management consultant and friend of the Clintons, as co-head of the Health Care Task Force. They produced a plan that would require businesses to provide health insurance for their employees. The "employer mandate" scheme aspired to guarantee universal health coverage for Americans, but it would also place a stiff burden on American businesses and require a monumental bureaucratic overhaul. The 1,300 page piece of legislation was far too complex and aggressive to win Congressional support. Health care was Clinton's greatest shot, and he misfired. Nothing of similar ambition would be proposed during his presidency.

Try as he might, Clinton could not steer America, or his presidency, away from the specter of developments abroad. Moved by images of starving children, President Bush had sensed popular support for a military-backed hunger relief mission to Somalia, a small, poor East African country with little strategic value to the United States. He mustered the resources and deployed the troops, but warlords fighting for influence impeded the humanitarian mission.

Frustrations reached a critical point as Clinton assumed office and inherited the mission. He sanctioned, with Colin Powell's consent just prior to his resignation, a military incursion aimed at capturing an offending warlord named Mohammed Farah Aidid.

The effort was a disaster. America's high-tech Black Hawks were ineffective in close-quarter, urban combat. Elite Rangers were trapped and killed. Months later, the image of an American Ranger's corpse dragged through the streets of Mogadishu would capture the attention of the American public.

Clinton would pull America out, but not before sustaining a political debacle of the first order. Aidid remained and so did the humanitarian crisis. The only result of the engagement was a rather large blemish for the United States, now recast as a meek giant, reluctant to back up its commitments.

At home, the disaster demanded political casualty. Les Aspin, the secretary of defense, resigned. The incident seemed further evidence of Clinton's fecklessness as a commander-in-chief, his ineptitude in managing foreign policy.

The wounds of Somalia cast an enormous shadow. A little more than a year later, one of the most efficient and brutal genocides in human history unfolded in Rwanda: 800,000 Tutsi were systematically and unsparingly executed in 100 days. The administration could ill afford another Somalia, a costly American "humanitarian" commitment for the lives of Africans. As the genocide unfolded, the Clinton administration would purposefully avoid using the "G-word" at all costs. Key policy makers shunned calls to engagement.

Smarted by the debacle, the administration placed a wager: Americans would not care about Africans dying. Rwanda would never register a blip on the public approval ratings screen. It was dead-on, a brilliant political calculation.

Meanwhile, true to his election pledge, the new president was adhering to campaign promises to move government policy on *domestic* AIDS. He increased funding and resources for research, prevention, and care programs substantially. He would press for consistent annual increases in the Ryan White CARE Program, which provided health care for low-income Americans infected with HIV. After a good deal of pressure from the AIDS community, Clinton also made good on a promise to create the Office of National AIDS Policy, or ONAP. Under the aegis of the White House, the office was meant to guide U.S. AIDS policy and serve as a White House interface with the AIDS community.

HHS Secretary Donna Shalala explained: "The president was very clear that he wanted to do lots of different things, but mostly domestic. . . . I cannot say that the White House, at that point, was concerned about the international dimensions. . . . He left the international leadership to me."

Shalala would attempt to make inroads on global AIDS. For the most part, though, she left policy on the global front up to her trusted deputy, Patsy Fleming. After serving directly under Shalala at HHS early in the administration, Fleming was offered the opportunity to become the second director of ONAP, a position that had become known as "AIDS czar." The first AIDS czar was a former nurse named Kristine Gebbie, who had attracted the unfortunate nickname "Nurse Ratched," from some in the AIDS community. Gebbie resigned after fifteen months, complaining of a lack of access to the president. Fleming was thus "a little trepidacious" as she accepted the post in November 1994.

A former aspiring artist, the petite African-American mother of three brought twenty years of legislative experience to the post. Fleming had worked directly on AIDS policy for much of the 1980s for Representative Ted Weiss of New York. She had earned a reputation for commitment and compassion from the AIDS community. Standing at a press conference with Shalala and Fleming, the president pledged that the issue would be a priority and that Fleming would receive "real access to the White House and a real chance to influence me and my decisions."

True to the president's agenda, domestic AIDS remained Fleming's top priority throughout her three-year tenure. After attending the global AIDS Summit in Paris, though, in the summer of 1994, and visiting Uganda around the same period—from which she came back "heartbroken and with renewed energy to make some changes"—Fleming became increasingly passionate about the global dimension, which she could see was coming to dwarf the U.S. situation. Eventually she would spend roughly 25 percent of her time on global AIDS.

At ONAP, Fleming was at the helm of a meek outfit. Ostensibly, the office was created to help devise and advocate the White House's AIDS policy. It did play a role, but by and large, the White House considered the office primarily a liaison with the AIDS community—almost a public relations arm. Fleming had a very small staff of four or five full-time professionals, and an emaciated budget.

Fleming had met President Clinton, but didn't have much contact with him prior to assuming her post. Shalala threw some weight behind Fleming, but for the most part empowered her to function autonomously, leav-

ing her, at least on global AIDS, the captain of a small ship with little political capital.

Galvanized to move policy, she decided that the Office of Budget Management was the place to start. The president's appropriations arm, OMB,
plays a central role in drafting the budget and apportioning funds to various issues and areas. Fleming began to make what would become semiannual pilgrimages over to the OMB offices on Seventeenth Street across
the street from the Old Executive Office Building.

At OMB Fleming was unable to get an audience with a senior official.
Mostly, she met with third-tier operatives, below the deputy director level,
who were not generally decision makers. Fleming persisted, though. The
once aspiring artist would "paint a picture of the dire situation." She would
express indignation at the paucity of funds the United States was committing and lobby for an upgraded effort.

Year in and year out, she met unyielding resistance. When Clinton assumed office, the White House distributed a book throughout the executive branch with a list of the president's priorities. AIDS was one, but not
global AIDS. In the bureaucratic underworld the book became "sort of like
a bible."

Fleming argued with her interlocutors at OMB. She told them that they
had to step back and look at the magnitude of the brewing crisis. "Look,
we've got to do something about developing countries and especially
Africa, where this epidemic is going to become a new plague," she insisted.
Officials at OMB responded, "This is not one of the president's priorities."

Of course, there were many issues that were not included in the president's book, things that had been overlooked, or things that would emerge
as time passed. Many would receive funding and attention. But the book
became a convenient shield to ward off unwelcome advocacy. It seemed to
Fleming that "they could turn to that list whenever they wanted to and use
it," and so it became "like hitting my head against a brick wall. . . . When
you go to OMB and it's not a priority on a list, then you're really between a
rock and hard place."

Increasingly frustrated, Fleming began to use some of her scant time directly with the president to speak with him about the pandemic. Early in
1997, Fleming's office produced a two-volume strategic plan for AIDS at
large. Entitled *The National AIDS Strategy*—under the heading "The
White House"—a significant portion of the plan was "globally focused." It
clearly outlined the most recent estimates and projections as well as the

amount of funding that had been going into the effort to date. It was "a vehicle to try and mobilize the government."

Fleming found the president struck by the plan, or rather, "restruck" by it. "It wasn't that we brought this to his attention for the first time," Fleming explained with a faint laugh of resignation. Over the course of the previous three years, in memos or briefings, Fleming had presented the president with several postings on the global pandemic. On each occasion, Clinton would say something to the effect of, "Yes, yes, I understand, I see the problem, let's see what we can do about it," Fleming remembered. He was clearly "sympathetic," he clearly "cared." But, "from there, it didn't go anywhere."

It appeared that Clinton's facility to charm was not lost on Fleming. "[He was] sympathetic. [He] realized the problem and [he] wanted to help," she said of her former boss. But at the end of the day, Fleming was left to her own devices, thrown to OMB with no political capital, during a time in which balancing the budget and reducing the national deficit was priority number one, and in which the issue had attracted virtually no domestic political traction.

At 1600 Pennsylvania Avenue debacles would define the first several years of Clinton's presidency. Even if his initiatives did not bear fruit, no one could argue that they were ad-hoc and feeble. An early attempt to confer equal treatment on gays in the military and his doomed health care proposal were both bold and ambitious. Initially, Clinton led by leading. He sought to push America on the issues he prioritized. He would be pulverized for it.

The midterm elections of 1994 marked Republican Congressman Newt Gingrich's ascent to political power. The so-called Gingrich revolution swept Washington and the nation. Fifty-two Democrats lost seats in the 1994 election. The Democrats lost ten seats in the Senate. It was a stultifying blow for Clinton and the administration. Gingrich, who emerged as Speaker of the House, and his cronies unified around two core themes: a deep enthusiasm for a conservative, Reagan-like agenda and a vociferous and visceral dislike of President Bill Clinton.

The election sent Clinton reeling. He would assume a defensive posture for the rest of his presidency. In the winter of 1995, lodged in a bitter and notorious impasse over the fiscal budget, the federal government would actually shut down.

During the shutdown, some operatives who were eager to find time on the president's schedule to move policy on an important emergent issue saw opportunity.

On a cold winter morning in 1995, with Washington in paralysis, Donna Shalala walked along the thick, plush carpeting of the West Wing on her way to the Oval Office. She was accompanied by many of the country's leading AIDS experts, including Anthony Fauci, the director of the National Institute of Allergy and Infectious Diseases, or NIAID; David Satcher, the surgeon general; Harold Varmus, Director of the National Institutes of Health, or NIH; and Helene Gayle, head of the international AIDS effort at the CDC. For Shalala, the shutdown represented a long-awaited chance to command a captive audience with the president, and to advance an erstwhile neglected issue of staggering import.

Over the course of a several hours-long meeting, Shalala and her team peppered the president with information and data on the pandemic. They went over the research effort. They talked about prevention, and the absence of infrastructure in the most acutely affected regions. They outlined the data, and explained that the disease was "spreading like wildfire." The president was always very committed domestically," Shalala explained, "the message was that we have to move internationally, [that] this was not a domestic issue. We were talking about a dramatic expansion of our commitment internationally."

With characteristic aplomb, the president seemed to grasp the message. He was responsive, engaged, and in agreement that the problem needed to be addressed. The president "was very into it," Shalala remembered.

Shalala, like Fleming and McDermott before her, was certain that she had moved the president. Clinton's "sympathy" was genuine enough. On several occasions, upon speaking about AIDS, the president would well up, even in public. He began to attend a smattering of White House events and even included AIDS on his agenda when meeting with certain heads of state. But following his noteworthy session with Shalala and her colleagues—as with each prior encounter on the issue—the president failed to expend one dime of political capital to move U.S. policy.

In an oft-noted episode, in the heat of budget negotiations during the government shutdown in November 1995, Clinton once pulled his nemesis Newt Gingrich aside, and in his cool monotonal raspy Arkansas drawl told him that he was a rubber doll; the kind that when you hit it it bounces right back up again.

From the midterm elections through the end of 1998, Clinton spent most of his time trying to survive, trying to bounce back up again. In 1995, Clinton was looking very much like a one-term president. He was "totally consumed with how to reposition himself in order to win," Stephen Morrison remembered. "[Global] AIDS was not a part of that strategy at all. If anything it is not where you wanted to move. . . . AIDS was having a hard time getting onto even the second tier of priorities in foreign policy at that period. It just wasn't a competitive issue." All the energy it took to keep bouncing back up afforded little to press forward. Uncomfortable emergent issues that offered no political benefit suffered neglect.

In Clinton's push to regain political terra firma, he would bring a unique brand of leadership to the presidency. No president would expend as much energy gauging public opinion on as wide a swath of issues. The Clinton administration spent more on polling than all the previous administrations in American history combined.

He would become a leader by following. He emerged an intuitive political master, able to read the public's temperature even in his darkest moments. Longtime friend and former labor secretary Robert Reich would say: "Bill Clinton operates by sonar. He emits a huge number of priorities, ideas, and initiatives and he sees what kind of response he gets. And where he sees an opportunity to move, he moves." The implied corollary: where he didn't see an opportunity, he stayed away.

———◆———

Only months before Clinton would wage an improbably strong second-place finish in the New Hampshire primary in February 1992, Dr. Paul DeLay was still tending to AIDS patients in Lilongwe, the capital of Malawi in southeastern Africa. A typical day for DeLay, then forty-one, would begin with rounds at Kamuzu (the word means "father" in Malawi's native tongue) Central Hospital. By 1991, DeLay had gotten used to the devastation, but when he first arrived in 1988, to begin a tour working for WHO's Global Program on AIDS—still in the Jonathan Mann days— DeLay could hardly bear the sights that confronted him daily.

The hospital was "one of those classic African hospitals," a complex of scattered small buildings connected by a series of little corridors with ramps and concrete floors. There were no elevators, and nurses would clean the facility by pouring buckets of water across the floors and against the walls. Wards were "completely overwhelmed," DeLay remembered. There were really only four or five physicians who covered most of the hospital. Most of the care was done by nurse practitioners. Patients lay strewn out on beds, often with grass or blankets in lieu of mattresses, doubled up, with one resting his or her head where the other's feet lay.

Meanwhile, because resources were so scarce, patients' families were almost entirely responsible for the patient's nonmedical care. Families would huddle outside by makeshift cooking stoves, heating up maize for their dying family member. They would come in and cover them with blankets when they had the shivers, or dab them with cold compresses when their fevers spiked.

DeLay would circulate, speaking to hospital officials and patients. He inspected patients unable to swallow because of fungal infections that went down their entire esophagus. He walked by as thirty- or forty-year-old women tended to their daughters, who at fifteen or sixteen were at death's door, entirely emaciated, looking twice as old as their mothers.

In most cases, patients suffered from simple opportunistic infections that could be easily treated in the United States, and would have been treatable in Malawi had essential resources and medicines been available. But they were not, and there was almost nothing DeLay could do. He described those years in Malawi as wrought with frustration, "but there was also a sense that [I] had to do something."

With his $2 million a year budget from GPA, DeLay could help support selected initiatives like inserting AIDS education in school curriculums, running media campaigns, and buying a limited amount of medical supplies—mostly things like Imodium, that could be bought over the counter in the United States, to ease the pain from diarrhea. With infection rates reaching 10 percent in Malawi, though, it was as if DeLay was chasing an inferno with a bucket of water.

Deeply frustrated, but still energized, DeLay was flattered, toward the end of 1991, to hear from Jeffrey Harris, then still running the Division of Global HIV/AIDS at the United States Agency for International Development, or USAID. By then, the division was supporting surveillance work and was funding small projects at missions and through NGOs. It was distributing condoms, educating thousands about the disease, and making initial attempts at building infrastructure and capacity to assist countries in tackling the pandemic.

Harris wanted to recruit DeLay, who had an excellent reputation as a highly competent and energetic "technical guy," to join his division. The timing was right. After three years in Malawi, DeLay was ready for a change. Starving for funds at GPA, DeLay was thrilled about the prospect of moving over to USAID. He knew that the agency was GPA's largest donor and presumed that the division's deeper purse would provide him with an opportunity to enact some effective, perhaps even transformative programs.

Shortly after DeLay joined the division, Harris resigned. The following year the division's budget would plateau at around $120 million per year. The division head post would turn over several times in the ensuing years, leaving it without an effective leader or vision. By the time DeLay became division head in February 1997, the budget was still languishing at $120 million. Throughout those years, the division—the locus of the U.S. response to the pandemic—would remain a marginalized actor ensconced in the redoubts of the agency's manifold bureaucratic layers.

Even as it continued to proclaim itself the "global leader" in the response to the pandemic, the Division of Global HIV/AIDS seemed acutely aware of its own inadequacy. In 1993, USAID's official biennial report asserted: "Clearly present and future needs for prevention and care are so great that they will outpace currently available resources."

By the time Brian Atwood was confirmed as USAID's administrator, its top post, in May 1993, he brandished an impressive foreign policy résumé. Atwood had joined the Foreign Service in 1966. He was an assistant secretary of state for Congressional Affairs for Jimmy Carter in the late 1970s. As head of the Democratic National Institute, a prominent Democratic foreign policy think tank, Atwood kept his profile relatively high while his party stood on the sidelines.

When Clinton won the presidency, Atwood, whose close friends included future National Security Council leaders Anthony Lake and Sandy Berger and the new VP Al Gore, was well positioned to nab a plum position with the new administration. It seemed assured when he was named to run the transition team at the State Department.

When Warren Christopher was named secretary of state, Atwood was hoping to get one of the undersecretary slots he favored. When those filled, he agreed to jump in as USAID administrator. He would have a chance, he thought, to tackle favorite issues like democracy promotion, human rights, and sustainable development.

Officials at the agency, even those like DeLay who were several rungs down the bureaucratic ladder, could tell Atwood had pedigree, commitment, and integrity. In whispers, many wondered if Atwood was more interested in playing secretary of state or using his post to leapfrog to an even more prestigious diplomatic position.

Upon his confirmation as administrator, Atwood would not appreciate the difficulties of the road that lay ahead of him.

By the early winter of 1995, it had become clear that two matters would define Atwood's tenure. The first was institutional reform at the agency. At the time, Atwood's good friend Al Gore was trumpeting the idea of "reinventing government." Leading bureaucrats like Atwood were encouraged to streamline operations using technology and whatever tools or insights they could muster. Atwood spent much of his time reorganizing his agency's structure.

In foreign assistance, issues go in and out of vogue, in large measure dependent on the preferences of those captaining the effort. Health was not one of Atwood's primary interests. His own senior advisor Nils Daulaire remembered, "It wasn't even clear that health was going to be mentioned as one of the key strategic objectives of U.S. foreign assistance."

Amidst institutional restructuring, the Division of Global HIV/AIDS would actually be demoted. When Atwood merged the Bureaus of Nutrition and Population with Health in 1995, the division had become, in Paul DeLay's words, "a division within an office within a center within a bureau."

Atwood had little contact with the division or the effort. For the most part it was Atwood's deputies, or their underlings, who kept tabs on the division. Sometimes it would take pressure from congressional leaders, like Nancy Pelosi, to move him to focus on the division. Pelosi and Atwood had a close, congenial relationship. He would visit her at her office in the Rayburn Building and she would pepper him with questions about USAID's activities. She expressed particular alarm at the turnover at the division head position and the agency's inability to fill it, such that at times it remained vacant for months.

The challenge that would define Atwood's tenure more than any other, though, was the battle that he would wage with Jesse Helms, the conservative senator from North Carolina. During Atwood's tenure Helms was hellbent on abolishing USAID altogether, and if he couldn't do that, then at least moving it under the aegis of the State Department, where it would become, it seemed to Atwood, merely a device of U.S. foreign policy.

Atwood didn't flinch at the challenge, determined not to let USAID fall under his watch. It was a formidable and, at times, excruciating fight, and it would take just about all the political capital Atwood could muster.

In what Atwood refers to as "my period of great aggression," he would lash out at Helms. He publicly accused the chairman of the Senate Foreign Relations Committee of being an "isolationist." He once suggested that Helms's ideas about foreign assistance were absurd and tantamount to flippant calculations on the back of an envelope.

The Helms camp was taking note.

In one round of the fight, Atwood declared that because of the cuts proposed, "children would die." The Republicans then outflanked Atwood by earmarking, specifically, additional funds for child survival programs. It made them look strong on children's issues, and it also handcuffed Atwood, who lost budgetary flexibility due to the earmark. It was a stinging political turn. He "learned a lesson from that." He would think twice before once again getting too far out in front on any one issue.

While Atwood managed to maintain USAID's survival, he had less success salvaging the foreign assistance budget. Following the Gingrich revolution in 1995, balancing the budget became the top political priority of the day. Foreign assistance would become a casualty.

It was an agonizing time for Nils Daulaire, the soft-spoken but tough-minded longtime public health advocate. A Vermont native with light brown hair and a beard, Daulaire had a degree from Harvard and had practiced medicine and public health in more than a dozen countries in the developing world.

The budget dynamic and deficit reduction initiatives had reduced the agency's health activities to stasis. Daualaire remembered: "It was an embattled agency. Jesse Helms was trying to shut it down. Every two days in *The Washington Post* there was something about how USAID was going to be done away with. It was a bunker and hunker down mentality." The agency's budget would be lacerated during the period. Besieged by Helms and the overarching budget initiative, at USAID during those years, "survival outranked responding to new challenges."

While Atwood was bogged down in a fight with Helms, and beset by other exogenous and contextual impediments, leadership at the division level was uninspiring. The division heads, who would turn over in brief intervals during the 1990s, were experienced, competent, and dedicated, but they were functionaries, not leaders. All of them, including DeLay, would remain mostly supplicant on the big question of funding and the U.S. response at large. At USAID, self-censorship continued to reign.

In a *Washington Post* article, one of Bart Gellman's sources called it "shameful demand management." Divisional functionaries sensed that the political obstacles, the plethora of other problems and impediments, real or imagined, were simply too great to be overcome. Speaking out, therefore, in terms that called upon the United States to increase its commitment from just over $100 million to a response that demanded political and diplomatic leadership and billions in resources would be futile—or at any rate not worth the personal and professional sacrifice.

DeLay recalled one episode in which colleagues assembled to model out an actual comprehensive global response. What would it cost to recalibrate the U.S. response? "There was a concern that if we did such a calculation that it would be so astronomical that people would just give up." When they went ahead anyhow, the price tag came to around $6 billion for the entire global community. The implied U.S. share would be roughly $2 billion.

Then, as Delay recounted, the team realized, "wait a minute. This isn't that much money coming from the global community. We should have done that much earlier. It's funny that didn't happen. How much money do you need? The classical political question." But, officials at the division were afraid to even pose the question for fear that it would be a nonstarter, or they were simply unwilling to champion the plan and hazard what promised to be a perilous fight.

Duff Gillespie was a senior level official in the Office of Nutrition, Health and Population in those years. Gillespie explained his position: "In a policy position you learn a healthy skepticism for all the [projected] numbers. . . . If you look at all the studies on [ideas for] reducing mortality and you add them all up, you've saved every life about three times over." Gillespie's "healthy skepticism" was no doubt acquired through years of tough lessons learned. But it was a dangerous tack—what happened when the projections were right?

In a December 1998 memorandum, Gillespie summarized the agency's position at large: "to buy time until a vaccine or some other yet-to-be-identified tool becomes available." Launching an effective prevention campaign, Gillespie's policy summation implied, would not be feasible. And he did not try.

•   •   •

For much of the 1990s, it was not deemed particularly cost-effective to devote resources to AIDS prevention in the absence of a vaccine. In 1997, Jonathan Quick of WHO commissioned an illustrative chart. With $10,000, the bar graphs depicted, 9,900 children could be saved from fatal bouts of dehydration; hundreds might be saved from pneumonia and tuberculosis; only one AIDS victim could be saved through drug treatment.

Prevention successes in Uganda, Thailand, and elsewhere were just becoming evident. They would repudiate the methodology and thinking behind Quick's calculation. Uganda, for example, had yielded outstanding results in prevention by spending roughly $18 million a year. That translated into about $1.80 per adult per year.

Of course, in Uganda it was more than just funds; the entire country had mobilized. Upon hearing reports from Fidel Castro of sickness among his soldiers in the mid-1980s, President Yoweri Museveni had engaged his entire government and all sectors of society. Through the late 1980s and '90s, Museveni instructed all national, regional, and local leaders to speak openly and vociferously about AIDS. When other African leaders would not even acknowledge the disease, Museveni was screaming about it, insisting that fighting AIDS was "a patriotic duty." His government enlisted thousands of community workers in a grassroots effort to modify high-risk behavior. Their approach, known as "ABC," called on people, first, to *abstain* from nonmarital sex. If they wouldn't abstain, they must *be faithful*, or adhere to what some leaders called "zero grazing." Finally, if they wouldn't be faithful, they must use a *condom*.

Nonmarital sexual activity, particularly among young people, dropped precipitously. Condom usage among those engaged in promiscuous behavior skyrocketed. HIV infection in pregnant women, as measured in three key urban areas, dropped by almost half from 1990 to 1996. In Jinja, incidence among pregnant women aged fifteen to nineteen went from 21 percent in 1990 to 5 percent in 1996. National incidence decreased markedly. Uganda proved what leaders like Jonathan Mann, Michael Merson, and Jeffrey Harris had been saying all along: with resources, vision, and leadership, the disease was combatable.

Across the Indian Ocean, Thailand was in the midst of its own AIDS crisis in the early 1990s. In 1991, 143,000 new infections accrued in a country of roughly 65 million people. When Anand Panyarachun became Thailand's eighteenth prime minister in that same year, projections held that Thailand would be host to 10 million HIV infections by 2010. Immediately, Panyarachun appointed himself chair of the National AIDS Prevention and Control Committee. He funded a massive public information campaign, mass condom distribution among prostitute rings, and a comprehensive needle exchange program. By the early to mid-1990s, behavior modification among prostitutes and drug users helped curb Thailand's annual rate of infection from 143,000 in 1991 to around 50,000 in 1995.

It would be harder to turn away after the evidence from Uganda and Thailand came in. Senegal and Tanzania offered additional evidence of success. But experts continued to debate the data through 1998, and others argued that the cases were unique. Saving lives by engaging other problems, or pursuing other avenues still seemed to most to be more cost effective.

Still others were concerned that pressing for resources would require the agency to cut back on other programs. Nils Daulaire noted that demand management "was driven by the fundamental realities of the political dynamics in Washington in those days. . . . If we came in and said what we really need is $1 billion per year instead of $120 million, OMB would have said, 'OK, what are you proposing to cut?' " In the perilous environment, those advocating for global AIDS anticipated that officials in other programs would cling tightly, if not ferociously, to their budgets and resources. Many presumed, perhaps rightly, that pursuing a reallocation would have been highly contentious.

At the same time, USAID was struggling to find its modus vivendi in the post–Cold War world. Dr. Kenneth Shine, former president of the Institute of Medicine, worked with the agency on several projects during the period. He argued "they were [really] an agency of foreign policy, not of health. They knew what they were doing when they were trying to compete with the Soviet Union. When that changed they were really confused."

The agency was similarly ambivalent about how to conceptualize its response to the pandemic. At USAID, issues are either met with a long-term developmental response or an emergency response. The "emergency" side of the agency has historically moved quickly and has had far greater success and effectiveness than the long-term developmental side.

Those who were focused on global AIDS argued that it was an "emergency," but their voices did not resonate in other quarters, or with senior leadership at the agency. Stephen Morrison, then with the State Department, suggested that conceptually the agency, "defined it at some level as an emergency that needs an accelerated response. Institutionally, [they] haven't. It's the slow moving developmental side of USAID that was handling this."

As a senior advisor, Nils Daulaire felt increasingly frustrated as he witnessed the division "function, unfortunately, as just about all the elements of USAID did—in a pretty slow and bureaucratic way. It's very hard to get a big, well-established agency of the federal government like USAID to see anything as being urgent." Rather, there was "sort of a take it as it comes" mentality and pace.

It certainly seemed that way to Terje Anderson. The prominent advocate had begun to work with the agency in the latter part of the decade on several projects in Africa. He grew increasingly exasperated as the agency's efforts to execute the projects dragged on and on, muddled in red tape and bureaucratic inefficiency. To Anderson's consternation, he would discover, "It takes about two years to move a dollar from Washington to the ground in Tanzania."

The division's intervention efforts operated on contract cycles. It would outline parameters for various efforts. It would then provide nongovernmental groups, or NGOs, like Family Health International and Population Services International the opportunity to "bid" on those contracts, which were awarded based on the NGOs plans and capabilities. Contracts generally had a five-year life cycle.

The contract system was fraught with inefficiency. To begin, USAID had to lay the groundwork with the recipient country, a cumbersome vetting process. Then, the agency set the auction process in motion with contracting NGOs. At the end of the process an NGO, or several NGOs were selected. Next, USAID and the NGO would have to iron out the terms of the contract and the strategy going forward. USAID would then go back to the country to finalize arrangements. All of those steps took months, if not a year or longer, and all had to be done before the NGO even stepped foot in the country. Once on the ground, it would usually take the NGO at least a year or two to set up and find its footing. And because of the five-year contract cycle, at the end of the fifth year, the effort was often dismantled and the project terminated. Then the process was set in motion all over again.

Of even greater frustration to many was the amount of funds lost in the bureaucratic morass. Stephen Morrison explained, "If you're working through Africare or FHI [two prominent, USAID-funded U.S.-based

NGOs], all of these developmental organizations, they have their over-heads." He estimated that probably fifty cents on the dollar never gets out of the United States. Instead, it goes to their headquarters overhead.

The work that was being done was important, but the agency and the division were operating inefficiently. The agency's senior leadership af-forded the issue little priority and the division's own leadership operated as functionaries when the response demanded vision and advocacy. With USAID at the helm, the U.S. response foundered throughout the decade.

In one senior operative's view, USAID was "just not built" to lead the U.S. response to the pandemic. "Given the resources they're given, they've probably done a large amount of good work on the ground, [but] they're just not the solution."

An Awakening of Sorts
(1996–1999)

—⚍—

SEVEN

Drugs Change the Landscape, A Mission Crystallizes

On an ordinary day in 1983, Paul Boneberg, a longtime gay political activist from San Francisco in his mid-thirties, fielded a call from a pioneering domestic AIDS activist based in New York named Larry Kramer. Kramer was leading an effort to put together candlelight vigils in major U.S. cities to memorialize those who had died of AIDS. Kramer had a broad vision and wanted to enlist Boneberg and his organization, Mobilization Against AIDS.

Boneberg recoiled at the suggestion. "I didn't think it was a good idea at first," he remembered. "The government's neglect required political activism and I didn't think the candlelight memorials had anything to do with political organizing."

Boneberg consented, though, and would find out that he was deeply mistaken. The vigils would drum up awareness and become a poignant symbol of the victims' suffering and the government's neglect. The vigils' success helped them grow in size and breadth. By 1985 they had caught on worldwide. The global phenomenon required planning, coordination, and leadership. The task fell to Boneberg, who reluctantly agreed to lead the charge.

With international responsibilities, Boneberg became one of the first U.S. activists to look at AIDS with a global perspective. "There was no international leadership" back then, he explained. "It's the classic volunteer fireman response." Activism percolates out of local need. "Nobody's thinking internationally, you're just thinking locally."

Boneberg's responsibilities put him in direct contact with activists from all over the globe. Over months and in some cases years, through correspondence, phone calls, and meetings, relationships began to form with colleagues from abroad, and many became close friends. They came from Brazil, Mexico, Thailand, the Philippines, and elsewhere. Many, if not most, were themselves people living with AIDS.

Poor, marginalized, and often abused, Boneberg's colleagues in the developing world were deeply dedicated, and they came to symbolize, for the San Franciscan, the very best in activism. Over time, Boneberg was increasingly struck by the inequities in health and social services and in human rights between the situation in the United States and those facing his colleagues and friends in the developing world.

As telephone calls went increasingly unreturned and obituaries crossed his desk with a painful regularity, the international dimension came to have a visceral resonance for Boneberg. He shared his impressions with others in the domestic AIDS community. However, when trumpeting the need for global awareness among fellow domestic activists in the mid-1980s, Boneberg found himself alone.

Just as the vigils started to take off around the globe in 1985, Eric Sawyer's worst fears were confirmed in New York. A tall, clean-cut management consultant in his early thirties, Sawyer looked the quintessential Manhattan professional. Underneath the veneer, though, Sawyer's life was in deep turmoil.

Sawyer's live-in boyfriend of several years had come down with Kaposi's sarcoma, a lethal form of cancer common in AIDS patients. In the preceding years, Sawyer himself had experienced deep swelling in his glands and had suffered from intermittent bouts of painful ailments like shingles, a sign of a potentially weak immune system. When the tests formally became available in 1985, Sawyer received official confirmation that both he and his boyfriend had AIDS.

At the time he was living in Harlem. On the partnership track at a prestigious firm, Sawyer was also renovating brownstones around his neighborhood. The avocation meant that Sawyer was saddled with additional mortgages along with onerous medical bills, and he could ill afford to lose his job.

He watched in fury as a colleague was granted leave to care for his wife, who had breast cancer; and his boss was allowed to work from home during a difficult pregnancy. Sawyer was not permitted to take leave, nor allowed to work from home to tend to his dying partner. Senior colleagues sympathetic to his predicament told Sawyer that some in the company's senior management were looking for excuses to let him go, and that he would have to tread carefully to keep his job. Torn, he decided not to press the matter.

When his boyfriend got on a flight to return home to say good-bye to his mother, Sawyer was at work and couldn't accompany him. He was unable to find anyone other than a twenty-five-year-old secretary to travel with him. Shortly after the plane landed, Sawyer received a call informing him that his partner had passed away on that flight.

It was a profound loss. His grief turned into rage: that he was not there to say good-bye, that the poor young woman was put through such a traumatic experience, but mostly, that he had not spoken up. He resolved at that moment: "I will never be silent again."

One of the most important careers in late-twentieth-century American activism had been set in motion.

In March 1987, at the Gay and Lesbian Center on West Thirteenth Street in New York City, Sawyer became one of the co-founders of a new activist organization called ACT UP. The group would sprout up in cities all over the world, campaigning and protesting to advance AIDS awareness, civil rights, increased research for treatment, and access to drugs. ACT UP employed highly aggressive, "in your face" tactics. The group's activists, many of whom were dying of AIDS, or "neglect" as they might say, called their method civil disobedience. To those on the receiving end, however, it seemed anything but civil.

As head of ACT UP's Housing Committee, which aimed to provide housing for people who were HIV-positive and homeless, Sawyer was predisposed to support social equity–type issues relating to AIDS. When he started hearing from women and other constituencies involved in ACT UP about the international dimension of the disease, Sawyer tuned in immediately.

A gay man with AIDS in the business world, Sawyer understood what it meant to be marginalized. As he learned more about the steep rise of the disease abroad and about the destitution, civil rights abuses, and the lack of access to treatment and care, Sawyer became increasingly interested and committed to broadening the U.S. activist agenda to include global issues.

On World AIDS Day, December 1, 1990, at around 5:30 P.M. on a freezing early winter evening, Sawyer stood on First Avenue outside of the United Nations building in New York City, accompanied by roughly 250

fellow activists. Unlike many of ACT UP's demonstrations, Sawyer anticipated that at this one there would not be excessive physical confrontation.
By late 1990, he had established a dialogue with city police, who had come
to know him well. He wouldn't deign to request a permit, but if police were
informed prior to the protests, he found they were less hostile and released
those arrested sooner.

It was not one of ACT UP's most stirring protests. Only fifteen or
twenty would get arrested. But Sawyer had managed to steward something
very important—it was the first serious protest among U.S. activists with a
predominantly global message. The protestors took aim at the UN, WHO,
and the U.S. government: "AIDS is not only a U.S. issue, [it is] a global
issue concerning people in poor and developing countries as well." Of the
protest, he said, "We were demanding global access to all AIDS drugs including AZT and antiobiotics to treat AIDS related illnesses."

Despite the police's attempt to shepherd the protestors off the street to a
nearby park, they poured onto First Avenue chanting for global access,
managing to block traffic during rush hour. Their antics secured them coverage on the evening news.

The protest marked an embryonic stage in the emergence of global
consciousness among domestic activists. Galvanized, Sawyer founded the
Global AIDS Action Committee of ACT UP in 1991. The committee of
around thirty regulars began meeting weekly and became active in fund-
raising. Many were women who were driven to the global dimension
through their interest in the plight of women's rights issues in the developing world. Even then, women's involvement heralded an early sign that
global AIDS would come to broaden the activist community well beyond
the predominately gay domestic base.

Through the early and mid-1990s, meetings swelled to around sixty attendees as the biennial International AIDS Conferences approached.
These conferences became the focal point of the committee's activities.
The committee would transport ACT UP activists to the conferences and
organize demonstrations. At the Amsterdam conference in 1992, Sawyer
helped organize a town hall meeting co-hosted by Jonathan Mann, who
had moved on to Harvard University but remained a player. The meeting
aimed to bring U.S. activists and other activists from around the world together to brainstorm ways in which they might coordinate and pool their
efforts to advance the global agenda.

Sawyer's efforts at ACT UP were notable and important early stirrings.

But the U.S. activist community remained focused on domestic issues. When Sawyer tried to enlist a senior activist from the Gay Men's Health Crisis to participate in the town hall meeting in Amsterdam, he found the response shocking: "Look, we can't meet the needs of clients in Manhattan, let alone Brooklyn or the Bronx. There is no way we are prepared to take on AIDS in the developing world or AIDS in Africa, especially since they don't have clean water or food in Africa. Until we get everyone who needs treatment in the Bronx or until they get clean water in Africa, don't talk to us about AIDS in Africa."

Among his colleagues, Sawyer was something of an anomaly during those early days. Considerably less than 10 percent of the U.S. activist community afforded meaningful attention to the global dimension.

He wasn't entirely alone, though.

Seven weeks prior to Clinton's inauguration, Paul Boneberg had found that the initial election-induced delirium had ebbed into doubt and unease. For ten years, he had waged a battle against a disengaged White House. Now that the landscape had changed, Boneberg found himself in unfamiliar territory, not sure precisely how to navigate the seemingly friendlier shoals.

With little time to spare before the inauguration, the AIDS community called a "State Summit." Meeting a month after the election in a conference room at a large hotel in the Washington, D.C., area, more than fifty leading advocates and activists, including Eric Sawyer, assembled for two days to draft a transition paper outlining what the new administration's AIDS policy should be.

At first, dialogue was somewhat disjointed. Hopes were high, but no one seemed to know precisely how high they should shoot. One of the Summit's co-hosts, David Mixner, a prominent gay businessman from New York and a key Clinton fund-raiser, set the tone early on. He exhorted the crowd: "Stop thinking like this is Reagan. We won the presidency. We can do this. We can do it!"

Boneberg heard the message loud and clear. After years of struggling, the time had come to address new challenges with fresh vigor. As the group was splintering into working groups to begin formulating policy suggestions, Boneberg stood up and took the floor. "Wait a minute," he said. "Does anybody want to talk about international AIDS issues? I think this should be on the agenda."

A longtime committed and articulate activist, Boneberg had a well-regarded national reputation among community leaders. But he was from San Francisco, not the Beltway, and many considered him a fringe voice from the West Coast. It quickly became clear that Boneberg's colleagues weren't receptive. One working group leader responded, "This is not on any of our agendas. It's inappropriate for us to create something in the transition document that none of us have ever worked on or know about, or [that none of our] constituencies have expressed any interest in."

Boneberg persisted. Time was scarce, though, and colleagues were becoming perturbed. Boneberg was getting "off-agenda." No one knew what to ask for, what to suggest. Any recommendations on global AIDS would "not have been as real as other parts of the document," Boneberg was told.

Boneberg was disappointed, but understood. He hadn't entirely thought through the global issues. He wouldn't have known, were he empowered to draft a several page policy paper, how to direct the administration to engage the issue. For Boneberg, the State Summit was a launching pad. He had broached the issue, and henceforth he would move to raise the profile of the global dimension and to formulate authoritative answers to the community's queries with a view to moving policy.

Eric Sawyer respected his colleague from the West Coast. In Sawyer's eyes, though, Boneberg was a "suit," and did things in more or less "polite, professional ways." Sawyer shared Boneberg's agenda, but diverged markedly from his colleague in approach. At a separate incident at the Summit, the ACT UP co-founder stood up and banged on the table, accusing people at the Summit of negligence, and of committing global genocide.

"We cannot ignore global AIDS," Sawyer shouted. The vast majority of people in the world with AIDS were living in the developing world. The United States was the richest country in the world and AIDS patients in the United States had enjoyed success in obtaining a social safety net, and in securing money for AIDS research. Sawyer argued that the country had an "obligation to bring the agenda of global AIDS to the president."

The domestic AIDS community had theretofore benefited handsomely from ACT UP's confrontational style. On global AIDS, Sawyer had now turned the table on his own colleagues, assailing their own inaction. They greeted his protests with the same bothered tone and dismissive refrain with which they responded to Boneberg. "Yeah, yeah, yeah," Sawyer remembered hearing. Activists said that they were sympathetic, "but our responsibility is to people in this country and until we get adequate funding for social services and health care and research and until we have a cure for AIDS, we really need to focus the AIDS agenda on this country."

Both Sawyer and Boneberg, operating independently, pushed the key decision makers at the State Summit to include global AIDS on the agenda. By the end of the proceedings they had gotten a mention, but by affording the issue only a few lines at the bottom of the transition document, the leading AIDS activists ensured that it would not register as a key community concern with the president.

"It's a pivotal moment," concluded Paul Boneberg. "That is the first time that the American leadership is confronted. They basically decline."

Sawyer's advocacy would intensify over the ensuing four years. Likewise, the AIDS community's abdication at the State Summit had piqued Paul Boneberg's resolve. He decided that there "was this missing piece" on the U.S. activist agenda. He started knocking on the doors of the nation's leading activists.

He found mostly excuses veiled in sympathy. As Boneberg made the rounds through 1993, most of the executive directors of the nation's prominent AIDS advocacy organizations would say something to the effect of, "I can't change my mission statement. I can't tell my board that I'm spending any meaningful resources on global AIDS." Few, even in the domestic advocacy community, had a proper appreciation for the true dimensions and magnitude of the global problem. It hadn't been part of their mandates, and it wasn't what they were hired to do. They weren't willing to rethink their institutional priorities and/or expend the political capital to fight for the issue.

Boneberg decided in 1994 that ignorance would no longer be an excuse. In response to the community's indifference, he founded the Global AIDS Action Network, or GAAN. The new group's mission was to be a clearinghouse for real-time information on the pandemic and the U.S. response to the pandemic. It was the first stand-alone advocacy organization exclusively focused on driving the U.S. response on global AIDS.

Even with GAAN's creation, progress was slow and hard to come by. Still, Boneberg did begin to make inroads. By August 1995, he had gotten a working group on global AIDS started at National Organizations Responding to AIDS, or NORA, the national umbrella group comprising the country's leading AIDS advocacy organizations.

Commissioning help from anyone and everyone he could find to drum up interest, Boneberg had been in contact with a Belgian doctor named Peter Piot, who had recently been named the executive director of a new global organization, headquartered in Geneva, though not yet officially formed, called UNAIDS. Piot had a keen appreciation for the role activists could play in moving the leading nations to play a larger role in the global response. As Mann had before him, Piot immediately recognized the importance of cultivating strong relationships with activists around the world. When Boneberg asked Piot to come and address NORA, he was thrilled to learn that the invitation would be accepted.

As two hundred leading AIDS activists, representing an array of national and local organizations, grabbed their boxed lunches and piled into the AIDS Action Council's conference center in Washington, D.C., for the weekly lunchtime session, Boneberg's excitement peaked. It was February 1996 and Piot had now officially become the world's leading voice and champion on global AIDS. Boneberg sensed another possible historic moment.

In addition to Piot, NORA's leaders had invited a congressional staffer to discuss the latest on Medicaid reimbursement for domestic AIDS patients. Nibbling on sandwiches just after noon, the crowd listened to Piot, who outlined the global dimensions of the pandemic, and the steep challenges and inaction framing the world's response. He waged an adamant appeal to the U.S. activists to engage in these problems.

Boneberg found himself becoming increasingly despondent as the talk went on. It seemed the crowd was more interested in the second speaker and Medicaid reimbursement.

NORA had decided that "Peter was not a significant enough speaker to speak alone, so they added another speaker. He's given twenty minutes— ten minutes to speak and ten minutes for questions. . . . It gives you an idea of the lack of priority."

———— • ◆ • ————

Dr. Seth Berkley was working at the Rockefeller Foundation in international health in 1993 when he started to field a steady stream of calls from a group of leading AIDS scientists. Berkley didn't believe what they were telling him.

In his late thirties, Berkley was an itinerant physician with extensive international health experience in Africa and Asia. Berkley hadn't yet found the time to settle down and get married. His passions were health and the developing world.

Like any U.S. physician in the 1980s, Berkley had followed the rise of AIDS in America. But he was interested in international health and other issues. By 1987, Berkley found himself stationed in Uganda on loan from the Carter Center—former President Jimmy Carter's influential not-for-profit—to the Ministry of Health, where he was overseeing the ministry's epidemiology efforts. He hadn't gone abroad in search of AIDS work, but in Uganda he couldn't escape the burgeoning epidemic.

Struck by the number of AIDS cases he was seeing, Berkley set out with colleagues to conduct Uganda's first national surveillance study. When Berkley's American girlfriend, Charlotte Puckette, brought the results of the study, completed in 1988, to Berkley's home in Entebbe, he thought that she had made an error. "You must have put the decimal point in the wrong place," he told her. It was 1988 and Berkley's study had found an adult 18.6 percent prevalence rate in Kampala, the country's capital, and a national adult prevalence rate of 12.6 percent. When she insisted that the decimal point was correctly placed and the tests were accurate, he said, "Oh my God, this is a Black Plague."

When Berkley returned to the States to take a job with the Rockefeller Foundation, he was still shaken by the weight of the crisis he had helped unearth in Uganda. So when leading AIDS scientists including David Heymann, Don Francis, Marcus Connant, and others began inundating Berkley with phone calls, he was eager to hear what they had to say. They had all been talking, and they shared a grievous concern. "The AIDS vaccine effort is dead," each would tell Berkley. He was incredulous at first. He presumed that a matter of such import had to have been fully attended to. He looked into it, though, and they were right. In 1994, the U.S. government was spending less than $100 million per year to research and develop an AIDS vaccine.

Under the auspices of the Rockefeller Foundation, Berkley convened what *Science* magazine called at the time the largest and most diverse gathering of AIDS scientists ever assembled. The conference was held on Lake

Como, Italy, in March 1994. Amidst Lake Como's splendor, the scientific luminaries brainstormed, attempting to chart a path forward. As the experts shared viewpoints, Peggy Johnston, who at the time was running the AIDS vaccine effort at NIH, stood up to alert Berkley and his colleagues to something shocking. The U.S. government was the largest single international donor contributing to the global effort to develop a vaccine. "[The U.S. government] can't do it," Johnston declared.

In 1984, when the HIV virus was discovered and HHS Secretary Margaret Heckler declared that the world was only two years away from having a vaccine ready for testing, vaccine development was, in fact, the number one U.S. policy priority in fighting the disease. Over the course of the 1980s, that would change. Through the decade, the policy agenda veered markedly away from vaccine development to treatment.

The virus's lethal design and evasiveness would be the single greatest impediment to finding a quick-fix vaccine. The scientific community needed time to learn about the virus and how the body's immune system reacted. The insights gained from pursuing treatment helped them to do that. Nevertheless, vaccine-specific research could have done with much more in the way of resources and priority. There was another critical factor at work.

During the 1980s, activists represented HIV-positive or AIDS patients. Many were HIV-positive themselves. A vaccine, of course, was not the main priority for these constituencies. They wanted to save their own lives. They demanded a cure.

When scientists told the activists, "We don't know how to manufacture a cure," the activists screamed back defiantly, "Throw money at it and do it." The Nobel Prize, in Berkley's opinion, should have gone to the activists. They would force policy makers to pursue a formidable path to discover treatment, if not a cure.

But there was a horrendous backlash as a result. "Everybody discounts their risk in the future," Berkley noted. "The people who are infected, of course, will do anything to stay alive," and they're going to drive a treatment agenda. Vaccine development was of course a long and costly undertaking that never held high promises for short-term reward—i.e., near-term political gain. Activists weren't driving it, and politicians weren't gravitating toward it. The net result: "Here was this weird situation where the community wasn't pushing forward, the U.S. and other countries weren't pushing forward, and so it was not on the agenda anywhere . . . The only thing that could stop the epidemic was a vaccine," Berkley said, "but nobody was working on it."

Johnston explained that in addition to the dearth of funds, there were other reasons why it was difficult for the government to coordinate and lead the vaccine effort. Most notably, much of the research and development would have to be done in the corporate sector. It was very difficult for the government to deal with the various leading pharmaceutical companies, already wary of making big investments in AIDS vaccine development because of the low economic reward and liability issues, in an impartial and expeditious manner.

After another two years of detailed planning and deliberation, the Rockefeller Foundation decided to lead the way in launching the International AIDS Vaccine Initiative, or IAVI, in 1996. It would be a not-for-profit working to accelerate the science and aiming to raise awareness and funds. It would serve as a clearinghouse for information, as a leader in global advocacy, and it would help to bridge the gap between governmental efforts and private sector initiatives.

The decision makers who founded IAVI were so impressed with Johnston and her command of the issues that they brought her on to start the fledgling initiative. In no time, IAVI made its presence known in the international political arena, drumming up awareness and interest among the world's most prominent scientists, health officials, and national leaders. IAVI implored the United States to lead the charge, and zealously lobbied the administration, Cabinet members, Congress, and the media.

At first, it appeared as if Berkley and his colleagues had chosen a long and punishing road. Then suddenly, on May 18, 1997, Berkley received astounding news. Delivering a commencement address at Morgan State University in Baltimore, Maryland, President Clinton announced that the United States would commit itself to discovering an AIDS vaccine within ten years, by 2007. Clinton compared the aspiration to John F. Kennedy's pledge, almost exactly thirty-six years earlier, that the United States would put a man on the moon in the next ten years. "He gave us a goal of reaching the moon and we achieved it," Clinton declared. "Today, let us look within and step up to the challenge of our time." It wouldn't be easy, Clinton made clear. "There are no guarantees. It will take energy and focus and demand great effort from our greatest minds."

It was no accident that what would later be dubbed "Clinton's man on the moon speech" was delivered at Morgan State, a predominantly African-American university. On the homefront, AIDS had risen sharply in African-American communities. By 1996, AIDS had become the number one killer among African-American adult males, and it was the number two killer among adult females. The Congressional Black Caucus had called on the president to increase his administration's efforts. And some, like Congressman Elijah Cummings of Maryland, whose own extended family had incurred the wrath of the disease, were particularly interested in vaccine development.

Berkley had been publicly demanding that U.S. national leadership take up some such ambitious plan. He had been calling on the global community to set a deadline of 2005. He was thrilled with the 2007 deadline, though. It was an unexpectedly bold pronouncement, and it appeared as if the U.S. response was poised to turn a corner.

In the days, weeks, and months following the Morgan State address, however, it became clear that the new AIDS vaccine research effort housed at NIH would receive only nominal additional funding and manpower. NIH funding increased from $130 million in 1997 to $148 million in 1998. The budget increased by an additional $34 million the next year. Eighteen months after Clinton's declaration, less than 10 percent of the overall U.S. research effort for AIDS would be directed at vaccine development. It would take the NIH one year to appoint a director to the Office of AIDS Research and almost two years to appoint a director to the Vaccine Lab.

Funding and attention would increase significantly in the final year of the Clinton presidency. However, measured against Clinton's promise at Morgan State and the enormity of the calamity, Berkley concluded, "in the end, they didn't follow through on the level of commitment," in both funding and priority, and it was a source of deep frustration for him.

Of greatest concern to AIDS expert Jon Cohen, the plethora of players in the effort—government, research institutions, big pharma, and biotech companies—were all moving in different directions. IAVI's advocacy notwithstanding, there was no one authoritative coordinating body to drive the effort to develop a vaccine for one of the worst pandemics the world had ever seen.

So, Berkley would have to keep plugging away, making the case for a vaccine. It was an uphill battle. In early 1996, the little that was spent on vaccine development was still very much driven by domestic concerns.

The U.S. global AIDS effort, therefore, consisted entirely of prevention efforts. AZT, the only treatment available at that point, cost roughly $15,000 a person per year in the West, and there was still little public discussion about pharmaceutical companies reducing their prices in the developing world for the treatment. As an option for fighting global AIDS, treatment was dismissed as not being cost effective.

If prevention and treatment were neglected pillars in the war to fight global AIDS, vaccine development was the pillar that had been almost entirely forgotten. IAVI sought to change that with a powerful advocacy message: "You're spending all this money on AIDS," Berkley would tell national policy makers around the globe, but "you're spending zero on AIDS vaccines. We don't know what the right number is. It sure isn't 100 percent, but it sure isn't zero either." Prevention and treatment were imperative, but "most critically, it's getting us a vaccine." It would be a daunting road, and many credible scientists were skeptical of the effort's prospects. Berkley remained undeterred: "In history there is no viral epidemic that has ever been eradicated without the use of a vaccine."

———•◆•———

Five months after Peter Piot's inauspicious introduction to U.S. activism at NORA and just as IAVI was being formed, the global AIDS community—scientists, activists, policy makers, and journalists—convened in Vancouver, Canada for the Eleventh International AIDS Conference. It was the most highly anticipated conference in the pandemic's history. A seismic development was to be announced to the tens of thousands of participants.

After more than a dozen years of backbreaking scientific research, activism, and public policy, a treatment had been discovered. The July 1996 conference would showcase the development and demonstrated efficacy of a drug regimen dubbed HAART, or Highly Active Anti-Retroviral Therapy. The antiretroviral, or ARV, drugs, scientists would explain to a jubilant international audience, had been proven effective in suppressing the virus, mitigating its impact on the body's immune system. Dubbed the AIDS cocktail, the treatment comprised several pills with high levels of toxicity, usually administered several times a day. They weren't pleasant, but the drug therapies offered dramatic improvements in life extension for most of the HIV/AIDS patients who took them.

There were still questions about HAART. The drug was relatively new. Just how long could it prolong life? Would the toxicity of the drugs wear away at some or most of the patients who would take them? Would strands of the virus impervious to the drug's efficacy mutate, rendering it useless? Despite the nagging questions, the development was received as an unmitigated triumph. Vancouver was a celebration.

HAART's discovery epitomized the best in science and medicine and the best in activism. Against deeply improbable odds, activists had insisted that the public and private sector pursue treatment development. Seven million people around the globe had already died of AIDS. An estimated additional 26 million had been infected and were living with HIV or AIDS. Now, there was hope.

Appointed the North American representative from the activist community to serve on the coordinating committee to help organize the conference, Eric Sawyer would have an opportunity to speak at the opening ceremonies in Vancouver. He knew in advance what Vancouver's headline would be. No one was happier than Sawyer. He had been living with HIV for fifteen years, or possibly longer. He had fended off intermittent bouts of serious illness, and he never knew what awaited him around the corner. He had been tossed in jail more than thirty times, spit on, shouted and laughed at, all in large part fighting for this moment. The new ARV treatment was Sawyer's best hope for living a longer, easier life. But it wasn't enough.

"Distinguished guests," Sawyer began his address to the capacity crowd at the GM Place arena, "I am going to be very blunt. I'm here to sound a wake-up call. . . . If you think a cure is here, think again. The cure is not here."

Sawyer acknowledged the proven efficacy of the new drugs. It was clearly a positive development. But he wanted to turn the glare of the spotlight to the remaining 95 percent of the HIV-positive people in the world. Most couldn't even get simple medicines like aspirin, or bactrum, a cheap but effective antibiotic treatment that helps ameliorate opportunistic and potentially lethal bacterial infection.

"The headlines that PWAs [people with AIDS] want you to write," he exhorted the journalists in the audience, would read: " 'Human Rights Violations and Genocide continue to kill millions of impoverished people with AIDS.' That is the truth about AIDS in 1996."

"Government promises don't save lives," he averred, "but government actions and funding for AIDS programs can." Sawyer launched a direct salvo at President Clinton: "Bill Clinton, if you care about PWA, ask Congress for $3 billion for international AIDS programs instead of $130 million." As he went on, Sawyer's pitch rose in intensity. As he finished, he began the chant: "Greed Kills—Access for All." It echoed throughout the arena, as the audience joined in.

Sawyer was not the only player at Vancouver for whom the recent development heralded not only hope, but profound and difficult questions. For some, like Ben Plumley, who was working for UNAIDS and spending time on the ground in developing countries, the wheels began to turn. At Vancouver, "a lot of us sat around and said, 'Oh shit!' How the hell do we bring this there?" remembered Plumley.

Journalist Laurie Garrett was struggling with the same dilemma. Garrett remembered walking out of a session, her head spinning. Researching her award-winning book, *The Coming Plague*, Garrett had spent time traveling through Asia and Africa and was deeply attuned to the horrors the pandemic was exacting in ill-noticed corners of the globe. As she left the session, she noticed Jonathan Mann sitting on the lawn with his girlfriend (later to be his second wife) Mary Lou Clements, also a prominent figure in international health.

At the time, a small vanguard of activists like Sawyer were already demanding that drug companies lower their prices in the developing markets. The drug companies were refusing to comment on their international pricing policies. Little in the way of progress had been made, and with much at stake for both sides, the contention promised to get worse before it got better. Even assuming the drugs were affordable, other questions regarding infrastructure and whether or not developing countries had the capacity to accommodate and administer these drugs remained.

Garrett asked her good friend Mann: "How long do you think it's going to be before African constituencies want these drugs?" Mann told Garrett that access would be a human rights issue. When she prodded, he couldn't get much further. "It was obvious to me," Garrett recalled, "that he hadn't thought of it. All of a sudden he was so flushed."

Details and practical matters such as access and implementation constituted a challenge from the outset. But Vancouver heralded a watershed moment in the U.S. activist movement. Vancouver's slogan was: "One World, One Hope." "I think we began realizing how hollow that was," said leading advocate Terje Anderson. "The Vancouver Conference was a real milestone for North American advocates because it became very clear that this intervention was going to be available to the people in the developed world and very clear that it wasn't going to be available to the people in the developing world. I think that allowed people to start thinking about the ethical implications. . . . We started turning corners there."

Nils Daulaire agreed that the advent of efficacious ARV treatment catalyzed change in the U.S. activist community. "The biggest thing that made a difference is that we ended up having effective drug treatment for the first time when protease inhibitors and combination therapy were started in 1996. It really pointed out the growth in inequity more than before, and it served as a mobilizing factor for activism around HIV internationally."

More than any other factor, the advent of effective drug therapy was the catalyst that helped galvanize the U.S. AIDS activist community to begin to fight the disease beyond America's borders. It was perhaps the single most significant development in turning the corner of the U.S. response at large.

If a corner had been turned at Vancouver, the velocity of the shift was hardly sharp and decisive. The activist community would need time to absorb the development. Among domestic activists there was still the matter of ensuring that their local constituencies got access to the drugs, and that they were proven effective on a much wider, national scale. Over the next two years, that became priority number one.

Before ARVs became accessible, the annual death rate in the United States had crested at around 50,000. By 1998, the death rate had dropped to just above 17,000. There was a 42 percent decline from 1996 to 1997, followed by a 20 percent decline from 1997 to 1998. By 1998 there had been a 70 percent decline since 1995, and, wrote Laurie Garrett, "in 1995 HIV was the number eight cause of death in the United States: by 1998 it didn't even rank in the top fifteen." The drugs worked.

At a meeting in Washington, D.C., two years after Vancouver, Paul Boneberg sat in a room full of prominent national advocates. One of them addressed the crowd, standing next to a chart exhibiting a powerful graphic. It was the number of AIDS deaths in the United States in the past several years. It looked sort of like the stock market after the tech boom, recalled Boneberg, chuckling: "Boom! Way down. . . . A complete sharp decline."

Under Boneberg's leadership, GAAN had been sounding the trumpet, championing the cause of global AIDS for four years. Looking at the chart, he turned to the executive director of a prominent national advocacy outfit sitting next to him, and pointing to the graphic, he said, "Look, this is the moment. . . . Everything has changed."

To Boneberg's chagrin, though, it wasn't going to be that easy. Even as the sands were shifting, the voices of the few were mostly drowned out by celebratory refrains. The United States and the world were clearly at an epochal turn and "end-ism" was in vogue. At the time, many leading thinkers were buoyant, predicting the end not only of communism, but war, or even history, as at least one analyst defined it. AIDS fell neatly into that complex. After fifteen years of coping with the disease, and enduring hundreds of thousands of deaths, billions in resources, and countless uncomfortable confrontations with sex and other dicey subjects, the United States was "fatigued." When the media heralded an end, it played well.

A *Newsweek* cover read: "The End of AIDS?" David Ho, who had led the way in discovering HAART was named *Time* magazine's Man of the Year in 1996. To great controversy, Andrew Sullivan, a prominent HIV-positive journalist wrote a provocative piece for *The New York Times Magazine* in November 1996, entitled, "When Plagues End: Notes on the Twilight of an Epidemic."

Rather than rally to a call to engagement on the global dimension, most Americans, and most in the activist community, were happy to make the comforting presumption that the AIDS threat was over. Dr. Ken Bernard, a senior HHS official at the time, said, "there was this time when antiretrovirals were becoming very effective, and then people's interest began to fade." As death rates started plummeting across the nation, "For a U.S. audience," said Stephen Morrision, "nobody's thinking about AIDS."

———•❖•———

In a Philadelphia prison, in 1986, Dr. Alan Berkman noticed that a young Puerto Rican inmate was sweating and coughing profusely. When he started having seizures, Berkman surmised that he had AIDS. Berkman made the diagnosis not as a prison doctor, but rather as a fellow inmate down the row.

Berkman, a 1960s radical who graduated from Cornell and then Columbia's medical school, was imprisoned for several years because of involvement with militant groups that had orchestrated a bank robbery in which two police officers and a security guard were killed.

Upon his release, Berkman spent the better part of the 1990s treating patients for mental illness or AIDS in low-income areas of New York.

Destitute and marginalized as they were, by 1998, many of Berkman's patients were making dramatic improvements in health. Strides in domestic AIDS policy had helped enhance access to treatment for all Americans. A trip to South Africa early in 1998, as a consultant to the Columbia School of Public Health, introduced Berkman to AIDS in Africa. At a village hospital, a flood of patients was overwhelming the hospital staff, whose ranks were thinning precipitously, also due to AIDS.

As the Twelfth International AIDS Conference rolled around in Geneva, Switzerland, that summer, Berkman thought the theme of the conference more than appropriate: "Bridging the Gap." The gap was more like a chasm. Roughly 32 million people were living with HIV or AIDS worldwide. Yet only a fraction, only the world's wealthiest, were afforded access to the new ARV drugs, which had actually exceeded expectations of efficacy in the two years since Vancouver.

Geneva was long on talk—about recalibrating the global effort and expediting drug accessibility to the developing world—but it was short on action. Berkman agreed with Eric Sawyer's assessment that at Geneva "nothing effective" was accomplished. "It [was] more PR, window dressing, lip service."

Following the Geneva conference, Berkman and his wife, also an AIDS doctor, visited friends in Germany, who took them to Dachau, the Nazi concentration camp. "It was a very moving experience for me to recall that . . . the world let genocide happen," Berkman recalled. Following the visit, he could not shake the images from Africa. He knew he had to do something.

As a physician, he had seen what the domestic advocacy community had done for drug access at home. He felt that the community needed to mobilize in much the same way to fight for global access, to truly narrow the gap. Berkman approached a longtime, prominent ACT UP member, Bob Lederer, and argued that global access had to be put on the domestic agenda. Their meeting in the late summer of 1998 marks the genesis of the formation of the HealthGap Coalition, an association of activist organizations united to fight global AIDS, with a particular focus on making drugs accessible around the globe.

In the preceding year or two, there had been a steady increase in activism directed at the multinational pharmaceutical companies that manufactured the ARV treatment. The "pharmas" seemed a logical target for the activists. The drug companies had by and large refused to entertain price adjustments for the developing world. Though price was only one impediment—though irrefutably a critical one—to ensuring global access, it was an obvious one, and rich corporations made for good targets.

The high-profile, well-financed Beltway-type national advocacy organizations began slowly to be drawn to the issue. They favored meetings, conferences, and planning sessions. In contrast, groups like ACT UP New York and ACT UP Philadelphia—whose ranks had been depleted mightily in the wake of the domestic success story, though a few core members remained—organized demonstrations, protests, and acts of civil disobedience.

They ran the gamut. Folks like Eric Sawyer, and Paul Davis and Asia Russell of ACT UP Philadelphia would organize pickets outside of headquarters of the multinational pharmas. They would chain themselves to corporate buildings and even storm inside, on occasion reaching CEO offices. Eric Sawyer remembered participating in one protest in 1998 directed at the Pharmaceutical Manufacturers Association in Washington, D.C. He and his fellow demonstrators marched in a somber procession, while some banged on drums in a funeral-like cadence as others carried cardboard boxes configured to look like coffins and threw out drug money caked in red paint, or even the protestors' own blood.

It was a high-stakes game. Many of these companies had multibillion-dollar market capitalizations. Their financial fortunes depended on the integrity of their patents and their ability to manage the prices of their drugs. Corporate leaders felt enormous pressure not to move on pricing policy, for fear, they would argue, that it would set a precedent, and start down a slippery and costly slope. Pharma's position certainly wasn't helping their image, but much was at stake, and they weren't prepared to budge without a serious fight.

In January 1999, an assemblage of fifteen or twenty core activists associated with HealthGap, then still a fledgling enterprise, met at the AIDS Treatment and Data Network headquarters on Broadway just north of Houston Street in New York City. Paul Davis and Asia Russell of ACT UP Philadelphia were there. So were Eric Sawyer and Paul Boneberg. Bob Lederer was running the proceedings. It was, for the most part, the usual cast of long-time AIDS activists. There was one newcomer to the group. No one knew him or knew what he was doing there. His name was Jamie Love.

Forty-nine years old, Love had dark curly hair and the sharp features and worn but ruddy complexion of someone who looked as if he hailed from the Pacific Northwest. Love's father had been the mayor of Bellevue, Washington, and was later elected as a city judge. He grew up in a civic-minded family and came of age in the era of the New Frontier, when "public service was still considered a pretty high calling."

Though his father had been a Republican, Love's political leanings diverged from his old man's as he navigated through a series of positions at nongovernmental organizations early in his career. Love received master's degrees from both the Woodrow Wilson School at Princeton University and the Kennedy School of Government at Harvard. After his forays in academia, Love looked forward to actually making "some real money" working for a big pension fund. But service beckoned again when he heard from his friend Ralph Nader, who wanted Love to join him in 1990 to work on intellectual property, or IP, rights issues with respect to drug treatments. Love spent years looking at IP issues pertaining to cancer drugs and became an expert in government policy and IP law.

Though there were countless lawyers who specialized in IP law and policy, Love became a leading voice in the nongovernmental sector, one in a very small universe of experts in a niche field. Love began publishing and appearing at conferences and lectures. By the mid-1990s developing nations were seeking him out. He traveled to Brazil and Argentina in 1994 and India in 1996. Governments and NGOs were suffering badly from a host of health crises. They wanted to know what rights they did and did not have with respect to drug patents.

It was only a matter of time before developing countries started to solicit Love's advice about drug patents for the new AIDS drugs. By the end of 1998, Love had become a key advisor to several developing countries, most notably South Africa. Each of his entreaties on behalf of his developing world colleagues was met with a stiff wall of resistance buttressed by the U.S. pharmaceutical lobby, the United States Trade Representative's, or USTR, office as well as other wealthy nations. Progress was glacial.

The losers in all of the interest-based jostling and politicking, it seemed to Love, were the millions perishing of AIDS simply because they could not afford the drug treatments that would save their lives. Having trained with some of the Ivy League's leading economists, Love harbored no illusions about a market-free utopia. There are simply things some people can't get access to, Love explained, like a Chevrolet or a Brooks Brothers suit. Those are things that cost a lot of money to make.

Drugs were different. They required financing, but mostly in the form of research and development, or R&D. On the ARVs, the drug companies made their profits in the developed world markets. Making the drugs available in the developing world would have carried only a nominal marginal cost for the pharma companies. But they were afraid of reducing prices for fear of setting a precedent. At developed world prices, the developing world couldn't afford them. Drug companies were, thus, keeping drug costs at an artificially high level. To Love it seemed fantastically cruel.

He began his advocacy a cool-minded intellectual, but by 1998, the magnitude of the suffering and the developed world's callous indifference had driven Love to despair. "There was a time when I couldn't even think about the infection rates without crying. It was just mind-boggling to me. I couldn't imagine there was anybody in America who could tolerate the situation we were in. . . . It's so horrible—you can't even have it in your conscious mind and function. So you end up blocking it out because it's just numbing."

In January 1999, Love received an invitation from Bob Lederer to come to a meeting with a small group of relatively radical U.S. AIDS activists. It was a foreign milieu for Love, but he was desperate for action and felt that there was little time to lose.

The fledging HealthGap Coalition was looking for a new plan of attack. The three-hour January meeting held just north of Soho in New York City adhered to a highly structured agenda. Each participant was given around ten minutes to speak. Love listened intently as they went around the room proffering suggestions. Big pharma remained everyone's favorite target. Some wanted to throw blood on drug company executives, some wanted more protests. Most suggestions varied only in the manner of attack or organization.

An unknown newcomer, Love was given a mere five minutes to speak at the end. As Love told the activists about the U.S. government's systematic application of pressure to restrict developing countries from pursuing lawful means to purchase or produce drugs at affordable prices, the activists appeared dumbfounded. The activists could rail against big pharma all they wanted to. "You can talk to the CEO of Pfizer until you're blue in the face and maybe he'll get religion and maybe he won't," Love said. The pharmas were accountable to their shareholders, who were in it for profits.

There was another angle, Love explained. "Patents are territorial and governments can override patents as a matter of policy." Love offered the activists a new target: the U.S. government, who would be none too thrilled at being accused of preventing tens of millions of poverty-stricken people in the developing world from getting access to lifesaving drugs. Politicians would be vulnerable in a way that executives were not.

Love was invited to a follow-up meeting the next month. This time, his agenda was the focal point for two and a half hours out of the three-hour meeting. There was much educating to do. Terms like "compulsory licensing" and "parallel imports" were new and foreign to the activists. There were many questions. As the meeting progressed, the activists became increasingly animated. The energy in the room became palpable.

Eric Sawyer was listening in rapture: "I immediately realized that Jamie Love had given us the key to unlock the door."

—ᴍ—

The Clash, A Forum

Vice President Al Gore wore a proud smile as Karenna, his eldest daughter, then eight and a half months pregnant, introduced him to the local crowd of eight thousand in Carthage, Tennessee. It was Wednesday, June 16, 1999, and in moments he would take to the podium to formally announce his candidacy for the presidency of the United States. The moment was a lifetime in the making.

Gore was the son of Albert Gore Sr., a well-known populist senator from Tennessee. He grew up amidst prominence and politics, groomed to elevate his family to the pinnacle of the American pantheon—the White House. Leaving no box unchecked, his résumé was impeccable from top to bottom: Harvard graduate, Vietnam veteran (he enlisted as a reporter in the army), congressman, senator, published author, and two-term vice president of the United States.

The economy was nearing the crest of an unprecedented boom. There was peace and prosperity. Americans seemed content with their lot. Everything seemed to have fallen into place. Still, the polls suggested that Gore would be in for a tough fight against formidable candidates.

His staff had labored furiously in the preceding months. The address and the occasion would help set the tone for the campaign to follow. After much speculation, it would be the first glimpse into Al Gore, the formal presidential candidate. Leaving nothing unattended, the event had been fastidiously scripted.

Set against the backdrop of the Smith County courthouse on Main Street in Carthage, his quaint all-American hometown, Gore's eighty-seven-year-old mother would be in attendance. His wife, Tipper, had lost her voice, and so Gore's daughter would introduce him to the local crowd. Wearing a smart dark blue suit, a white shirt and a light colored tie, hair neatly combed, and looking confident and earnest, Gore began to deliver the carefully crafted twenty-five-minute address.

He highlighted the country's economic progress and other Clinton administration successes. He cautioned his audience not to let America slip into the problems of old. His vision for America in the new century involved progress and family. In the background, Gore's staff and handlers seemed pleased.

Unbeknownst to the candidate or his team, the night before a group of about a dozen and a half men and women had boarded a van in New York to make the fourteen-hour trip down to Carthage. They were all associated with a new organization called HealthGap. The ragtag group was led by Mark Milano, a longtime HIV-positive ACT UP activist. They carried whistles and furled banners that read: "Gore's Greed Kills: AIDS Drugs for Africa."

Global AIDS was Al Gore's sort of issue. Over the years, he had rightly earned a reputation as a progressive, forward-thinking internationalist. He was hardly a dove. He had helped lead a Democratic bloc in favor of U.S. military action in the Persian Gulf War of 1991. But he was also a well-noted humanitarian. Together, he and his trusted foreign policy advisor, Leon Fuerth, had long made the case that humanitarian and moral considerations abroad were part of, rather than antithetical to, the national strategic interest.

Following his son's near-death in an automobile accident, Gore wrote a book entitled *Earth in the Balance*, published in 1992. Unlike most of his published colleagues in the Congress, Gore researched and wrote most of the book himself. It was a detailed and incisive examination of the depletion of the environment, and a passionate call for policy reform. A cerebral, wonky policy maker, Gore took to other "nontraditional" issues like genocide, terrorism, transnational crime, and even space junk. "Anyone who knows anything about Al Gore knows that he is a cutting-edge thinker," said Bob Orr, former director of the Council on Foreign Relations in Washington, D.C.

One of the most notable moments in Gore's public career came at an

Oval Office meeting in 1995 in which key policy makers were deliberating upon ordering military strikes in Bosnia to quell the genocide.

The weekend before, an extended feature article in The Washington Post had profiled a young woman in Srebenica who had, using her own belt and shawl, made a noose and hanged herself, in despair over the genocide decimating her homeland. After reading the article, Gore's youngest daughter asked her father how the administration could do nothing.

As the foreign policy players went back and forth, weighing the pros and cons, Gore interjected. In a very unusual turn at the senior policy making level, Gore posed a personal, highly moralistic question: "Why is this happening and we're not doing anything? My daughter is surprised the world is allowing this to happen. I am, too. I want you tell me how to answer her—my own daughter."

Gore's colleagues were taken back. His emotive entreaty resonated, though, and, according to David Halberstam, helped swing the pendulum in favor of U.S. intervention.

The vice president played an unusually significant role in the administration's foreign policy. As part of his responsibilities, Gore was appointed to chair several binational commissions with important states undergoing transition. It was in the context of these commissions that global AIDS would emerge on his radar screen.

Few foreign policy priorities were more important early on in the Clinton administration than the success of Russia's economic and political transition from communism. At the Vancouver Summit in April 1993, Yeltsin and Clinton agreed to create a U.S.–Russia binational commission. Gore was appointed the U.S. co-chair. Heeding the counsel of his senior foreign policy advisor, Leon Fuerth, Gore pressed to insert public health into the agenda. Russia's mortality rate was disturbing, and the prognosis was worsening. Fuerth estimated that the country's health would be seen as a critical benchmark of the new leadership's effectiveness. There was a clear health-stability nexus, and therefore health became a U.S. priority.

Still, matters deemed more pressing, such as trade, continued to consign health to a lesser priority on the commission's agenda. Even within the context of health, AIDS, at first, was only one of a wide array of issues. By the commission's final years in the late 1990s, the Gore camp afforded AIDS equal priority with drug-resistant TB.

Gore would address it, and so would Fuerth. They would bring in HHS

Secretary Donna Shalala for a detailed presentation. They implored their interlocutors to acknowledge the threat and to mobilize public education and resources. They applied no diplomatic pressure, however, nor did they offer anything above nominal aid and modest levels of technical expertise.

If the Russians refused, Gore and Fuerth had higher hopes for South African mobilization against AIDS. They pressed the matter in the context of the South African binational commission, also chaired by Gore.

Gore's co-chair was South Africa's then Deputy President Thabo Mbeki. Like Gore, Mbeki was western educated, and the son of a prominent national politician. The two developed a strong mutual respect and an amicable rapport. Their friendship paved the way for the commission's success in resolving several long-standing trade disputes. The United States also played a critical role in aiding South Africa's rural electrification project and privatization projects in its telecommunications sector.

Fuerth had been briefed on AIDS in South Africa at least as early as 1993 by Michael Merson, and he had subsequently received data from intelligence that he found "staggering." He entreated Gore to include AIDS on the agenda. He was "certainly willing to do so," remembered Fuerth. The issue came up intermittently in the commission's semiannual meetings during its first years.

With political stability and a peaceful transition to post-apartheid South Africa accomplished, issues previously deemed of secondary importance could be given increased attention. By June 1997, at a commission meeting in Cape Town, Gore directly engaged Mbeki on the AIDS situation in his country. "South Africa is in the beginning stages of a full-blown AIDS crisis," he reportedly said to Mbeki. The United States had "waited too long" to address its own AIDS crisis, and he implored South Africa not to make the same mistake.

Aware that most of the South African cabinet would be in attendance, Gore had also brought Donna Shalala to the meeting. After listening to Gore "confront Mbeki and just beg him to move" on the issue, she took the floor to hammer home her case. Across the table from most of the South African cabinet, Shalala outlined what she believed to be the scope of the problem.

Leon Fuerth listened, pleased to have Shalala force the issue. He grew disconsolate though when, upon the completion of her presentation, he scanned the reaction among the South Africans, who were eerily silent, all looking down at their notes. Following the meeting, on the way to the airport, Shalala expressed her own frustration to Fuerth. The issue was still mired in deep taboos, and she couldn't crack it, even at the cabinet level. The prognosis was frightful, and Fuerth could see it in Shalala's face.

Increasingly, the vice president began to use his correspondence to highlight AIDS, and to press Mbeki to move on the issue. In short order, South Africa called the Gore camp on its admonitions. In 1997, South Africa's national leadership was mulling over legislation to pursue "parallel trade," which would enable it to buy the life-extending antiretroviral drugs from other countries where they were sold for less. In the course of their legal research, South African officials stumbled upon an expert from the United States named Jamie Love.

Upon consulting with South Africa's minister of health, a forceful woman named Dr. Nkozasana Zuma, Love advised the South Africans to take the measure a step further, suggesting that the government consider importing cheaper "generic" drugs. He even suggested that South Africa endorse "compulsory licensing," whereby South Africa would grant licenses to manufacturers to produce "generic" drugs at home, making them cheaper still.

Parallel imports and compulsory licensing were the two primary weapons of attack in Love's arsenal. Though abhorred by drug companies, the practices were not restricted by international law. The United States, European countries, and Japan had employed these measures at certain times of need. But South Africa was keen to maintain its good international economic standing and wary of risking the ire of multinational pharmaceutical companies, foreign investors, or the USTR, the U.S. government's trade office. Love remembered, "They thought compulsory licensing too radical. They didn't want to piss off the Americans. They wanted to do things that were pretty safe."

The Gore commission, which included Charlene Barshefsky, the chief U.S. trade negotiator, was averse to considering even the idea of parallel trade. "The U.S. made it clear that the drug companies were unhappy with what they were doing," said Love. The Americans suggested that by pursuing these measures, South Africa was putting its ability to attract U.S. foreign aid and foreign investment at risk. It was meant to intimidate South Africa, to get them to back off.

The issue was a hot potato in discussions at the July 1997 bilateral commission meeting, held at the infamous Watergate Hotel in Washington, D.C. Dr. Zuma and her colleagues were unversed in international intellectual property rights. When the Gore team insisted that she negotiate directly with drug company lawyers and U.S. trade negotiators, she asked that Love and Rob Weissman, Love's colleague, come in to the conference room and sit with the South African delegation, to advise them through the negotiations.

When the United States got wind of the invitation, it insisted that Love and Weissman be prohibited from participating. The two were not well liked by the USTR. "They were tough like that," Love said. "Gore and Barshefsky were really beating the crap out of them. They preferred to negotiate with developing countries when they have as little information as possible."

The South African parliament went ahead and passed the Medicines Act in the fall of 1997. It was hardly a cure-all. It didn't address the need for a vaccine, care, or prevention. It did not seek to address the country's dearth of infrastructure and capacity, which would impede the drugs' administration. And even if it did lower drug prices, the act did not allocate funds to help subsidize the vast majority of infected South Africans, who would still be too poor to afford them.

But it was a critical first step. It would lower drug prices, saving lives. And perhaps even more importantly, it may have helped open the floodgates to acknowledgment, leadership, and mobilization on a much larger scale.

The pharmaceutical companies were aggrieved. As early as May 1997, the head of Johnson & Johnson and key industry representatives began writing to Charlene Barshefsky, the chief negotiator at the United States Trade Representative, and William Daley, the head of the Commerce Department. A $350 billion industry, the pharmaceuticals had a tremendous amount of clout. The industry's connection to the Gore camp was noteworthy. Two of Gore's former senior aides—Peter Knight and Roy Neel—received significant consulting fees from the pharmaceutical lobby. In 1997 and 1998, still prior to the stage in which fund-raising would really heat up, the industry had already donated close to a third of a million dollars to either a Gore political action committee or the Democratic party. Jamie Love and other activists were keenly aware of the connections.

When Gore met with Mbeki in his office in the West Wing on August 5, 1997, he said to his visitor, "You know, Thabo, the American pharmaceutical industry . . . exerts an influential voice in political circles."

Mbeki retorted, "Yes. All over the world."

Gore would need pharma's electoral and financial support in the upcoming election. He wanted to have a solid record advancing U.S. trade interests and not look weak to big industry. Yet, sympathetic and pressed by Fuerth, he was ready to consider revisiting the U.S. position. He was willing to put parallel trade on the table. In turn, he made clear, the United States would need to reserve the right to approve of those trades.

"This is a tough one," he told Mbeki. He risked bearing the brunt of a great deal of animosity from one of America's biggest, most influential industries. Nevertheless, "We are prepared to enter that fray," he pledged, "and mix it up with them because we believe strongly that this proposal best addresses their needs for patent protections and people's needs for affordable medicines."

It was a significant step for Gore. The U.S. proposal clearly demonstrated that he was still trying to straddle the humanitarian imperative and U.S. economic—and perhaps his own electoral—interests.

A western-trained economist and a deeply proud man, Mbeki found the proposal unpalatable. The U.S. provision would deny South Africa autonomy, and that didn't sit well. South Africa would continue to pursue the legislation through the judicial process.

That fall when Gore hosted Mbeki at the vice president's private residence, he listened to his guest's concerns about pressure from the pharma industry. Over a working dinner, Gore "urged Mbeki's continued 'cooperation with concerned U.S. pharmaceutical companies' to modify the new law."

By early 1998 roughly forty pharmaceutical companies had sued South Africa over the Medicines Act. Barshefsky and the USTR had brought a good deal of pressure to bear, if not overtly, then certainly at least by holding out the threat of trade penalties and other tough measures. Gore seemed to hold the pharma line.

During the ensuing months, pressure from big pharma began picking up steam. Rodney P. Frelinghuysen, a congressman from New Jersey, home to some of the country's largest pharmaceutical companies, lambasted South Africa in the House. He successfully sponsored an effort that threatened to withhold all foreign aid from South Africa. On February 5, 1998, the State Department formally acknowledged that there was an "assiduous, concerted campaign" to repeal the Medicines Act.

Around this time, the USTR also placed South Africa on its "watch list" of states, diminishing its stature as a desirable trading partner. It was a tacit signal to the international economic community, imperiling South Africa's ability to attract foreign direct investment and impugning its international economic standing.

Weeks later, at another meeting with Mbeki in the presidential suite of the Table Bay Hotel in Cape Town, Gore told his South African counterpart: "I want to make you aware of the strong and growing domestic pressure being brought to bear in Washington." Reappropriating the recent negative developments as negotiating leverage, he cautioned: "I'm concerned that, without significant progress toward a resolution, a single trade issue could overshadow our bilateral relationship."

It was more than a warning shot across the bow. Gore seemed to be telling Mbeki that if he wanted U.S. support at all for parallel trade, he had better agree to the U.S. proposal. Otherwise, he risked not only the dissolution of an agreement, but the very standing of the "bilateral relationship."

The way *Washington Post* journalist Bart Gellman saw it: "What for South Africa was an exploding health emergency . . . the United States treated mainly as a problem of trade."

———————•◆•———————

It was precisely the point that Jamie Love was making to his new colleagues at the second HealthGap gathering in February 1999 held in New York City.

Love had been working on the Gore commission and the USTR for almost two years on drug accessibility for Africa. Ignored, Love watched as South Africa's aid was suspended, and its economic standing denigrated when it was put on the infamous "301 Watch List."

That fall, he met Gregory Pappas, a senior HHS official, who would become the activist's first Clinton administration ally. After listening to a presentation by Love, Pappas told him that his position made a lot of sense. The staunchly pro-pharma USTR hadn't made that sort of information and data available to officials in the administration.

A newfound ally, Pappas told Love that he had heard from a reliable source in the White House that Gore had assured Bristol-Myers Squibb that he would advance their interests on the issue. In return, the giant pharma company would provide campaign contributions. It was a third-hand account and he had no proof, but Love bought in immediately. He was incensed.

Love's outrage now had a forum and a sympathetic, newly converted audience of roughly twenty activists. By the end of Love's comprehensive February presentation, the key question outstanding was how to proceed. It was clear that the activists would now set their sights on the U.S. government. But, they still needed to decide who, precisely, they would go after, and how they would do it.

The USTR remained the primary governmental actor advancing pharma's agenda, pummeling away at the South African government. The activists agreed that Charlene Barshefsky and the USTR would be a target.

Barshefsky, though, wasn't accountable to an electorate. She wasn't running for office. The activists wanted to make a real splash. They wanted to inject the issue into the media and the national discourse. Protesting the USTR wasn't going to do it. Love pointed out that there was an election coming up. And Al Gore happened to be running for president.

The activists recoiled at the suggestion. Love's organization, the Consumer Technology Project, was a Ralph Nader–backed group. The activists suggested that Love was trying to manipulate the agenda to serve his boss's political ends.

Love denied the accusations. He made the case that it was the best plan to effect change: "You're all going to vote for Gore a year from now anyhow, this is just the primary season, this is your little window of democracy when you get to go out there and make your case. This is what primaries are for. Relax. Believe me, everyone will forget about this by the time the election comes around. But, you have to go for it. This is too important, you just can't tolerate this." Eric Sawyer was a Gore supporter. But, listening to the debate, he found Love's argument persuasive.

Others needed more convincing. Paul Davis, from ACT UP Philadelphia, noted that there was a demonstration coming up in the next few weeks, scheduled around legislation pending on development in Africa. He had developed an in with Jesse Jackson Jr. on the Hill, and targeting Gore would threaten the protest. The momentum was clearly coming around to Love's position, but the group agreed to accommodate Davis's concerns and wait until his demonstration was complete.

About a month later, Davis managed the Herculean feat of shepherding roughly one thousand protestors—mostly poor black, welfare recipients—from Philadelphia for the demonstration. As Davis's crowd marched, Jamie Love sat with Eric Sawyer at a press conference at the Carnegie Institution on P Street in D.C. eager to field queries from all the reporters they were expecting the demonstration to attract. Waiting behind a table piled with clippings, documents, and fact sheets, after several hours it became clear that no one was coming to cover the press conference. They were furious. "We get zero, bupkis, not even a school newspaper."

It was mid-spring. Sawyer and Love were unaware of the Gore camp's efforts to reach an agreement on the Medicines Act with Mbeki. More important, with the exception of a few dozen government officials, the world was entirely unaware that Leon Fuerth had set in motion an ambitious interagency group to entirely recalibrate U.S. policy on global AIDS. Movement from the U.S. government seemed nonexistent, and the two men were fed up with being ignored. Millions were dying and becoming infected. They were now hell-bent on taking the fight to Gore.

Boarding a flight at Dulles airport in Washington bound for Australia via Los Angeles in the early summer of 1999, Jamie Love was nearing his boiling point. He had been working on the U.S. government for roughly two years, and he could not account for one iota of tangible progress. He had become convinced that the Gore camp was in the pharmaceutical industry's purse. Working around the clock, traveling around the globe trying to advance the cause, Love could think or speak of little else.

On the plane waiting for takeoff, for a moment Love thought that he might be going delusional. A woman who looked exactly like Tipper Gore was walking down the aisle of the plane, and seemed to be heading straight for him. The blond lady drew closer—it was the vice president's wife. Tipper stopped at Love's row and began speaking to the man seated next to him, who turned out to be Clark Ray, her longtime senior aide.

Love couldn't believe it. By then, he had become "like a broken record." It was "all I could talk about to anyone, [even] my barber." He now had a captive audience with Tipper's "senior guy" during a six-hour flight.

When Tipper left, Love introduced himself to Ray. He explained that he had been working on this issue for several years to little avail. Recently, he had met some activists, he explained. And in a matter of weeks, they were going to go after the vice president. "I don't want to make Tipper's husband miserable during the campaign," Love told Ray, "and it's kind of strange because actually they are probably going to vote for him. They're not his natural enemy, they're his natural constituency."

Ray seemed to take it all in. "I don't know who he thought I was," Love said. "Maybe he thought I was a lunatic or something." Ray told Love that he should get in touch with Sandy Thurman, the president's AIDS czar. But, by then, Love and his new activist associates were no longer interested in second-tier bureaucratic meetings. They had their crosshairs fixed on Gore.

When Mark Milano and his crew arrived in Carthage for Gore's announcement on June 16, Love was in Australia following the wires for any sign of news. Eric Sawyer had stayed back in New York, to run the media campaign and feed inquiring journalists information. None of them knew that just weeks before, the Gore camp had sent a Gore staffer named James Babbitt, an Army officer specializing in African affairs, to begin negotiations on a trade deal with the South African embassy, aiming to "find a formula to settle the dispute."

By June 14, two days before the Carthage event, Leon Fuerth's office presented a settlement deal to Charlene Barshefsky's office. The deal called on South Africa to "reaffirm" its commitment to international patent laws. In return, the United States would withdraw objections to the Medicines Act.

As Mark Milano and his comrades stood anxiously across from the steps of the Smith County courthouse, the settlement sat unsigned on Charlene Barshefsky's desk. None of the activists were aware of the behind-the-scenes developments. Nevertheless, by that time the activist agenda had broadened beyond the South African Medicines Act. They wanted the United States and the rest of the developed world to make drugs accessible to HIV/AIDS patients in Africa. Had they known about the proposal, it most likely would not have stopped them.

As Gore declared his candidacy, the activists sprang into action. They stripped a layer, revealing T-shirts that read: "Gore's Greed Kills." They unfurled their banners, started blowing on their whistles, and threw out "blood money."

It all happened very quickly. There were only a dozen and a half or so activists. Most of the crowd didn't know what was going on. A handful of rowdy hometown Gore supporters began muscling, pushing the activists. In doing so, they did the activists a huge favor. The tussling and shouting generated even greater commotion, which in turn startled Gore in the middle of his delivery. Briefly stunned, he regained his composure. Trying to appear unrattled, he said, "I love free speech."

Within moments, the local police pounced on the activists and escorted them from the ceremony. They were told in no uncertain terms that they were not welcome back in Smith County. Gore continued his address, per-haps somewhat less enamored of free speech than when he began.

Back in New York, Eric Sawyer was working the phone. The media had noticed the protest. Sawyer explained what the hubbub was about. He had folders of information and fact sheets prepared. The story hit, and got men-tion in *The Wall Street Journal*, *The Washington Post*, the *Los Angeles Times*, CNN, and PBS. In Australia, Jamie Love caught a few lines in an Associ-ated Press blurb. A few days later *The New York Times* ran an editorial, sup-porting the activists' position on the issue.

The activists had scored a direct hit. In a few chaotic moments, they had managed to leave a nettling blemish on the long-anticipated, tightly scripted event. It was only the opening salvo, though. The activists made it clear that they planned to continue to follow Gore on the campaign trail, dogging him until he saw to it that U.S. policy would change.

True to their pledge, Milano packed his troupe back into the van and headed up to Wall Street in New York City, arriving that evening. Deftly avoiding security, the activists slept underneath the bleachers that were al-ready set up for the next morning's campaign event.

The next day, in the middle of Gore's speech, the activists once again held up banners, blew their whistles, and jumped in front of the press cameras. The protest, this time with even fewer than a dozen protestors, disrupted Gore's speech again. "I love this country. I love the First Amend-ment," he yelled over the noise. "Let's give a hand to those who are exer-cising their First Amendment rights. . . . Let's give them another hand. Make it louder," he implored his audience, hoping to rouse them to drown out the protestors as the NYC police shuffled them away. "Now I'd like to have my say," Gore said as they were removed from sight.

Later that afternoon, venturing into primary country in Manchester, New Hampshire, Gore, though clearly prepped on a response, was visibly perturbed when the activists struck yet again at an event at a university gymnasium. Bounding onto the stage behind Gore, brandishing a banner made from a bedsheet reading "Gore Kills, AIDS Drugs for Africa," the ac-tivists forced Gore, once again, to depart from his prepared remarks to ad-dress the incident.

This time, he played directly into the activists' hands: "Let me say in re-sponse to those who may have chosen an inappropriate way to make their point, that actually the crisis of AIDS in Africa is one that should command the attention of people in the United States and around the world," he said. Attempting to turn the issue into a positive, and no doubt alluding to the initiatives under way led by his camp, Gore continued: "This epidemic was ignored for too long in the United States of America and I'm proud our nation is taking the lead to try to do something about it."

A keen photographer, Tipper Gore snapped pictures of the activists as they were once again led away by security. At this point, the protests had come to represent a minor crisis for the campaign. "In his first week or so of campaigning [the activists] put themselves in his picture or disrupted his speech sufficiently that it was written about. This is very bad news for the campaign," said journalist Bart Gellman. "This is so not what they want."

After the protests Gore would call Leon Fuerth back in Washington. The "deal," then on Barshefsky's desk, was still being negotiated with the South Africans, according to Fuerth. "We were on tenterhooks, waiting to find out if someone in the South African Cabinet would object. We were convinced if it got out . . . they would blow it up." Fuerth said that Gore commanded his camp to "keep our mouths shut about it."

The protests were clearly having an impact. Gore asked Fuerth how much longer he thought it would take and implored him to do everything he could to reach an agreement—"obviously he very much hoped that we would get there quick."

The Gore camp clearly felt egregiously wronged by the activists. Global AIDS was an Al Gore–type issue. It had come on their radar screens early on. U.S. economic interests were involved, after all, and given the pressure brought to bear, they considered themselves out in front—prior to the media and the rest of the public's arrival—on the issue. They were pushing Mbeki to step up his leadership, and pushing the USTR to reach an accommodation with the South Africans.

To add to the tension, in the midst of the protests, Fuerth received a visit from a staffer from the Hill. The staffer told Fuerth that he had heard claims that the protests were politically driven. No doubt, the staffer had gotten wind of Jamie Love's role in galvanizing the protests, and his relationship to Ralph Nader. Fuerth was "incredulous." Nevertheless, the report shook him and piqued his concern, which had already reached a level of alarm.

On June 20, 1999, only days after the Gore protests began, and after years of economically driven tunnel vision, Barshefsky signed the trade deal. The next day Fuerth tried to connect with the South African embassy to establish a formal acknowledgment of the deal. A few days later, Donna Brazile, soon to be Gore's campaign manager, had "back-to-back meetings" with a cohort of activists at the White House and at Gore campaign headquarters on K Street.

Immediately thereafter, she reportedly contacted her old boss, Congresswoman Eleanor Holmes Norton, the representative from Washington, D.C., and a notable member of the Congressional Black Caucus, which was then becoming increasingly vocal about AIDS in Africa. Brazile intimated that it might be a good time for the Caucus to write to Gore to inquire about his formal position on drug pricing policy.

The next day the Gore camp wrote a lengthy reply stating that he supported both compulsory licensing and parallel imports, "so long as they are done in a way consistent with international agreements."

Presuming that they had met the activists' demands, and that they had insulated Gore from any further attacks, the Gore camp breathed a huge sigh of relief. That's not how the activists saw it, though. Gore had made an important announcement, but Barshefsky was still negotiating the details, and the USTR had yet to reach a formal agreement with South Africa. The USTR and the drug companies still held an enormous amount of influence over the South African government. And just how the agreement would be executed remained to be seen.

The protestors relented, giving Gore some reprieve, but progress with the USTR remained slow. In the meantime, the activists' demands escalated. It was no longer enough for Gore to relent on South Africa's drug pricing policies. Eric Sawyer now wanted Gore to champion a plan to produce AIDS drugs cheaply. That meant not only lower prices, but assistance in buying them. The activists wanted more than consent, they wanted leadership.

After several weeks of ostensible quiet, Eric Sawyer wanted to start things back up. He led a small cohort of activists at a fund-raiser featuring Tipper Gore in mid-July in New York City.

At the end of the month, another group of protestors targeted another Tipper fund-raiser. An activist would blow his or her whistle. Then he or she would get escorted out. Tipper would take a few moments to regain her composure, and then another activist would repeat the exercise. The disruptions were severe, and the candidate's wife was clearly flustered. "I'm telling you this was really not going over well with Tipper," said Jamie Love.

After one of the protests, Sawyer was invited to meet with Tipper. They met for about fifteen minutes while Sawyer made his case. Tipper said that she was certain that the vice president would meet with Sawyer for a discussion and she hoped that there would be no further outbursts.

There would be, though. On August 8, 1999, with the U.S.–South African trade agreement still formally unannounced, Eric Sawyer and another eight or so activists made their way up to Laconia, New Hampshire, for a family-style picnic fund-raising event for Al Gore. Rain moved the event indoors, to St. James Episcopal Church.

Sawyer and his associates—all paired off to look like run-of-the-mill churchgoing New Hampshire couples—filed into the quaint church around 11:30 A.M. so as to be sure to be well positioned among the crowd of about one hundred Gore supporters. Sawyer's pretend-wife had lagged behind to fill out nametags.

While Sawyer waited, a wholesome-looking family of four was ushered up to the front of the church next to him, right in view of the twenty or so news camera plastered against the wall. The young father struck up a conversation with Sawyer. He proudly declared that they had been selected to meet the vice president for a photo op and that the VP would pick up his children, young boys, two and four years old. He handed Sawyer his camera, and asked him to capture the moment for posterity. Sawyer agreed, "Oh, yeah sure," then turned and whispered, "Oh fuck."

The activists had a well-scripted plan: the other couples would take turns interrupting. They would be thrown out. Because Tipper had assured him that Gore would meet with him, Sawyer and his pretend-wife would not interrupt and would stay after to try and meet with Gore.

Sawyer's pretend-wife arrived with his nametag, which she had filled out: Eric Sandman. By 12:30, the VP entered the church to a good deal of fanfare. When Gore started heading in his direction, Sawyer began to get nervous.

Standing between Gore and the young family who had been preselected for the photo op, Sawyer started fidgeting, and thought he'd better move. Then he remembered that he had the young father's camera and had agreed to take their picture with Gore.

Gore approached Sawyer and said, "Well, hello there, and what is your name?"

"Eric," he replied skittishly.

"Eric what?" Gore asked with campaign-feigned interest.

Sawyer had forgotten what fake name appeared on his nametag. He looked down, but the cell phone in his jacket pocket created a bulge so that he couldn't make out the last name without moving his jacket. Seconds passed as Sawyer babbled.

"What's the matter?" Gore said. "You don't know your last name?"

Sawyer paused for a second, and said, "Actually, I'm Eric Sawyer."

Gore took a few seconds to process the name. Sawyer watched as it registered. He was one of the ringleaders who had terrorized his campaign, and badgered his wife only days before.

"Well, Eric Sawyer," Gore said. "Now correct me if I'm wrong, but Eric Sawyer isn't from New Hampshire, is Eric Sawyer?" Gore stiffened, trying to hold his smile in place.

"No, I'm from New York City," Sawyer replied.

"My, Eric Sawyer, you've certainly come a long way to see me, haven't you?" Sawyer could sense Gore's blood beginning to boil a little now. "He was clearly pissed, but trying to keep it together because he's surrounded by cameras—TV and print—and there are a million flashbulbs going off."

"Yes, I have," Sawyer replied, "and you may be surprised to know that I really do hope that you're our next president."

Gore gave him a stern look, and shot back: "You know, I bet you do."

By then, the Secret Service, aware of Sawyer from prior disruptions, had identified him and picked up on the tension between the two. As Gore turned to greet the young family, Secret Service agents began pushing Sawyer out of the way.

The father, oblivious to the dynamics underpinning the moment, called out, "No, he's got my camera. Can't Eric come and take my picture? He's got my camera."

With the media looking on, and Gore cozying up to the young kids, it seemed as if Sawyer had stumbled into a Norman Rockwell painting in which he was not welcome. In a bizarre moment, Gore—who had to know that he was moments away from yet another protest, this time in a quaint New Hampshire church—managed to muster the words, "Let Eric come and take the picture."

Only minutes later, Gore found himself the target of yet another protest. Like clockwork, the activists stood up, one pair after the other, chanting "Gore's Greed Kills." In what was now a familiar routine, they began throwing out large, empty pill bottles and "blood money" with Gore labeled as a "pharmaceutical industry puppet."

"Let's hear it for free speech," Gore announced in what had now become a canned reply. "I'd like to talk to you about a risky Republican tax cut," he said, hoping to add some levity.

"What about the future of Africa?" shouted one activist as he was led away, blowing his whistle.

As Sawyer was led out by his collar, he yelled at the VP: "Twenty-two million will die without these drugs in South Africa. Why are you trying to kill twenty-two million people?"

Gore replied that he would be glad to meet with them privately.

When the activists' shouts continued, the crowd tried to outshout them, cheering Gore on. "I have asked repeatedly to talk to these people," Gore said. "They don't want to talk. I'm proud the United States of America is doing more than any nation in the fight against AIDS," he exclaimed to the invigorated crowd.

Outside the church, the Secret Service suggested not so subtly that Sawyer and his comrades make themselves scarce. "Tipper promised us that we could speak to Al," Sawyer tried to explain, to no avail. "We're going to wait here until we get to speak with Gore," he said.

Exiting out of a side door after his speech, Gore was quickly whisked away out of sight of the activists waiting to speak with him.

In the fall of 1999, the activists redirected their sights on the USTR. They stormed Charlene Barshefsky's office. Several handcuffed themselves to the building's balcony. They organized a steady stream of protest marches outside USTR's offices, with oversized, twenty-foot puppets and more "drug money."

Barshefsky conceded that before the activists began speaking out, she did not fully appreciate that there was a staggering catastrophe rumbling through Africa. Until then, she said, "I was certainly not aware of this at all. . . . In years past, this [pharmaceutical] issue was treated purely as a trade issue and an intellectual property rights issue."

On September 17, 1999, the USTR released a press statement finally announcing an agreement with South Africa over the drug issue. The USTR would formally endorse the South African Medicines Act, in return for South Africa's affirmation that it would adhere to all formal international agreements going forward, including TRIPs, or trade-related aspects of intellectual property rights. The same press release noted that the Pharmaceutical Manufacturers Association of South Africa had agreed to drop all its pending litigation on the act a week earlier.

That December, amidst violent protests at an infamous World Trade Organization gathering in Seattle—including, among hundreds of others, a HealthGap crew—President Clinton announced that the United States would not pursue punitive measures against *any* sub-Saharan African country endorsing parallel imports or granting licenses to produce generic AIDS drugs. In May 2000, the president signed an executive order formally broadening the agreement to include all sub-Saharan African countries.

———•◆•———

On December 3, 1999, just weeks before thousands of activists would take to the streets of Seattle in riots protesting, among other things, the inaccessibility of AIDS drugs in the developing world, Ambassador Richard Holbrooke found himself milling about outside of a teacher-training center in Windhoek, Namibia. It was an early event in Holbrooke's thirteen-day trip to Africa. After being held in confirmation limbo by the Senate for fourteen months, Holbrooke had finally been confirmed as the United States Ambassador to the United Nations in August 1999.

Flanked by two large suburban vans, a coterie of colleagues, reporters, and diplomatic security, Holbrooke noticed a van heading in the direction of his entourage. As it drew closer, he saw that the van's windows were covered with curtains. Six women disembarked, their faces covered. They were ushered into the training center, and into a meeting room hung with curtains. They were afraid that if they were identified, they would lose their jobs and incur severe ostracism.

The scene struck a powerful chord with the American delegation. They had just been briefed that in regions of Namibia, the AIDS infection rate in the adult population was between 20 and 25 percent. As many as one in five or more adults were HIV-positive, and yet, those infected were shrouded in literal and figurative veils of stigma. Given the sheer magnitude of the crisis, and the societies' inability to deal with the issue openly and actively, Holbrooke foresaw that there would be profound social, economic, and even security implications.

Later on the same trip, Holbrooke and his wife, Kati Marton, a noted author and humanitarian, were the guests of honor at a special ceremony at a day school for AIDS orphans in Lusaka. The school's children treated the entourage to singing and dancing. When Holbrooke and Marton learned that every afternoon the school turned hundreds of children into the streets because they had no resources to afford them shelter, and that most were resigned to begging for food or even selling themselves for sex, they were crestfallen. "We are surrounded by breathtaking beauty," Marton wrote home during the trip, "marred by an overwhelming fact: AIDS is killing this paradise and much of the continent."

The AIDS visits had become "polarizing events for Holbrooke," said a senior aide. The ambassador had come to Africa with a robust agenda: de-mining, refugees, conflict, and other important issues. On the plane returning home, with his wife and Senator Russ Feingold from Wisconsin, who'd been a part of the delegation, Holbrooke couldn't stop thinking about AIDS. Flying over the Atlantic, Holbrooke picked up the phone and dialed the United Nations. He asked for Secretary General Kofi Annan, with whom he had spoken intermittently via cell phone during his trip.

The timing was propitious. The United States would be in the presidency of the United Nations Security Council in January 2000, the first month of the new millennium. Holbrooke wanted to devote the month to Africa. He also told Annan that he wanted the first session of the Security Council to be devoted to global AIDS. It was a bold break with precedence. Holbrooke and his team anticipated that there would be staunch resistance—from U.S. policy makers, UN officials, and other nation-states. "It was at that point," recounted Senator Feingold, "that he just started doing what Richard Holbrooke does."

Though by the end of the 1990s he would not hold the post he had long coveted, secretary of state, Richard Holbrooke was still the most compelling and perhaps the most effective U.S. diplomat during the Clinton administration. By the time he was nominated to serve as the U.S. ambassador to the United Nations in the early summer of 1998, Holbrooke had put together a dazzling and eclectic résumé. He had been a Foreign Service officer in Vietnam during the war, a managing editor of *Foreign Policy* magazine, an assistant secretary of state for Asian Affairs overseeing the normalization of relations with China in the Carter administration, a senior executive and vice chairman of two leading Wall Street investment banks for much of the 1980s, then U.S. ambassador to Germany during the first two years of the Clinton administration.

When the seemingly insoluble crisis of civil conflict and ethnic genocide in Bosnia had finally drawn serious U.S. engagement, Holbrooke was recalled to Washington as assistant secretary of state for European Affairs to oversee the negotiations for a peace settlement.

Holbrooke was a voracious reader and a fiercely independent thinker.

Sometimes confrontational, his confidence in his abilities and his aggressive manner ruffled some feathers. But there was no one better suited in the U.S. foreign policy establishment to sit across the table from Slobodan Milošević. At an army base in Dayton, Ohio, in November 1995, Holbrooke masterminded and oversaw the execution of a complex peace settlement, quelling, at least for some time, the violence in the region. The Dayton Accords won Holbrooke seven Nobel Peace Prize nominations.

Still, Holbrooke's forceful style and general UN-skepticism held up his confirmation for more than a year. During that period, Holbrooke had put together a small staff of bright young up-and-comers to flesh out an agenda for their high-profile boss. Several considerations underpinned their deliberations. At the time, Congress, under Jesse Helms's leadership, had halted its dues payments to the UN, crippling U.S.–UN relations. Holbrooke's first task was to reform the financial structure of the UN, lowering U.S. dues, and mending the relationship. In addition, Holbrooke was eager to identify a neglected isssue that he could utilize the UN forum to advance.

At a New York City dinner party in the mid-1980s, Holbrooke and his then girlfriend, high-profile journalist Diane Sawyer, had listened as Dr. Mathilde Krim, a social friend and leading AIDS researcher, shared a prescient analysis: the disease's epicenter would be in Africa, where mobile populations of truckers, migrant laborers, and refugees were transmitting the disease via heterosexual contact. Sawyer went to Kenya and Uganda and did a moving story on it for 60 Minutes.

When, in 1998, Holbrooke's good friend Kofi Annan shared his grave concern about the pandemic that was closing its grip on his home continent during a conversation at Annan's Sutton Place residence, Holbrooke immediately recalled the conversation with Krim, almost a decade and a half earlier. Annan would broach the subject with Holbrooke regularly, no doubt calculating that the issue could use Holbrooke's advocacy. Shortly before Holbrooke's formal confirmation, Annan brought up the issue again, and urged Holbrooke to take it up at the UN.

Bob Orr, who quickly became one of Holbrooke's most influential aides, had spent years in Africa, and was well attuned to the continent's problems. He also helped direct Holbrooke to the continent. For the most part, though, Holbrooke needed little help. A constellation of factors began lining up, all pointing toward Africa.

Most important, there were real and devastating problems on the continent that had been ill attended to. Africa needed the attention; the world needed to get engaged. In addition, the continent represented more than fifty votes in the UN. They were votes Holbrooke needed for support for his dues realignment agenda.

The first order of business was organizing that African trip in early December 1999. Bob Orr took the lead. Holbrooke would cut a swath across the continent on his ten-country tour, meeting as many national leaders as he could, enhancing his credibility on continental issues and shoring up support for dues realignment. It was decided that the focus of the trip would be the bloody civil war raging in the Congo.

Meanwhile, Peter Piot, executive director of UNAIDS, had also been in touch with Holbrooke on AIDS. In prepping for the trip, Holbrooke conferred with a series of officials and policy makers. Among them, Ken Bernard, then the Senior Advisor for International Health at the NSC, and Helene Gayle, head of international HIV/AIDS at the CDC, were invited up to Holbrooke's twelfth-floor office at the U.S. Mission, across the street from the UN on First Avenue.

In the expansive office featuring a wall of books and pictures of Holbrooke with various dignitaries and statesmen, Bernard and Gayle briefed the ambassador on the pandemic. They told him that a quarter of southern Africa's adult population was likely to die of the disease, which was also spreading at explosive rates in South Asia and the former Soviet Union. His interest was piqued even further when an up-and-coming GOP senator from Tennessee named Bill Frist came to discuss his concern. Frist was chairman of the African Affairs Subcommittee, and a key congressional contact for Holbrooke.

The pre-trip advocacy helped to focus Holbrooke on the issue. Though the focus was supposed to be on the Congo, he instructed his team to schedule AIDS visits in each of the ten countries he would visit. Later, Holbrooke recalled that the visits were "horror shows," and the issue came to have a visceral resonance. He resolved to inject AIDS into the world's most visible forum.

RP Eddy, Holbrooke's twenty-eight-year-old aide, an up and coming diplomat, also a former defensive tackle at Brown University, became the ambassador's point person on his plan to devote the new millennium's first Security Council session to AIDS. Eddy would have his hands full advancing the agenda.

First, he called to check in with U.S. Principal Deputy Assistant Secretary of State for International Organization Affairs Bill Wood, a resident UN sage. Wood told Eddy, "This is not a security issue. This does not constitute a threat to international peace and security. It should not be in the council."

When Eddy reported back to his boss on his conversation with Wood, Holbrooke explained, "RP, one of the only UN entities that ever gets anything done is the Security Council. That's where decisions are made, that's where attention is focused." Issues relegated to other areas of the UN tend to languish in debate and inaction. "If we get AIDS in the Security Council, that will begin to break down the stigma; that will begin to get more money to the issue; that will bring more leadership to the issue, and that will lead to a solution." Holbrooke had a genuine conviction that global AIDS was a security threat, but he was less hung up on the semantics of the issue, than the practical efficacy of inserting the issue into the forum in which it would command attention.

Holbrooke received a similarly negative initial response from Nancy Soderberg, the U.S. alternate representative to the UN. He was undeterred. "Everyone said you couldn't do these things," Holbrooke said. "Of course you could do them. All you had to do was do them."

But even if Holbrooke was prepared to circumvent his colleagues in Washington, he still needed support from other nation-states on the Security Council.

At the UN, Eddy tried to advance the notion that AIDS would overwhelm nation-states, begetting violence and disorder and possibly war. Only days before the planned session, Eddy found himself pitching the issue to an assemblage of African military attachés. The African generals took the presentation personally. They were offended that the United States would suggest that a disease was threatening to overwhelm their ability to rule their own countries. Walking out with a sinking feeling, Eddy thought the issue's prospects were bleak.

When he checked back in with Holbrooke to relay the encounter, his boss assuaged his concerns, telling him that the meeting didn't really matter; the critical body was the Security Council. But Holbrooke and his team were having trouble convincing the members of the Council to give global AIDS a forum. "People were really scared to talk about this issue in a public setting, on the record, with implications," Bob Orr said. Russia, China, and France were all intransigent. "Nobody's like Richard Holbrooke," Princeton Lyman explained. "When Richard Holbrooke wants something, he just drives you crazy day and night until he gets it. It's very effective." Unrelenting, Holbrooke spun the issue around.

Years before, in 1992, on a trip to Cambodia, Holbrooke had heard anecdotal accounts of UN peacekeepers who were infected with HIV, and had written a letter to the senior UN representative there, to which he received no reply. In some parts of the world, UN peacekeepers have a dubious reputation for engaging in prostitution and drugs. Peacekeeper activity was under the purview of the Security Council and was an issue that the body could not appear to skirt. Holbrooke said that if peacekeepers were getting infected, and were in turn passing on the virus, it was an issue for the Security Council.

It was true, Eddy said, "but a little overblown. . . . It is the ultimate irony," though, and "that was our hook, [that's] how we got it into the Security Council."

With Holbrooke's prodding, Paris and Beijing fell in line. Then, in what Holbrooke called "a classic act of old-time Russian heavy-handedness," the remaining holdout agreed to the Special Session, but declared that it would not speak. "This had us rolling in the aisles," Holbrooke later told the *Village Voice*. "I was tempted to say, 'Do you promise?' "

In breaking with precedent by showcasing a health issue at the Security Council, Holbrooke embarked on a difficult swim upstream. But he had made up his mind, and he forced the issue through. In Ken Bernard's estimation, without Holbrooke's efforts, the UNSC Special Session never would have happened. "He said, the first meeting of the UNSC in the new millennium is going to be on Africa and health, because that's the way it's going to be." And so it was.

A few weeks before the historic meeting on the morning of January 10, 2000, Leon Fuerth's telephone rang in his White House office. It was Holbrooke asking if the vice president would come and chair the session. "Leon got it immediately and made it happen," Holbrooke said.

It was the first time that a sitting vice president would chair a Security Council session. Holbrooke had purposefully arranged Gore's participation to showcase the pandemic and U.S. commitment. It just so happened, as well, that Gore was running for president and if—as expected—he won, would be naming the next secretary of state. It was a further coincidence that in the preceding months, the vice president had been pummeled by activists protesting his "negligence" on AIDS in Africa. In one masterful stroke, Holbrooke managed to confer prestige on his event, and also alleviate a debilitating political liability for the VP, thereby tightening his already very strong relationship with Gore, and cementing his standing as the front-runner to become Gore's secretary of state.

The stars seemed aligned, indeed, when Holbrooke and Gore walked across First Avenue together, on that frigid January morning, news cameras flashing, on their way to the 4,086th meeting of the UN Security Council. Inside, Holbrooke had gotten the UN to open up the galleries to the public. With throngs of visitors looking on and cheering, there was an unusual air of exuberance in the chamber.

Later that morning, the vice president of the United States stood facing the most visible forum in the world. Gore proceeded to deliver a finely crafted speech, both emotive and conceptually sophisticated. Laying to rest lingering doubts about the security-AIDS nexus, Gore said: "The heart of the security agenda is protecting lives, and we know that the number of people who will die of AIDS in the first decade of the twenty-first century will rival the number that died in all the wars in all the decades of the twentieth century." It was a stultifying metric. The issue not only deserved but demanded consideration by the Security Council.

Gore guided his audience through the human element of the pandemic. He profiled the ineffable statistics and finally placed the historic event in a larger context. He declared: "This meeting demands of us that we see security through a new and wider prism, and forever after, think about it according to a new, more expansive definition."

Kofi Annan, World Bank Director James Wolfensohn, and ministers from many other nations followed Gore. The historic session injected the issue into the international political discourse at its highest level. A resolution pressing for national leadership and engagement was passed. The session and the resolution affirmed that the world was watching and national leaders would be accountable. They were critical catalysts in galvanizing many around the world to action.

In the United States, the special session helped gain the issue wider press play and prominence with legislators and policy makers. In its aftermath, Holbrooke was asked about global AIDS on *The NewsHour with Jim Lehrer*. "People always ask me, 'What's the biggest problem in the world?'" His answer: "There are dozens of big issues, but the level of the AIDS crisis, its potential to destroy economic achievement, undermine social stability and create more political uncertainty and the inability of the rest of the world to contain it on one continent, because it can't be sealed off in Africa . . . is so enormous. . . . So, that's my considered judgment."

For Holbrooke, the UN episode illustrated a critical truth: "The simple line is that America makes a difference. When people dig in . . . it makes a difference. This is a take no prisoners issue. You can compromise politically and bureaucratically on many issues," but not global AIDS. "This is a life or death issue."

Evidence-Based Advocacy,
Start the Press

In early 1995, five years before Richard Holbrooke would appear at the
UN Security Council, Peter Piot's life was about to take a radical turn.
The Belgian prodigy who had collaborated with Joe McCormick on the
Ebola outbreak of 1976 in Zaire was now in his mid-forties. He had
emerged as one of the leading figures in the world of international health
and disease. When he joined McCormick once again on that first AIDS investigation at Mama Yemo Hospital in Kinshasa in 1983, Piot had been a
key member of the vanguard examining the disease's international dimension. He played a leading role in collaboration with Jonathan Mann on
Project SIDA, and he spent much of the 1990s at the Global Program on
AIDS, or GPA, as director of research and intervention development.

Piot was well aware of the trials that both Mann and Michael Merson
had faced as the leading figures in the global response. At GPA, his work
was technical, even tending toward the academic. So when he was offered
the reins of a new international vehicle, yet unformed, called UNAIDS, he
was ambivalent: "I wasn't sure I wanted to do this."

Upon its formal inception in January 1996, UNAIDS would become the
world's leading vehicle in combating global AIDS. It would advocate for
an upgraded global response, serve as a clearinghouse for technical expertise, and emerge an authoritative global source of information and best
practices.

Unlike GPA, it would not be housed at WHO. Hiroshi Nakajima, the
agency's director general, had thoroughly discredited his agency and had
lost the trust of leading donors like the Americans, the British, and the

Dutch. It was also becoming clear to donors that each of the UN's disparate agencies—WHO, UNICEF, UNDP, UNFPA, UNESCO, and the World Bank—had their own AIDS initiatives. With their own distinct strategies, the agencies weren't talking to each other or coordinating. As a result, the aggregate response had become mired in overlap and inefficiency. In addition, some donors were adamant that the pandemic's magnitude required a multisectoral global response that engaged all of the dimensions and capabilities of the UN. For a variety of reasons, then, it made sense to pull the response out of WHO.

Instead, UNAIDS was formed as a stand-alone secretariat. Officially a Joint United Nations Program, the UN's various agencies were its cosponsors. UNAIDS would coordinate all of those disparate agencies' efforts, attempting to provide strategic vision and a more effective, comprehensive global response. In structure and mandate, the effort would be without precedent.

Still, in early 1995, UNAIDS was merely an idea. "I didn't fully understand what this was about," remembered Piot. If the new program's efficacy was uncertain, Piot knew that regardless, its new executive director would be on the hook.

Piot had spent more than ten years working on global AIDS. He had spent much of that time in the field, at hospitals and care facilities. He had studied the disease inside and out, and still patients were dying in masses, and still the world seemed to take no notice. For Piot, the time for studying the pandemic had come to an end. "I wanted to switch from studying AIDS to doing something about it."

The challenge of coordinating the different agencies and the vast array of efforts scattered throughout the UN leviathan would fall to Peter Piot. It was clear what his real mandate would be from the outset: "Making sure that the UN agencies are doing more on AIDS, and that they do it in a better way, qualitatively, and that they do it in a coherent way." Piot would be the conductor, attempting to "harmonize policies."

He also grasped the underlying political dynamics framing the challenge. "There was really a war between UNDP, or the United Nations Development Program, and UNICEF and WHO and the World Bank. They were spending so much time fighting each other, rather than fighting AIDS. Ending that was the first mission. You won't find it on any document," but "that's what it came down to."

The irony that UNAIDS was now supposed to "coordinate" the very agencies that co-sponsored the new program did not go unnoticed by its new executive director. It would not be easy.

In the mid-1990s, anti-UN sentiment, which had been long fomenting, was reaching a boiling point in the United States. Though the UN was Franklin Roosevelt's brainchild, the organization had been subsumed, and largely discredited, by the bipolar order of the Cold War. Even as the UN failed to meet its loftier expectations, it had swelled into a bureaucratic behemoth. A leading U.S. diplomat spoke of "bureaucratic arthritis." U.S. ambassador to the UN, Madeleine Albright, at the UN's Fiftieth Anniversary in 1995, said that the UN would have to "reform or die."

To compound matters, by 1995 post–Cold War insularity had crept into U.S. foreign policy. At the same time, the country had been mired in a nasty economic recession. All of these factors had the effect of dampening U.S. enthusiasm for funding international, and certainly UN-based initiatives.

As U.S. ambassador to the UN in Geneva, Dan Spiegel was at the forefront, or more aptly, in the crosshairs of developments for much of the decade. "Despite the emphasis on the epidemic," he recounted, "[UNAIDS] was still a UN program, and we didn't have the money to fund the UN. . . . I was worried about closing agencies in Geneva and running out of money because we were badly in arrears."

In addition, USAID had a vested interest in keeping funds for its own efforts. The agency was more than happy to dismantle GPA, which had clearly come to function as an "operational" outfit, funding in-country efforts and supporting national AIDS plans. Replacing it with a sleeker, leaner secretariat would also provide USAID cover to pull back its financial commitment. Upon UNAIDS's formation, U.S. funding dropped by over 50 percent compared to its support for GPA, from around $40 million to $20 million.

After cannibalizing his own program, and nobly ceding his own bureaucratic power, Michael Merson could only sit on the sidelines and watch in dismay as donors pulled back. UNAIDS "shouldn't have been an excuse to drop what they were giving. They should have maintained their contribution and given more."

Upon its official creation on January 1, 1996, UNAIDS emerged the child of myriad cross-cutting considerations, interests, and agendas. Amid all the driving factors, the one commonality among donors was a willingness to break the mold. Hans Mulkirk, the Dutch representative and head of the governing counsel of GPA, was convinced that the program needed to be gutted and dissolved. Others agreed.

According to Dr. Thierry Mertens, an insider during the deliberations, the new effort was "perceived as a trial for UN reform . . . a field test." Everyone seemed to want to try something new. The appetite for constructing a new prototypical global vehicle had piqued, and, as another insider remembered it, "AIDS just happened to be there."

Some were hopeful that the new vehicle would yield results. Given its dubious origins, though, many predicted disaster.

In retrospect, many consider UNAIDS's inception a seminal moment in the U.S. response. Princeton Lyman opined: "The decision to switch from GPA to UNAIDS is the point where the U.S. and everybody else recognized that this was a problem bigger than we've been able to handle. . . . The decision then that this was too big, and it was more than a health problem: I think that's the turning point. I would mark it there."

In 1996, however, few outside of the global health or the UN communities were even aware that the unprecedented new program existed. Susan Rice served as the National Security Council's director for African Affairs, and later as the assistant secretary of state for African Affairs. The positions made her one of the highest-ranking U.S. officials to focus on the region. During its infancy, the program didn't seem to register with Rice. "I don't know when UNAIDS started, but I don't recall it in 1995, 1996, or even 1998."

Piot and his deputy, Ambassador Sally Grooms Cowal, a longtime U.S. and UN diplomat, did their best to knock on doors, but they weren't getting access to senior politicians or policy makers outside of the realm of health. The media was not yet focused and domestic political constituencies had not yet arrived. Moreover, several strategic and internal problems handcuffed the program through 1998.

UNAIDS was an experiment. Its mission was ambitious, its budget exiguous, and its leader a novice in the realm of international political advocacy. It was disappointing, if not surprising to Michael Merson to see the program stumble out of the blocks. "There's no question that there's some confusion and some slowing down of the response. You can imagine dismantling a program that had 500 [staff people] and building it back up," with a diminutive budget, a disinterested donor base, and weighty expectations.

The GPA and UNAIDS staff labored tirelessly, doing all they could to make the transition seamless, but the logistics and the shift in mandate and scope yielded difficulties early on. "You had an eighteen-to-twenty-four-month period in which it [still was not] effective operationally," Stephen Morrison said.

While it was a trying time for Piot and Merson, it was a disastrous time for affected countries. GPA had been overseeing, supporting, and even funding national programs and had been providing all sorts of technical assistance. With GPA's demise, that support was withdrawn. UNAIDS had neither the funding nor the mandate to fill in the vacuum. At the same time, USAID was shifting its backing from national governments to NGOs. "So, now the governments are just stranded because the donors are pulling out from supporting them and GPA pulled out," said Sheila Mitchell, who experienced much of the disarray on the ground in Africa. "So that was a tough time, a tough period . . . all that was going on at about that time."

Of course, the program's architects were hoping that GPA's extraction would be more than offset by an upgraded, coordinated effort among the UN's "operational" agencies. Piot knew from the get-go that bringing the agencies in line would be one of his greatest challenges. In short order, his fears were realized.

UN agencies were not interested in being "coordinated" or managed by an upstart, newfangled program with few resources to offer. They had their own programs in place, their own strategies and agendas, and their own manner of operating.

Pressure from the secretary general's office might have helped bring the agencies in line, but none was forthcoming. "The sad, unbearable truth is that the UN responded far too slowly," said Stephen Lewis, a former UNICEF official working as an advisor to Piot. "We all responded way too slowly, and I include UNICEF. We just never took it as the desperate reality it was and is. . . . There was just never the sense that what we were facing was the obliteration of a continent and that you just had to move heaven and earth to respond."

The UN agencies' obstinacy became Piot's greatest frustration. "The transition was not smooth at all. Co-sponsoring agencies didn't really get their acts together until a few years later. The creation of UNAIDS didn't mean that they should stop dealing with AIDS. On the contrary, the idea was that there should be more and better [coordination]—that they would work in their area of expertise, but that didn't happen," Piot lamented.

The co-sponsoring agencies' financial support waned almost immediately. World Bank loans dropped from $50 million to less than $10 million; WHO's support dropped from $130 million to $20 million; and UNICEF's dropped from $45 million to $10 million. Though the decline was precipitous, it was somewhat expected, and might have been fine, had the funds gone to a larger UNAIDS-coordinated effort.

Agency leaders looked at the upstart agency as a paper tiger. Their own agencies, on the other hand, had established programs under their control. Being "coordinated" seemed tantamount to being managed and controlled to most agency leaders.

The net result was that coordination foundered terribly. "The UN community was happy doing what it was doing about AIDS all along," said Ambassador Sally Grooms Cowal. They were not eager to have "some little fly" come along and reconfigure and manage their efforts.

One of Cowal's first tasks as deputy director was to chair a meeting with several of the "co-sponsoring" agencies. The issue at hand was HIV transmission through breast-feeding. By then the evidence suggested that about 50 percent of babies breast-feeding from HIV-positive mothers would acquire the virus. From UNAIDS's perspective, mothers needed to be told. But because babies receive various health benefits that come with breast-feeding, WHO's policy was to promote it. Elsewhere, UNICEF had waged a ten-year-long battle with baby formula manufacturers defending breast-feeding. They were not eager to reverse their position. "I can't tell you what an incredible fight this was. It went on and on," Cowal said. After much time, the groups were able to hammer out an agreement. It was a "lowest common denominator" solution, but incorporated UNAIDS's concerns.

Several months later, Cowal was walking through the corridor in Geneva, and spotted a book about baby nutrition put out by WHO. She purloined a copy and took it back to her office. To her exasperation she saw that it "was all about breast-feeding and it didn't say a goddamn word about certain circumstances, etc. So, despite the fact that it had taken us I don't know how many meetings to hammer out an agreement, six months later they put out whatever they wanted to put out."

Cowal took it up with WHO brass and insisted they pull the books. But the episode was emblematic of the turf wars and the competing agendas that consigned the global effort to stasis during UNAIDS's first two years of operation.

With the going painfully slow, it appeared as if Piot might have been the wrong man for the job of leading the world's response. His scientific credentials were unassailable. But with global disinterest high, UNAIDS needed a Machiavellian statesman, not a do-gooder scientist. "When I started, since I came from a scientific background I thought that it would be enough to present the evidence, the data, and say this is bad," and then "the funding and so on would come. I see now that one has to use very different arguments."

Piot had not accepted the job to fail, though. Relentless, he embarked on a probing examination of the challenges facing UNAIDS, including his own role and performance.

Prodding and cajoling the UN agencies, Piot insisted that the global effort had to transcend petty feudal conflicts. It soon became clear to Piot, however, that the agencies would fall in line only when he had amassed political power. He began building his staff and deploying them in-country, where they would assist national governments in surveillance and strategic mobilization against the disease. The initiative would help broaden UNAIDS's role as well as its political network.

Importantly, Piot also recognized that UNAIDS's credibility would in large part be a function of his authority as a global spokesperson for the disease. He traveled constantly. He spent a good deal of time in the United States and other Western countries lobbying for resources and trying to raise awareness. He also spent a good deal of time in Africa and the developing world.

Appealing to world leaders became Piot's number one agenda. After all, he says, "We could have done a super job in making the UN more efficient, but if the political reality was still one of denial of the AIDS problem, then we could forget it."

In addition, he worked to position UNAIDS as the clearinghouse for best practices and as the axis of an international collaborative network of scientists, public health people, and activists fighting the pandemic.

When he became a professor, the legendary former CDC director Dr. Bill Foege shared a key dictum with his students: "Tie the needs of the poor with the fears of the rich," he told them. "When the rich lose their fear, they are not willing to invest in the problems of the poor." It was perhaps a sad commentary, but by 1998 Piot was beginning to grasp its kernel of truth.

"The evolution of my thinking is that more than ever, I [was coming to believe] that we needed to keep AIDS at the top political level. By political I mean not only the professional politicians, but the top business leaders, the top religious leaders—those who really shape society." To appeal to those strata, Piot would have to repackage his advocacy pitch. Slowly, he started talking about the social issues, as Mann had, then the economic issues and even the military issues. AIDS was not just a health problem, it was a catastrophe that touched on every dimension of national and international society.

To insert AIDS on the global political agenda, Piot knew that he would have to fire a very loud shot, and that would require ammunition.

When UNAIDS began two years earlier, it had been clear for at least ten years that the pandemic represented a crisis of monumental proportions. But since the contentious conference in Atlanta in 1985, the epidemiology and the estimates had been scattered. As the pandemic swelled, various actors offered disparate estimates of its magnitude. Mann's group at Harvard had a set of global and regional estimates. Karen Stanecki's group at the U.S. Census Bureau had estimates, as did the CDC, WHO, and others. Some offered global estimates, some regional, and some estimated for specific countries or locales. The methodologies driving the epidemiology, which fed into the disparate groups' models, also varied considerably. Revisions were rampant and estimates ran a sizable gamut.

The dissonance generated confusion among policy makers, the media, and the public. With various numbers being lofted around, it was unclear which source to believe, which numbers were the most credible. Without a single authoritative set of numbers, the pandemic seemed to most to be some kind of terrible, but nebulous threat.

To redress the predicament, Piot made, in the fall of 1996, perhaps his most important hire, enticing noted epidemiologist Bernhard Schwartlander from the German government. When Schwartlander arrived, the program's epidemiology effort was weak. GPA's in-country surveillance efforts had been disbanded. Countries did not have the resources or knowhow to sustain those efforts. As a result, the pullout left a gaping hole

in global surveillance for over a year. Building up the epidemiology, establishing credible estimates, and doing it all under the aegis of UNAIDS—
ensuring its role as global authority—became Schwartlander's driving
mission.

The first step was bringing the disparate groups together. Schwartlander
made sure that the various players would compare and synthesize data-
bases, providing his team with the most accurate detailed information
available. In addition, recognizing that the epidemic was driven by distinct
factors in each country and that each would require unique strategic interventions, he concluded that his team would have to focus on national estimates.

The effort would require important reforms. Schwartlander would build
up the surveillance effort by putting epidemiologists back in the field in the
developing world. He called on the CDC and other leading technical players to help rebuild national efforts.

Then, with all the key players at the table, Schwartlander focused on
building a new, sophisticated model with hundreds of key driving variables.
The U.S. Census Bureau became a critical partner. Their comprehensive
database and detailed analytics helped shape the new more robust model.

Finally, Schwartlander realized that in order to really understand the dimensions of the pandemic and its growth, his team would have to delve
into what he called "second generation" HIV surveillance. That is, rather
than making generalized, blanket assumptions, Schwartlander and his
team would have to explore sexual behavior from region to region and
country to country.

By 1998, having captained the program's effort for almost two years,
Schwartlander was exhausted. He had been working at a fevered pace formulating the first authoritative country-by-country global estimates. His
effort was woefully underfunded, and despite general cooperation and collaboration among the disparate players, there were moments of acrimony.
All the while, Schwartlander had to fend off "fanatics" who argued that
the numbers coming out were way too high, or way too low. Debunking
their criticism took up a lot of his time, and they were a thorn in his side
throughout.

Even as he labored, Schwartlander was losing some of his friends and
colleagues in the developing world to the pandemic. He suffered from intermittent bouts of depression. "For somebody who wants to get it right
like myself, there are phases where you question whether you can continue

and whether it's worth your effort. It's extremely tiring." The chance to score a breakthrough kept him going.

At the Geneva Conference in June 1998, UNAIDS—under Schwartlander's leadership—presented the world with the first set of consensus-backed global country-by-country estimates. The major groups—Harvard, the U.S. Census Bureau, WHO, and others—were all on board. Finally, the world had authoritative numbers.

With a bold stroke, those authoritative numbers washed away much of the confusion and discord. Schwartlander's persistence had now laid bare the chilling magnitude of the pandemic. In the preceding three years, twenty-seven countries had seen their HIV infection rates double. One out of every four adults in Botswana and Zimbabwe was infected. There were 8 million AIDS orphans around the world and 16,000 people were becoming infected with HIV every day.

The breakthrough would have a profoundly galvanizing effect on the U.S. response. Until UNAIDS was able to establish itself as the global authority on estimates, Sally Grooms Cowal explained, "Everybody was looking at one piece of the elephant and deciding that was the elephant. So you had people looking at the trunk and people looking at the tail." They were not "focusing on the entire elephant." In the summer of 1998, at Geneva, the elephant had begun to come into focus.

Peter Piot's thinking was also crystallizing. Just like Alan Berkman in New York, Piot realized in the aftermath of the Geneva conference that the response to date, business as usual, wasn't working. Piot called a confidential retreat. He amassed a group of leaders and experts, not just on AIDS, but from various corridors of international power: industry, the media, foreign policy, and politics. "The main question," Piot said, "was how to put AIDS on the really big agenda."

He asked the participants: "What do people take seriously in the world?" In the context of the UN, they concluded, "it's the Security Council and that's about it." War and peace, the military, economics, and security attract attention at the top political levels. "So, if they would only deal with AIDS that would make a big difference. . . . So, that's the conclusion we came up with: Moving from a public health strategy to a political strategy."

Armed with credible estimates, a more resonant message, and a refined advocacy strategy, Piot and Cowal began to employ what they called "evidence-based advocacy." They traveled exhaustively, trumpeting the catastrophe unfolding. Increasingly, they linked the pandemic to economic and security considerations.

Cowal addressed the Council on Foreign Relations, where she showcased the pandemic as a foreign policy issue with great economic and security import. Piot and his colleagues at UNAIDS fought to get the issue on the G7 Agenda, in which the finance ministers from seven of the wealthiest countries in the world address global economic issues, and as an agenda item at the World Economic Forum, a collaborative meeting place in Davos, Switzerland, for world leaders to address pressing global issues.

More and more, doors began opening. At the Office of National AIDS Policy, the new AIDS czar, Sandy Thurman, met with Piot and Cowal in 1998. Her deputy, Todd Summers, explained: "That was really a pivotal point because it was the first time that you had a generally agreed-upon set of numbers that showed the magnitude of the epidemic. . . . When those numbers became available and all of a sudden the world went, 'Oh, wow!' "

By the end of 1998, the authoritative estimates presented at Geneva had begun to circulate among the international community with increased velocity and salience. Piot had emerged a savvy international figure, with a serious network and a trunk full of political capital. Responding to the magnitude of the pandemic and Piot's stature, the UN agencies began to come in line. All in all, UNAIDS was beginning to hit its stride.

It had been more than eight years since Jonathan Mann's departure from GPA, and the reemergence of a credible, high-profile global advocate. As 1999 rolled around, another authoritative global advocate had emerged to shine the spotlight on the pandemic. The advocacy from above was complemented by a forceful groundswell from the domestic activists who had awakened with a vengeance, from below.

Suddenly, the pandemic was news.

———•◆•———

Late one night in February 2000, sometime past nine o'clock, Steve Coll, the managing editor of The Washington Post, strolled into Phil Bennett's office. Both relatively new in their posts, Coll and his friend Bennett, the paper's assistant managing editor for foreign news, had spent much time brainstorming about how they could best devote the paper's resources to dig deeper into the defining challenges of the day. Referencing a large map affixed to the wall of Bennett's office, the two newsmen paced back and forth, throwing out big ideas.

"Thirty years from now," Bennett asked out loud, "what will history record as the single most important issue that we failed to take stock of?" Studying the map, his eyes pulled focus on Africa. Bennett answered his own question, "Global AIDS." He had a follow-up: "How'd it get this bad? Who could have stopped it?"

Days later, Bart Gellman was summoned to meet with Coll and Bennett in a glass-encased office by the north wall of the paper's newsroom.

Thirty-nine years old, with short dark hair and glasses, Gellman was a twelve-year veteran at the paper. His primary focus was foreign affairs. He had already been nominated for a Pulitzer Prize, and was one of the *Post's* star journalists. He knew about global AIDS and was deeply concerned, but it wasn't a particular focus. When Coll and Bennett made their pitch, it was a no-brainer. "I'd love to do this, it sounds fantastic," Gellman replied immediately.

Coll and Bennett were hardly the first newspeople in the U.S. media to awaken to the pandemic. In fact, in the preceding ten months, through most of 1999, there had been a marked upsurge in media coverage. Of course, the media hadn't been entirely silent on global AIDS before that. Some of the nation's preeminent journalists—like Larry Altman of *The New York Times*, Laurie Garrett of *Newsday*, and Jon Cohen of *Science*— had all covered global AIDS in detail.

"We all know each other. We all saw each other at the same meetings," said Steve Sternberg, a *USA Today* reporter, who had also covered AIDS since the early 1980s. To varying extents, their pieces touched on the disease's social, economic, and geopolitical implications, but that was not generally their primary point of embarkation; and it was not, for the most part, what their core readership expected. They were science or health journalists. Their reporting, while detailed and prescient, remained for the most part consigned to their papers' health/science sections, where it would not reach mainstream policy makers or the general public.

Two years later at a conference at the Columbia School of Journalism, Dean Arlene Notoro Morgan proclaimed: "AIDS is a story that calls on us to take down the silos of the newsroom. It is a story that demands that we bring the different disciplines together and break down the divisions in our newsrooms." AIDS touched so many dimensions of the human experience, and it could have been covered from a plethora of angles. It was a humanitarian issue, a social issue, it had profound economic and developmental implications, it was a foreign policy issue and clearly had security or geopolitical ramifications. Until 1999, however, it had fallen through the structural cracks of the U.S. media and remained almost exclusively a health/science story.

In addition to the structural deficit, there was a powerful macro-trend working against the issue in the U.S. media through the 1990s. U.S. insularity and the increasingly profit-driven nature of the media industry enervated the level of serious foreign news coverage in the United States through the decade.

Of the 1990s, David Halberstam, a seasoned foreign affairs journalist, wrote: "Nothing reflected the changes in American attitudes towards foreign policy more clearly than the way the three main television networks—ABC, CBS, and NBC—had gradually been moving away from serious foreign coverage in the eighties . . . the networks had become essentially isolationist, or neo-isolationist, both reflecting and at the same time increasing the nation's self-absorption." He continued, "America was only interested in itself. The rest of the world had become far more distant, less important, indeed more foreign." Statistics support Halberstam's claim. From 1989 to 1996 total foreign coverage on network nightly news declined from 3,733 minutes to 1,838 minutes at ABC, and from 3,351 minutes to 1,175 minutes at NBC.

Television stations, magazines, and newspapers were increasingly becoming subject to the profit-driven conglomerate. In addition, new technologies such as cable, satellite TV, and the Internet turned the erstwhile consistently profitable "television marketplace," as well as print media, "into a competitive cauldron in which journalism must increasingly compete with entertainment programming."

As a result, the media sought to strap its operations in "high-cost, low-return" efforts. Foreign coverage generally required a news organization to have foreign bureaus. That meant overhead and high costs. Domestic coverage was cheaper. Even cheaper still was "recycled" news, covering the same story over and over again from different angles; hence, OJ and the Lewinsky scandal.

It was a punishing decade for media professionals. Around 2000, a Harris poll indicated that journalists were held in the lowest public esteem of any professional group. In the cacophony of chiming cash registers and loud flashy news banners, with foreign news bureaus shutting down all over the world, important international issues would suffer neglect. Global AIDS was one of them.

Still, nothing is as powerful, it has been suggested, as an idea whose time has come. And with UNAIDS's authoritative estimates in wide circulation, Piot's advocacy, and—perhaps most important—the visibility of domestic activists, who were awakening to the global dimension, the dam of media neglect burst in a flurry of coverage in 1999.

In May 1999, Steve Sternberg, the longtime health reporter from *USA Today*, accompanied Clinton's third AIDS czar, Sandy Thurman, on a trip to Africa. It was a struggle to convince his editors, whose focus was on domestic issues, to fund the trip. Sternberg pressed hard. The paper printed several of Sternberg's pieces, and one made the paper's front page.

With domestic activists sounding an alarm, and creating a stir during the first week or two of the Gore campaign in June, coverage picked up markedly. Bob Davis of *The Wall Street Journal* covered the protests and the aftermath in detail, as did other mainstream papers. The protests really started to "get the newspapers interested," said Bart Gellman.

During that summer and early fall, a handful of journalists ventured to Africa to learn more. Their pieces, published later that fall, would make a big splash.

In October 1999, Wil Haygood and Kurt Shillinger wrote ten stories in the course of a four-part series published in *The Boston Globe*. Beginning with Shillinger's piece on October 10, "A Continent's Crisis," the series framed the magnitude of the pandemic, examined African leaders' silence, and profiled some of the suffering.

A month later, Mark Schoofs's eight-part series entitled "The Agony of Africa" began running in *The Village Voice*. Schoofs had spent months researching the series in South Africa, Nigeria, and elsewhere. His in-depth profiles brought to life the horror of the pandemic, humanizing the suffering. He explored the stigma and denial attached to the disease, its origins, the science, and the dynamics behind its transmissibility.

The January 17, 2000, cover of *Newsweek* featured a child with a blanket wrapped around his head. The title of the cover story was "10 Million Orphans," and the subtitle read, "The AIDS Epidemic in Africa is leaving a generation of children without parents." All along, Altman's coverage in *The New York Times* and Garrett's in *Newsday* continued and picked up steam, leading the charge from the health/science side.

Television coverage began to take off as well. In 2000, the BBC News did a five-part series on the issue. PBS was covering it with increased attention. The major networks all took their turn. In June 2000, Ed Bradley did a piece for 60 *Minutes* entitled "Death by Denial."

Bradley's hour-long piece won the Peabody. The Schoofs series in *The Village Voice* was awarded a 2000 Pulitzer Prize. The awards were certainly a ringing affirmation of the import of the subject matter. They were also an implicit indictment that so little had been done previously.

By February and March 2000, it was clear to Coll, Bennett, and Gellman that they were not the first to home in on global AIDS. The uptick in coverage was well under way. Intent on making their mark, the three began deliberating upon a fresh angle from which to attack it. Reviewing the existing body of journalism, it became clear that it had a common theme. Much of the coverage was excellent. But, "so much of it was vast descriptions of [a] train wreck." The pieces had the effect, it seemed to Gellman, of directing the reader to the "twisted wreckage" and imploring them to "look how awful it is."

For the most part, it was what Gayle Smith, former NSC director for African Affairs, called "soft, feature" coverage. The bulk of the reporting attacked the issue from a human-interest angle, profiling people—a story would feature a local woman and her children, for example—who were suffering. The approach sought to humanize the crisis, and bring the reader beyond the numbers and the body counts, allowing him or her to identify with the pandemic's victims.

To policy makers like Smith, it was a point of great frustration. "The bulk of the media coverage is feature coverage. . . . It's not really covered as news; it's all mushy. . . . That just reinforces the notion of this being a soft issue." *USA Today* gave as much or more space to the photographs or images as it did to the text of Steve Sternberg's pieces, illustrating Smith's point. It frustrated Sternberg, who returned from his trips with notepads full of material and deeper themes.

The pandemic had critical economic and geopolitical consequences, all but ignored in such coverage. Framed solely as a "humanitarian" issue, Smith and other champions found it harder to use the coverage to move the issue on the policy front.

By showcasing the statistics, the human dimension, and the local context, the "soft, feature" reporting had no doubt covered a key element of the catastrophe. There was another way to cut it, though, Gellman postulated, and his editors agreed. "Let's draw some concentric circles around this problem," they decided, "and look at various issues of responsibility."

Laurie Garrett had taken aim at the same question at points in time, and from various angles. But Gellman was the first to take it head-on from a political and individual accountability perspective. He planned on investigating the institutions and people that had the money and the responsibility. His questions: "What did they know? And when? And what did they do about it?"

It was a challenging mission. Gellman was a world-class foreign policy expert. Eventually, in 2002, he would win his Pulitzer for breaking a story on a missed opportunity to attack Osama bin Laden. However, he knew little about science, public health, and AIDS. It was also clear that Gellman was after a story that was not going to flatter his subjects. He anticipated, rightly, that access would be a problem.

Gellman started with what he knew. His best contacts were in the national security realm. Researching his story, Gellman noticed that the National Security Council and security types were now focusing on the pandemic, and increasingly designating it a threat to U.S. "national security."

On April 30, 2000, Gellman "broke" the story for the *Post* in an article entitled, "AIDS Is Declared Threat to Security." The article reported that the Clinton administration had "formally designated the disease for the first time as a threat to U.S. national security." It was certainly true that some policy makers—most notably Leon Fuerth, Al Gore's chief foreign policy advisor—had been treating the pandemic as a "national security" threat. Whether the designation was in fact "formal" remained a point of contention. When asked about the "national security" designation, press secretary Joe Lockhart reportedly replied, "I don't know if we've declared this, *The Washington Post* has declared this."

Despite the confusion over the designation, Gellman's article drew attention to the "national security"–global AIDS nexus, and had the effect of promoting the issue in the public discourse. On a talk show the Sunday the story broke, Senate Majority Leader Trent Lott declared that it most certainly was not a security threat, and that it was yet another instance of the Clinton administration's "appealing to certain groups"—by which he seemed to mean gays and/or blacks.

Days after Gellman's piece, Ray Suarez asked Clinton's NSC director,

Sandy Berger, about it on *The NewsHour with Jim Lehrer*. Berger implicitly acknowledged the designation. Before the end of his presidency, Clinton himself would make the declaration.

Having planted a stake in the discourse on the pandemic, Gellman proceeded to pursue his story. He traveled to Geneva twice. He also went to South Africa.

Visiting Kwazulu-Natal, in northeastern South Africa, Gellman witnessed AIDS in Africa for the first time. Moving around from hospital to hospital and orphanage to orphanage, he could see that the resource-starved health and social workers were at the end of their ropes. After days of travel, Gellman came to a small hamlet called the Village of Hope, where he was told of an AIDS outreach program for orphans. The staff of the program seemed to have boundless energy. Impressed by their determination, Gellman spent some time with them. In the course of his reporting, Gellman encountered an emaciated woman, clearly within weeks or months of death. She had no idea what would become of her children. Later in the day, he met a beautiful eleven-year-old girl, an AIDS orphan, named Siphiwe—which he was told means "gift" in Zulu. Innocently, he asked her through an interpreter, "How's school?" She answered that she couldn't go to school. He learned that the government charged $15 a year, too much for Siphiwe to afford.

In July 2000, *The Washington Post* published Gellman's flagship piece, entitled, "The Belated Global Response to AIDS in Africa." Gellman wrote it long, almost eight thousand words, expecting his editors, as was their wont, to cut it down. After reading the story, though, Gellman's editor implored him to flesh out the already lengthy piece even further. He was delighted to do so.

It was the first in-depth political examination of the world's response to the pandemic. In one of the nation's most high-profile newspapers, it was a ringing alert holding policy makers in key international and U.S. bureaucracies and centers of power accountable. Many were reading.

One of them was Richard Holbrooke. During an interview on *The NewsHour with Jim Lehrer* on July 13, a week after Gellman's piece appeared, a moderator asked Holbrooke: "How did this problem, which every day we're hearing more about. . . . How did this remain unaddressed internationally for so long?" For Holbrooke, the media itself was part of the answer. "You'll have to ask yourself that question," Holbrooke shot back. But by July 2000, there was also some good news: "The media is finally paying attention to this," he added. "I congratulate you and your colleagues for doing this."

John Donnelly was reading as well. In the kitchen of his comfortable suburban home in Chevy Chase, Maryland, Donnelly, the five-foot-six, thin-framed journalist with short brown hair and glasses, couldn't put Gellman's piece down.

A dear friend of Gellman's, Donnelly had been in Washington as senior foreign affairs correspondent for *The Boston Globe* for about a year. Donnelly and Gellman had both been stationed in Jerusalem covering the Middle East from 1994 to '98. Thrown into the foreign milieu, the two journalists bonded immediately. Their wives became close, too, and Donnelly's kids became friendly with Gellman's triplets. Over dinners, at cocktail parties, and out together on stories, the two developed a strong personal affinity and a mutual professional admiration.

Finishing Gellman's piece, Donnelly was of two minds. He was pleased for his friend, who had clearly broken an extraordinary story with exemplary journalistic deft. As a competitor, though, he wouldn't have minded seeing his name on the byline. Turning to his wife, he asked, "Have you seen this article by Bart? I hate him," he added jestingly.

Later that morning, Donnelly sent his old friend an e-mail: "You did it again. You did a great job."

Like Gellman, Donnelly had been following the ascent of global AIDS for some time. He knew that AIDS was one of the biggest stories of the 1980s and '90s. He presumed that there was a wide swath of journalists all over global AIDS, that most of the big stories had been unearthed, and that the barrier to entry would be enormous.

But he had been rearing to cover the pandemic, and after Gellman's story, Donnelly decided to jump in. "To me it was a seminal work," he said of Gellman's piece. "Not only was it a great story, but it showed how asleep journalists were to this story."

With characteristic intensity Donnelly dug his reportorial heels into the issue. "And then I realized that all those presumptions I had were wrong. There weren't that many people covering it well. There were a lot of things going on that no one knew about.

"This is one of the most important foreign policy issues, and not only that, no one is covering it from a political perspective," Donnelly pitched his editors. In short order, John Donnelly became one of the leading journalists covering global AIDS.

Most of the reporters who had broken stories in 1999 and even 2000 would move on. Gellman was one of them. "We promised ourselves we weren't going to do a huge package and [said] that we weren't going to tell our readers that this is the biggest calamity in the world right now and then drop it," Gellman explained. After Gellman spent most of 2000 on global AIDS, his editors passed the issue on to another journalist.

To policy champions like Richard Holbrooke, it was a great fear realized. "The problem is not going to go away," he said on the *NewsHour*, "and I hope the media doesn't go away either because you, you are the key to breaking through on this issue."

The Washington Post stayed with global AIDS through much of 2001, but then "9/11 came along and that was the end of it," Gellman said. "That's the tough thing about being a newspaper and being driven by recent events."

At the *Globe*, John Donnelly stayed with the story. He went to Abuja, Nigeria, in April 2001 to cover a summit on AIDS in the continent. When the conference broke, Donnelly left Abuja, the country's capital, for a plateau area in central Nigeria called Jos. He wanted to see the toll the disease was taking away from the capital and the political noise. The seasoned journalist was shaken by what he encountered. At a local facility and around the town, people were dropping like flies.

Not long before, a generic drug manufacturer in India named Cipla had begun to sell generic ARV treatment at a very low cost, only several hundred dollars per year per person. Donnelly was floored when locals circled him asking him about the drugs. "When would they be available?" they wanted to know.

A local physician, John Idoko, had received a small shipment of drugs for a clinical trial, and was struggling with the ethical dilemma of whom to provide access to. One of those denied access was a woman named Hajara Abubakar. She was clearly dying and about to orphan several children. She had tried to get access to drugs so that she could stay alive for her children. She had $147, $139 short of the amount needed. Donnelly had spent time interviewing and visiting with Hajara and her family. He had hundreds of dollars on him, enough several times over to help her pay for the drugs, enough to help her survive.

It presented a wrenching journalistic dilemma: he wanted to help, but Hajara was a subject. It would make Donnelly part of the story. After a grueling deliberation, Donnelly, with profound pain, told her son that he couldn't help, but that he was going back to America to write a story about his mother, and he would raise the money to help her pay for the drugs.

Donnelly wrote a searing piece in the *Globe* a short time thereafter. At the end he wrote that concerned readers could send donations along. Within days Donnelly received $10,000 in contributions. Immediately, he got in touch with Dr. Idoko.

It was too late. Hajara had gotten on a bus to return home—to die.

The episode drove Donnelly's personal and professional commitment. He covered virtually every major international and U.S. conference and development after that, showcasing the political, diplomatic, and personal dynamics and dimensions of the issue. From 2001 on, even through 9/11 and the war in Iraq, Donnelly stayed with global AIDS, one of the very few U.S. journalists not from a health or science background to stay with the issue for an extended period of time.

Following the flurry of coverage in 1999 and 2000, Donnelly expected journalists to swarm to the issue. Laurie Garrett, Larry Altman, and a handful of other leading science/health journalists remained stalwarts. But the foreign affairs and political people had come and gone. "Even at the Barcelona Conference," in the summer of 2002, Donnelly said, "I didn't meet anyone else who covered foreign affairs—it was all health and science writers."

Receiving an award in 2002 for outstanding coverage of the pandemic, Donnelly spoke extemporaneously: "I'm a very competitive journalist," he told the crowd. "But this is one area in which I wish that I'd have more competition. This is one area in which I'd love to have more competition."

Opportunities Squandered
(1998–2000)

—⚏—

Continental Abdication,
The Ultimate Crutch

L ate in 1999, activist Paul Boneberg received a call from Hillary Rod-
ham Clinton's office. More than any of her predecessors, the first lady
had spent much of her husband's tenure traveling the world speaking out
on women and children's issues. Late in the second administration global
AIDS had come to command her concern.

She was convening a White House meeting and her office extended an
invitation to Boneberg and advocate Terje Anderson. Several Cabinet offi-
cials were to be in attendance, including Donna Shalala from HHS and
Larry Summers from Treasury. Brian Atwood, the administrator from
USAID, was coming; as were Peter Piot, Jim Wolfensohn, director of the
World Bank, and Sandy Thurman, director of the Office of National AIDS
Policy.

Seated off to the side of the table right behind Mrs. Clinton, next to
Anderson, Boneberg was relishing the grandeur of the Roosevelt Room,
and thrilled to witness deliberations at such a senior level.

He sat quietly, intently taking in each facet of the proceedings. AIDS
czar Sandy Thurman opened the meeting with a presentation on the state
of the pandemic and highlighted a recent increase in U.S. funding that
she had championed. Peter Piot spoke next, then Donna Shalala. All three
spoke with conviction about the horror of the pandemic. Then the foreign
policy arm of the government chimed in. In short order, Boneberg's enthusiasm turned into frustration. Both State and USAID shared everyone's
concerns, but they weren't advocating an upgraded U.S. effort. Instead, the
foreign policy people told the first lady and the esteemed participants that

they were doing the best they could, but "these countries don't want us to do more. They don't want it to be a priority issue. They don't want us to do it."

Boneberg and Anderson bristled, listening as the direction of the conversation veered from a discussion of U.S. policy to a lamentation on the negligence of national leaders in the developing world. "This goes on for basically an hour, and I'm realizing this is going to be the message," Boneberg said. "No one's ever going to challenge this," and everyone's going to leave the meeting without having accomplished anything substantive.

Sitting directly behind the first lady, feeling as if he was there merely for window dressing or to appease the advocacy community, Boneberg finally interjected, "Mrs. Clinton, can I say something on behalf of the community?"

"Of course you can," she replied.

Boneberg addressed the esteemed group and noted that there were protests under way on this very issue (by late in 1999, no one at that table needed to be reminded). Boneberg explained that the protests under way were driven by activists' anger about the absence of activity around U.S. global AIDS policy. Boneberg asserted: "The problem is not entirely around [developing world countries]. The problem is also the developed nations of the world. The fact is that the U.S. has not prioritized global AIDS issues."

Boneberg's colleague, Terje Anderson, then chimed in, echoing Boneberg's plea for U.S. commitment.

Boneberg recollected the first lady responding that her husband had recently traveled to Africa, and he did not profile AIDS—in fact, he gave it nary a mention—not so much because he didn't want to, but because he was told that the subject was not welcome.

Others made similar points. As the exchanges continued, Larry Summers, the blunt-spoken secretary of the Treasury, thought that it was about time to explain the facts of life to the activist guests. Boneberg recalled him declaring: "Americans need to realize that they can't care more about another country's issue than the government of that country itself cares."

Whether on the subject of human rights abuses, or in cases of civil conflict or humanitarian disaster, the U.S. government has a long history of advancing an agenda contrary to the ones promulgated by foreign governments. When U.S. domestic political constituencies promote a position, or when U.S. economic or strategic interests are deemed to be at stake, it is a matter of course for the United States to engage differing foreign agendas or responses to a given issue with approaches ranging from diplomatic overtures to direct intervention.

When an issue does not register, and when pressure from domestic constituencies is scant, pressure from leadership from the regions affected naturally emerges as a critical component of the policy calculation. Absent powerful foreign leadership, in such cases, the imperative for U.S. action is softened.

Through the 1980s and the 1990s leadership in the developing world was abysmal. Leaders—with several rare, but notable exceptions—oscillated between denial and the "ostrich" approach. Even in 1999 and 2000 when African leaders began to acknowledge the disease and awaken to its devastation, leadership remained mind-bendingly negligent. Still struggling to cope with denial and stigma, leaders could not bring themselves to raise their voices and solicit much-needed assistance from the United States or the developed world.

By the middle of 2001, the African continent's leadership had joined in a chorus rallying for U.S. relief and assistance. Their awakening would help punctuate the wasteful negligence of their silence and abdication. They had foregone their moral and political responsibilities by not engaging the developed world in the problem. They had also unwittingly provided the United States and those who cared to look away the ultimate crutch for their own inaction.

Africa's were not the only national political leaders to cast their gaze away from the pandemic through the late 1990s. A handful of interested U.S. policy makers watched the leadership of the "next-wave" countries—India, China, and Russia—representing roughly 40 percent of the world's population, mirror their own government's earlier discomfort and unwillingness to engage the disease in its incipience.

For a select few U.S. policy makers, national leaders' abdication represented a grave concern to be redressed. For most, though, it made their own inaction rest that much easier.

In 1997, roughly forty miles outside of Moscow, at a conference room in an old resort village where former members of the Communist apparatchik used to assemble for work and leisure, members of an Al Gore delegation, including Leon Fuerth and Donna Shalala, sat down to discuss matters of health with their Russian counterparts in one of their Binational Commission meetings. There were several items on the U.S. agenda. Donna Shalala was particularly concerned about Russia's burgeoning AIDS epidemic.

The primary mode of transmission in Russia was IV drug use. Rampant in prison, drug activity in the general population increased precipitously when the new post-Communist government released hordes of prisoners in a series of large-scale immunity conferrals. Onlookers like Shalala and her colleagues in the U.S. public health establishment foresaw disaster in an emergent state that was already coping with daunting economic, health, and demographic issues.

Fuerth found it hard to connect with the Russians on the issue. There was enormous turnover in their Ministry of Health. His team would work on one minister, only to see him replaced by the time that they had their next meeting.

As the meeting turned over to Donna Shalala, Fuerth was pleased to note that the better portion of the Russian cabinet was in attendance. Shalala made a detailed and comprehensive presentation. When then Vice Chairman Viktor Chernomyrdin asked her in front of the full delegation: "Can you get it by kissing?" Shalala was aghast.

In one of the commission's last meetings, in 1998, Fuerth was pleased to note that the Russians had become more "open" on the issue; however, he was perturbed at their unwillingness to meet the threat with a tangible policy commitment. Sensing Fuerth's frustration, a mid-level Russian bureaucrat, with whom Fuerth had developed a strong rapport approached him after a break in one of the sessions. The Russian official explained: "One of the reasons we are not being responsive is that we can't figure out what the point of alarming the Russian people is, if we don't have the resources to deal with the problem."

At the time, Fuerth pointed out, the Russians were "up to their ass in alligators." Their currency, the ruble, had just collapsed, they were in a financial free fall, prime ministers were shuffled in and out of office, and the country's health in general was very poor. Indeed, the Russians had grave and pressing matters to contend with, and little in the way of resources with which to combat them.

Overwhelmed, the Russians chose the "ostrich" approach. Fuerth tried to explain to the Russian delegation that, even without resources, acknowledgment and an open public discourse was perhaps the most effective preventative measure anyhow. "This is a mortgage on your whole country," Fuerth and his colleagues would say in the course of these meetings.

By the close of the administration, the Gore team had forced their counterparts to, at the very least, join them in an open dialogue on the issue; no mean feat, but by early 2001 Fuerth, who continued to follow the situation closely, remarked, "I don't think I ever really saw much evidence that they had seriously engaged the issue. . . . There was a lack of knowledge, denial, and a kind of panicking."

Meanwhile, late in the Clinton administration, a group of officials from the Department of Health and Human Services approached Fuerth about the AIDS situation in China. Gore co-chaired a U.S.–China environmental forum, and thus had a direct line of communication with Li Peng, the Chinese premier. Though health was not a part of the agenda, the officials hoped that he would take up the issue.

AIDS had been spreading at a rampant rate in certain Chinese provinces. In many places the virus had gotten into the blood supply. Prostitution and drug use marked other critical vectors where the disease was becoming increasingly prevalent. Yet the disease remained veiled in taboos about deviant behavior, and a rigid government was unwilling to address the problem. China's notoriously closed public health establishment had essentially taken no measures to manage the blood supply, or to promote public education and awareness.

"The Chinese leadership is not dealing with this," the officials told Fuerth. He agreed to have Gore send a letter to Li Peng outlining U.S. estimates of infection in China. The letter asserted that the United States believed China was still at the early stages of its epidemic, and, with "drastic government action," China could still avert a full-blown national catastrophe.

"I don't recall a response on the subject," Fuerth said.

The crisis was harder to ignore in India. On December 12, 1998, at a speech in New Delhi, India's conservative Prime Minister Shri Atal Bihari Vajpayee made his first comprehensive public address on India's AIDS crisis.

The disease had been present in India at least since the early 1980s, transmitted primarily through heterosexual contact. Migrant labor, truckers, crowded slums, and India's pulsing black market in prostitution all catalyzed the spread of the virus in the world's most populous democracy.

Indian officials had shunned acknowledgment and public discussion about the disease for years. Part of the reason was a fierce national and cultural pride that prevented national leaders from believing that the stigmatized disease could explode in their own country. India's deeply conservative mores served to further stifle an open public discourse. Bollywood, India's burgeoning cinema industry, remains comparatively reticent about dealing with sex, even kissing. Further, India's frightfully low per capita GDP made it difficult to muster the resources to treat many of its infected. Turning away seemed an exigent solution.

It came as a grave shock to many Indians to hear their conservative prime minister concede that their nation was already home to 3 to 4 million HIV infections. Some experts put the number at 5 million, even then. "I shudder to contemplate the numbers," the prime minister said in his rather lengthy speech.

"There is no reason why we should not be able to control HIV/AIDS in India," he proclaimed. "It requires all-out efforts by both government and the community: let us make a beginning towards this goal today."

They were clearly the right words, but little followed in the way of action. The country's technical leadership, abetted a great deal by several hundred million dollars' worth of World Bank loans made intermittently in the 1990s, was excellent. And there were patches of strong provincial leadership; places like Maharashtra, Tamil Nudu, and West Bengal all recorded successes in their HIV programs.

However, political leadership, even after the prime minister's fiery rhetoric, remained abysmal. India's AIDS budget remained roughly flat through the 1990s. India's then health minister dismissed U.S. National Intelligence Council estimates, generally viewed as credible, as "completely inaccurate." Even late in 2002, when Bill Gates traveled to India to announce a $100 million grant to help India fight AIDS, the minister snidely commented that Gates was "spreading panic." The prime minister's staff downplayed Gates's visit and the announcement.

According to an account in The Washington Post, the Indian government's planning commission put a ceiling on certain national programs, including AIDS. "That puts India in the seemingly bizarre position of refusing some of the money that donors are eager to give," wrote John Lancaster.

In all three of the leading "next-wave" countries, even as they each face distinct and perilous challenges to their own prosperity and stability, the virus is poised to explode to astronomic dimensions.

Feeding off of the apathy and negligence of their counterparts, the United States sought to pry open slight avenues rather than sprawling thoroughfares. The CDC supplied some degree of technical expertise. There was indirect support in the form of World Bank loans and UNAIDS attention. And the Gore team used their access to promote the issue.

By the late 1990s and into 2000, there were already at least hundreds of thousands of infections in Russia and in China. As many as 5 million infections had accumulated in India. All of these countries were critical strategic priorities for the United States. National leaders' unwillingness to lead on the issue helped tacitly abet U.S. inaction.

———•◆•———

Even as the disease was tightening its foothold in the "next-wave" countries, it had set off an undeniable conflagration in the pandemic's epicenter: sub-Saharan Africa.

By mid-September 1999, as Peter Piot ventured to Lusaka, the capital of Zambia, for the Eleventh International Conference on AIDS in Africa, it was estimated that 11 million people on the subcontinent had died of AIDS. An additional 23 million were living with HIV/AIDS. Between 20 and 26 percent of the adult population in Southern Africa was already carrying the virus. The region was home to more than 80 percent of the world's AIDS deaths and almost 70 percent of infections worldwide.

Piot was desperate for leadership from the continent, and he had high hopes for Lusaka. Then he got some disturbing news. Zambia's president, Frederick Chiluba, whose office was all of five minutes away from the Mulungushi International Conference Center in Lusaka, would not be attending the conference. In his stead, he sent the country's vice president to read the opening remarks.

Insiders like Piot were deeply despondent. The day before the conference, word had leaked that Zambia's powerful housing minister, Bennie Mwiinga, had died. Though the government was oblique, insiders were certain that he had died of AIDS. The minister's death could have served as a poignant backdrop for Chiluba to ring a loud alarm bell about the pandemic's grip in the subcontinent and the need for African leadership. Instead, like the other fifteen national leaders invited, Chiluba opted to stay away, officially explaining that he was detained by "unavoidable circumstances."

The conference proceeded nevertheless. A smattering of national health ministers and other mid-level officials, as well as scientists, doctors, journalists, and a few activists were among the crowd of roughly six thousand in attendance. They milled about at the conference, outraged at the leaders' absence.

In addition to the standard speeches and presentations, the conference featured a heart-wrenching art display with paintings like "Africa Fire," showing the continent engulfed in a raging inferno, with a man in the middle of the African map crying. Some of the pieces tried to convey a sense of hope, but by and large, the display echoed the artists' despair and fatalism. The paintings reduced some Cabinet-level officials to tears.

Incensed at Chiluba's absence, Piot went to pay him a visit at the presidential palace. Hoping to engage him in the issue, Piot instead found himself on the receiving end of a heated lecture from the Zambian president about the effects of malaria. Spouting a familiarly chilling refrain, Chiluba insisted to Piot that AIDS is God's punishment for deviant and irresponsible behavior.

Piot left Lusaka dejected. The conference produced a ministerial statement saying that "AIDS is a disaster and must be fought at every level." In the course of the preceding seven years, though, African leaders had passed no less than ten similar statements or declarations, each emptier than the one before.

By the late 1990s, ten times more Africans were dying of AIDS each year than of war. In 1997, it was reported, sub-Saharan African countries spent only $160 million, roughly $145 million of which was provided via foreign assistance, to deal with the subcontinent's millions of new annual infections. In contrast, the United States spent roughly $8.5 billion per year, and had 44,000 new infections.

Even as the World Bank's HIV/AIDS coordinator, Dr. Debrework Zewdie, cautioned late in 1998: "All of the progress of the last 20–30 years on the development front in Africa is now in jeopardy," World Bank lending for HIV/AIDS in the subcontinent decreased precipitously during the latter years of the decade. The Bank's funding commitments for HIV/

AIDS–related projects in the region fell from $67 million in 1994 to $48 million in 1995, to $2.3 million in 1996, and finally to $1.7 million in 1997. Dr. Zewdie insisted that the funding had not decreased because the World Bank was any less willing to lend. Rather, "The funding has been going down . . . because there are no new projects in the pipeline. . . . To my knowledge, no country that has requested funding for HIV/AIDS has been turned down."

Zimbabwe spent roughly seventy times more financing a foreign war in the Democratic Republic of the Congo than it did on HIV/AIDS prevention. While national spending on HIV/AIDS remained nominal, defense expenditures among fourteen leading Southern African countries rose 37 percent from $6.5 billion in 1998 to $9.8 billion in 2000, even as 20 to 30 percent of national populations had become infected with the lethal disease. Many pondered what exactly would be left for Southern African governments to protect.

In 1999, African leaders would finally begin to acknowledge the disease.

In March 1999, Sam Nujoma, the cattle herder turned military revolutionary who became the first president of the Namibian Republic in 1990, officially launched a national campaign against HIV/AIDS. Even after losing two sons and a daughter-in-law to the disease, the seventy-year-old leader with a wide pearly smile and a long gray beard could only muster $3.5 million for the new five-year effort.

Robert Mugabe, the seventy-five-year-old strongman who came to power on the back end of a military revolution in Zimbabwe, addressed a crowd of roughly twenty thousand countrymen at the national sports stadium in Harare on April 18, 1999. It was the nineteenth anniversary of his country's independence, and the first time Mugabe acknowledged that 1,200 Zimbabweans were dying of the disease every week.

The government had already quietly acknowledged that roughly 20 percent of the country was infected with HIV. Yet it was the first time the despot, and ruler of a notoriously corrupt regime, had made a national address on AIDS. "It is reversing the gains which the country has made since independence," he conceded to the crowd.

In late November 1999, Daniel arap Moi, in his mid-seventies and in his twenty-first year of national leadership, declared the Kenyan AIDS situation a "national disaster." Only a year prior, though the disease had already claimed well over half a million lives, infected an additional 2 million people, filled more than 70 percent of the nation's hospital beds, and taken a weekly average of fourteen students and teachers at the University of Nairobi, the conservative, devout Christian could not bring himself to use the word "condom" in public.

Even as Moi finally set the wheels in motion to mobilize his nation's government, declaring, "In today's world, condoms are a must," the Catholic Church, which wields strong influence in Kenya, rebuked him, suggesting that Moi's position, on which he would subsequently equivocate, would only serve to increase promiscuity.

In late November 2000, on the "Day of Affirmation" for people living with AIDS, Zambian President Frederick Chiluba, who had not bothered to attend the conference hosted by his country only a year before, issued a statement about the AIDS pandemic now overwhelming his government. The "human catastrophe" had undermined the gains made during his nine years in office. With one in every five Zambian adults infected, Chiluba declared, "So overwhelming has been the scale of the scourge that our medical, social, and traditional structures are unable to cope with the human cost exacted by the pandemic."

In Africa's most populous country, also one of the most important to U.S. interests, Nigeria found itself with a new president in May 1999. Olusegun Obasanjo, a former military leader in his mid-sixties, was democratically elected to lead the northwestern African country, vowing to fight corruption and poverty after years of despotic military rule. In short order, Obasanjo began speaking out about AIDS, a disease many Nigerians had written off as a Southern African problem.

By World AIDS Day on December 1, 1999, Obasanjo acknowledged that 2.6 million adult Nigerians were infected, and pledged that the government would introduce a new, comprehensive national HIV/AIDS policy. Even as the country's finance minister proclaimed the situation a "national disaster," though, the oil-rich country had set aside only $300,000, which would be earmarked "for publicity." Four years later, Obasanjo's "national plan" was still being formulated.

Perhaps Southern Africa's most vocal and articulate voice on the pandemic was Festus Mogae, the soft-spoken, Oxford-educated economist who rose to national leadership in Botswana in March 1998 at fifty-nine years of age. Grasping the relationship between the disease and economic development, Mogae was outspoken about AIDS in Botswana early on—fielding strong criticism.

Rich in diamonds, Botswana's relatively high GDP per capita and its prodigious economic growth rates—in the high single digits—in the latter half of the 1990s masked the looming crisis. Securing his political footing through reelection in 1999, Mogae insisted that combatting AIDS must be Botswana's "number one priority."

It would take Mogae until the end of 2000, however, to have amassed sufficient national mobilization and credibility on the issue to solicit U.S. and global assistance. At a conference at the Harvard AIDS Institute, which would honor Mogae for his leadership, he declared that the U.S. government had made "sympathetic noises," but had done little of substance "while African nations reeled on the edge of economic and demographic implosion." By the time of Mogae's remarks, more than one in three adults in Botswana was HIV-positive. Mogae had already spoken globally about the possibility of the "extinction" of his people.

Mogae was at the vanguard of this new wave of acknowledgment among African leadership. By June 2001, during a United Nations General Assembly, sub-Saharan leaders and some others joined Mogae in a unified front, all making a strong case for U.S. and global assistance.

It had taken twenty years, 17 million deaths, and an additional 25 million infections on the African continent for leaders to complete the flight from abdication to advocacy.

Taking aim at an explanation, Nelson Mandela commented in March 1999: "HIV/AIDS is one of those critical issues which demand visible leadership. . . . [How do we] understand why there is this silence? It is because transmission occurs primarily through sex, which is not openly discussed."

Discussion of sexual behavior in public has been deeply taboo on the subcontinent. Cultural mores and the unwillingness of leaders to take them on helped erect walls of silence and denial. When Sheila Mitchell's NGO, Family Health International, contacted national and local leaders about conducting interventions with prostitutes, she would often hear, "We don't have prostitutes here," or rape, or teenage sex, or extramarital affairs.

By the late 1990s, most of the subcontinent's leaders were in their late sixties or early to mid-seventies. Though several of them were corrupt and/or violent, most of these leaders had pretensions of religious piety. Most had been in power for some time, insulated from changes in cultural mores around them. Stephen Morrison said, "These guys are generationally incapable of dealing with an issue like this."

Acknowledging the magnitude of their country's AIDS crises, most leaders felt, would have serious economic and security implications. Doing so would detract from their ability to attract foreign direct investment. It would diminish their international economic standing. It would hurt tourism. Of even greater concern to many of the military-minded leaders, it would be viewed as a sign of instability, signaling military vulnerability to domestic rivals, others on the continent, and the international community.

To compound the problem, the subcontinent, despite signs of economic vitality in the late 1990s, was still deeply impoverished. Leaders found it difficult to muster new resources for an emergent threat. Most of these countries were deeply indebted. Zambia, for example, paid $170 million in interest payments in 2000, yet it allocated only $76 million to its entire national health budget. The absence of resources to confront the threat provided all the more impetus to turn away from it.

And, for a good portion of the decade, leaders could. The virus's several-year incubation period meant that even as infections skyrocketed, the number of deaths, though enormous, lagged behind the more prolific infection rate. Because no one ever officially dies of AIDS—they succumb to infections or sickness due to the weakening of the immune system—reporting on causes of death is notoriously deficient, making it easy for leaders to turn away.

Assailed by a multitude of other pressing health threats such as malaria, tuberculosis, and even dehydration, which produced more deaths than AIDS on the subcontinent until the late 1990s and were deemed more cost-effective to prevent and/or treat, leaders found further cause to turn away from an emergent, stigmatized disease.

In addition, each leader's response to his nation's AIDS crisis was driven by particular, contextual factors. In Kenya, for example, organized religion's strong political hold made it especially difficult for Moi to address the pandemic until no one in the country could continue to ignore the staggering death toll and the orphans lining Kenyan streets. Deep-rooted corruption framed the Mugabe regime's negligence. The Zimbabwean president increased administration salaries several-fold the same week he passed an "AIDS tax," ostensibly to raise money to fight AIDS, though few Zimbabweans had any illusions about where the money would in fact go.

For the United States and the rest of the developed world, the country that stands out as the continental beacon and bellwether is South Africa. The continent's most advanced nation industrially and politically, it is the

United States's most important ally in Africa. The country's long fight and successful transition from apartheid ignited the American imagination, and further strengthened U.S.–South African links.

By the end of 2000, South Africa was also home to the largest number of HIV infections in the world, roughly 5 million. No case of abdication emerges more enigmatic, troubling, and consequential—or more important in framing U.S. inaction—than that of South Africa.

———◆———

If there is a single thread coursing through the story of South Africa's AIDS crisis, it is the legacy of apartheid, the country's decades-long system of racial separation.

Through the 1970s and 1980s, apartheid forced thousands of freedom fighters into exile in neighboring northern countries. Away from their families, it was in places like Zambia and elsewhere that hundreds of South Africans were introduced to the virus. "By 1989," remembered an ANC minister of health in Lusaka, "we could see AIDS all around us in the countries where we were in exile and we were already seeing some HIV-positive comrades."

Apartheid also helped institute a system of migrant labor in which masses of black workers would leave their townships for months at a time, seeking employment far from their homes and families. Many gravitated to the mining towns—built around South Africa's rich resource base of diamonds and other minerals—for 10 to 11 months out of the year, where prostitution flourished.

By the early 1990s, as exiles returned home and the virus had been introduced to populations of migrant workers and the prostitutes who serviced them, the instability and movement created a perfect petri dish for the virus's proliferation. The mining communities, in particular, proved to be cauldrons for HIV transmission. Upon their return home, workers often spread the disease to their wives or girlfriends, who, destitute and alone much of the time, sometimes turned to prostitution to make ends meet, further propagating the disease.

Though they were enmeshed in a political revolution, the country's emergent leadership had not failed to notice the spread of the disease. At a conference in 1992, Nelson Mandela gave the keynote address about AIDS in South Africa. An activist who attended remembered, "There was very little to add. He knew all the issues, everything that had to be done."

Even as he emerged one of the most credible and beloved political leaders on earth, from that early moment on, Nelson Mandela remained practically silent on AIDS until he addressed it at the World Economic
Forum—notably in Davos, Switzerland, not his home country—in 1997.

In 1993 when an advisory panel recommended that the government allocate $64 million to combat AIDS, Mandela reportedly proposed only
$15 million. Hein Marais, a South African journalist, wrote, "Indeed,
minute by minute, during his presidency, Mandela probably spent more
time with the Spice Girls and Michael Jackson than he did raising the
AIDS issue with the South African public."

Part of the reason was that, like his colleagues to the north, Mandela
was a septuagenarian, and deeply uncomfortable talking about sex. He
was also presiding over a tremendously important and fragile political and
social transformation. The task was replete with onerous and daunting
challenges.

In addition, the legacy of apartheid loomed large. The country's public
health establishment remained mostly controlled by whites. There was
a deep racial sensitivity, particularly about the stereotype of the super-
sexualized black African, and a sense that the South African public would
not be receptive to a public campaign. Sensitivities about the white power
structure's credibility were not without some basis. The apartheid government, wrote Samantha Power, had in fact "sponsored a clandestine germ-
warfare program that was accused of targeting ANC officials."

Few leaders had a more daunting agenda in the 1990s than Nelson
Mandela. Still, the fact remains that the AIDS epidemic burgeoned on his
watch. He knew about it, and knew of measures that he could take to stop
it. "I get so angry," Mandela's physician and personal friend told journalist
Mark Schoofs. "I give him hell. . . . The response by the previous apartheid
government was a national disgrace. The response by my government . . .
has also been disgraceful."

In June 1999, when Mandela passed the torch of national leadership to
his deputy, South African denial would come to be identified with a new
face. It belonged to Thabo Mbeki.

The son of a prominent dissident family, Mbeki was groomed for leadership from an early age. He was selected to lead a prominent student political organization at the age of fourteen. Because of his dissidence, Mbeki
was forced to spend much of his adult life in exile, in England, where he re-

ceived a master's in economics from Sussex University; and in Moscow, Botswana, and Zambia.

Handpicked as Mandela's deputy in 1994, Mbeki proudly declared to parliament in 1996 upon the ratification of South Africa's constitution, "I am African." Western-trained and very well read, Mbeki was cerebral, and did little to downplay his image as an urbane intellectual. He was also fiercely anticolonial, espousing an "African Renaissance" as the bedrock of his governing philosophy. The mantra was: African solutions for the African people.

Because of its wealth and its prominence, South Africa was the natural candidate to lead the continent against the impending conflagration. Mbeki seemed the right leader to assume the challenge. He was an independent thinker, and had an abiding passion for African economic development. He was certainly aware of his country's AIDS problem. As co-chair of the Gore-Mbeki Commission, his American interlocutors had continually pointed him to the crisis.

Indeed, through 1998 and part of 1999, Mbeki appeared to be emerging as the strongest continental leader on the issue. From 1994 to 1999, the Health Ministry had in fact increased condom distribution from six million to ninety-eight million. Mbeki had publicly castigated western pharmaceutical companies for keeping drug prices too high for African consumption. Similarly, he had lambasted the USTR, and had lobbied Gore to drop U.S. opposition to the South African Medicine Act, which aimed to make these drugs more affordable and accessible.

After working on Mbeki for five years on AIDS, in 1999, right before a joint press conference, Gore received a beaded AIDS ribbon from his South African counterpart. He put it on, and the two went into the press conference together wearing their matching AIDS ribbons. Gore was pleased, and took it as a symbol that Mbeki was on the threshold of emerging as a global leader on his continent's most pressing crisis. The prognosis was positive.

A few years earlier, in 1997, Mbeki had received reports that there was a new African drug called Virodene, and that it had demonstrated some efficacy in curing AIDS patients. In no time, the deputy president got behind the new miracle drug.

It soon became apparent that the drug included "an industrial solvent that caused severe liver damage." The South African press took Mbeki to task for his public demonstration of support for the lethal drug. But it was what Mbeki craved: an African drug for an African problem. He exhibited no apparent remorse. Instead, the initial criticism, and the subsequent waves to follow, seemed only to stiffen his resolve to formulate an independent viewpoint on the disease.

When a high-ranking official at the national Health Ministry gave Mbeki a book entitled *Debating AZT*, which suggested that the western drug was toxic, Mbeki launched a private investigation into the matter. He spent hours, sometimes late into the night, on the Internet investigating the disease on his own. In the course of his research, he stumbled onto a series of individuals known as AIDS "dissidents," who argued among other things that AIDS was caused by "lifestyle" factors such as poverty or malnutrition, not the HIV virus, which they contended was a harmless "passenger virus."

By October 1999, Mbeki publicly expressed doubts about the efficacy of the drugs. Much of the scientific literature claimed that AZT was "a danger to health," he said. He argued further that it was therefore incumbent upon the South African scientific establishment to investigate.

Over the course of Mbeki's investigations—most of which he conducted either independently or via e-mail correspondence with "dissident" scientists who were derided by almost all of the mainstream international medical and scientific community—he had come to espouse a decidedly "iconoclastic" view of his country's greatest calamity.

"The reality is that the predominant feature of illnesses that cause disease and death among black people in our country is poverty," Mbeki pronounced publicly in the spring of 2000. He would be careful to avoid official statements asserting that HIV was not the direct scientific cause of AIDS. Rather, as he would say in Durban when his country hosted the International AIDS Conference in the summer of 2000, "It occurred to me that we could not blame everything on a single virus."

Mbeki's fierce national and racial pride, his almost messianic drive for African economic sustainability, and his notion that a purely western-centered solution would merely pin his country in a position of dependency on foreign pharmaceutical companies had all coalesced to shape his new viewpoint on the disease: the country's underlying poverty created the conditions that led to the disease's fomentation. Long-term development was the key. Poverty was what needed addressing. In Mbeki's new schematic, HIV was, as Ambassador Princeton Lyman put it, "a diversion."

There was, of course, a profound kernel of truth in identifying the relationship between the disease and the economic conditions on which it feeds. And there was vision in the notion that economic development was the key to Africa's long-term ability to cope with its myriad crises and hardships.

Having embarked on his own independent forage for answers, however, when critics emerged to point out the empirically validated scientific truth that HIV causes AIDS, and the importance of that truth's recognition as the requisite building block of any effective national program to battle the disease, Mbeki only dug his heels in further.

In May 2000, he convened a conference to which he invited the "fringe" dissident scientists as well as more credible figures, reportedly giving each of them roughly equal time. Mainstream leading scientists were aghast. Nevertheless, their testimony at the conference did little to move Mbeki from his unorthodox position.

It was as though, in looking for a cover for his larger concern about development, Mbeki—too proud and too "intellectually arrogant"—had appropriated wildly errant and discredited arguments about the fundamental toxicity of the antiretroviral drugs and the science behind AIDS.

As a result, the public discourse about the disease was dominated by speculation on these matters and the attendant controversy. As Mbeki and his obstinate minister of health "investigated" what the rest of the world had long since accepted as validated fact, much less was devoted in the way of resources to prevention. Although it would have been a powerful symbolic gesture, Mbeki refused to take an AIDS test himself, suggesting in a television interview that the idea was a half-baked "publicity stunt."

Even after the United States dropped its opposition to the South African Medicines Act, and some pharmaceutical companies had agreed to drop their drug prices by 90 percent or more, in 2000, the South African government still refused to help provide its people with the lifesaving drugs, as neighboring Botswana had begun to do. Particularly egregious, his government refused to help make nevirapine, a drug with a very strong rate of success in reducing mother-to-child transmission, available to pregnant mothers. The South African Supreme Court had to overrule the administration, still pursuing its independent "investigation" into the drug's toxicity.

• • •

Ambassador for Global HIV/AIDS Jack Chow felt that African leader abdication played an enormous role in governing U.S. policy. "Obviously,
having more leaders who are out in front and are seized with the issue saying 'I want America to be a partner with us' is one of the fundamental
steps."

For Stephen Morrison, a State Department official during much of this
period, the role of African leaders can't be underplayed: "The fact that nobody was pounding the table was a huge disincentive. If you've got a crisis
happening and the people who are leading the country who are experienc-
ing this are unwilling to get on board or push this, it's an immediate out."
Morrison suggested: "If more leaders had come forward and said, 'Look
we're facing a national emergency we need your help and this is an unprecedented moral challenge,'" there's no doubt, "it would have stirred a
[U.S.] response earlier."

By the late 1990s, it was clear that something of an unprecedented magnitude was afoot. Twenty to thirty percent of the adult populations of most
nations in Southern Africa were infected with a lethal, insidious disease
that would lead to their demise in a few short years. As many as 10 million
children had been orphaned by the disease.

According to former Assistant Secretary of State for African Affairs
Susan Rice, for U.S. policy makers, African abdication in and of itself was
hardly an immutable roadblock. "There may have been a lot of things that
they may not have wanted to talk about and deal with, but we would be
worried about," and U.S. officials would press them on those issues. With
hard diplomatic pressure, U.S. policy makers could have moved their
African counterparts to engage the issue much earlier. With meaningful financial aid, technical assistance, debt relief, high-priority diplomatic attention, or any number of forms the U.S. carrot might have taken, the
situation would no doubt have appeared decidedly less hopeless for African
leaders. Such steps would have been likely to spur them to address their
epidemics with greater openness, force, and ingenuity.

By the middle of 2001, African leaders would finally call upon the
United States to enter the fray and to help combat the pandemic. The
United States would respond with a recalibration of its effort. The initiatives, from both sides of the Atlantic, demonstrated that leadership need
not have come so late.

—⁓—

ELEVEN

A Failure to Recalibrate,
Turf and Neglect

I t was a historic trip. For the first time in twenty years a sitting U.S. president was to travel to sub-Saharan Africa. The twelve-day tour through six favored African countries in late March 1998 offered the Clinton administration a rare opportunity to profile the continent and its challenges.

In the planning sessions in the months preceding the trip, all hands came on deck. Foreign policy officials, treasury, the president's political people, and others spent countless hours devising the president's itinerary. One of the key voices in the planning sessions belonged to Susan Rice. Only months earlier, in October 1997, at thirty-two years of age, Rice had been sworn in as the youngest regional assistant secretary of state in U.S. history. As assistant secretary for African Affairs, Rice was the administration's senior ranking official to focus exclusively on the continent.

Rice's ascent to the upper echelons of the foreign policy establishment was part of a lifelong pattern of achievement and precocity. Born into a prominent African-American Washingtonian family, in which political debate was a matter of course at the family dining table, Rice attended the prestigious National Cathedral School. At Cathedral, Rice was a three-sport letterwoman, president of the student council, and the school valedictorian. She also became well acquainted with the children of a woman who was close to her mother. The lady's name was Madeleine Albright.

By the time Rice had been recruited by Tony Lake and Sandy Berger to assume a directorship at the National Security Council, she brandished a host of formidable distinctions. A Phi Beta Kappa graduate of Stanford,

Rice had won the Rhodes and earned her doctorate in international relations at Oxford.

With director responsibilities at the NSC, Rice was the archetypal new
generation Clinton White House official. She was young, fresh, confident
and—in the image of her NSC mentor, Dick Clarke, the head of counter-
terrorism—disarmingly direct.

After a reshuffling at the NSC in 1995, Rice was appointed to direct
African Affairs at the council. Somalia and Rwanda had already delivered
the administration a frightfully checkered record on Africa. The administration's mild-mannered, longtime Africanist George Moose had had a
punishing tenure as assistant secretary for Africa. Already wounded, Moose
struggled for influence with the self-assured and strong-willed Rice. With
only a few years of experience, she had already effectively become the administration's leading African specialist.

At the NSC, the reports began to trickle in to Rice throughout 1995.
The U.S. Foreign Service was employing in the vicinity of five thousand
African nationals all over the continent. Particularly proactive, Rice kept
in close contact with the U.S. embassies throughout Africa. In increasing
numbers, she was hearing anecdotal reports about secretaries or drivers
simply not showing up to work one day, never to be heard from again.
Through 1995 and the ensuing few years, as the disease spread and latent
infections turned in to full-blown AIDS, embassy employees were dying in
large numbers. The disease, Rice remembered, "was beginning to hit home
in a personal way at our missions."

She began hearing about it from respected ambassadors, leading Afri-
canists, like her Deputy, Johnny Carson, a senior official who had been
U.S. ambassador to Uganda and Zimbabwe, and she started seeing it for
herself during her frequent travels to the continent.

When the assistant secretary position opened at State, in 1997, Rice's
position at the NSC had already automatically put her on the short list for
the spot. The arbiter of the decision, as it turned out, was the new secretary
of state, Madeleine Albright.

Rice's swearing-in on October 14, 1997, was a family affair, with her
husband, Ian, a college sweetheart, at her side, and her mother close by. A
gleeful Albright turned to Rice's mother at one point and said, "I feel like
I'm swearing in family." The unusually ebullient tone of the ceremony
helped stoke false rumors that Albright was Rice's godmother.

Several key diplomats and African specialists looking on had serious reservations about the appointment. They worried about Rice's youth and inexperience. Would she overcompensate by being overly aggressive or obstinate? Or would she prove too timid to see through a big fight? Would her ambitions compromise the integrity of her policy decisions? How would the dynamics of her relationship to Albright play out in the policy-making milieu? The questions were floating in whispers behind closed doors and in bull sessions over scotch. Similar doubts had marked the trail of her ascent.

More concerned with the tasks at hand, Rice wasted little time in outlining her own distinct framework for U.S. policy for the continent. There were two main foci. The first was enfranchising Africa in economic globalization. Africa was a source of oil and key minerals. There were pockets of economic vitality, and Rice promoted the continent as an underappreciated export market, and a potential opportunity for foreign investment, untapped and brimming with potential. Enhanced economic exchange would benefit both the United States and Africa. Her second major priority was sharpening U.S.–African cooperation on transnational security threats, like terrorism, transnational crime, and arms sales. Such security threats would define the post–Cold War world, and Rice knew that no continent could be left unattended.

Rice was one of a swath of senior administration officials to formulate the themes and the messages of the president's historic 1998 trip. Her agenda had a powerful impact in shaping the direction of the deliberations. Rice and her colleagues wanted to raze the misconceptions of Africa as a breeding ground of poverty, famine, conflict, and disease and to cast a spotlight on the continent's economic and political progress. "We were trying very hard to change the way the American foreign policy community, the Congress, and the press viewed Africa."

As the policy makers brainstormed about the trip, one or two brought up the continent's AIDS problem. "How should we feature the issue on the trip?" a few wanted to know. They discussed it on a few occasions. No one pushed hard. There was little support to profile the issue. As Stephen Morrison remembered, "The president's tour," it had already been decided, was to be "a good news trip."

New York Times journalist James Bennett pointed out that the president's policy people had clearly "underestimated Clinton's signature willingness to empathize with suffering." Though he fell short of making a formal apology, Clinton expressed deep remorse about the U.S. role in propagating the slave trade centuries ago. He expressed contrition about past U.S. support of African despots.

A few days into the trip Clinton and his coterie—roughly eight hundred strong, of administration officials, businesspeople, congressmen, political supporters, handlers, and Secret Service officers—landed at the airport in Kigali, Rwanda. Under a light drizzle, Clinton sat among a crowd of diplomats, Rwandans who had been mutilated in the 1994 genocide, and victims' family members. He listened to stories of machete-wielding executioners, of a survivor sliding along a floor of victims' blood to escape his captors.

During the genocide the Clinton administration was irresponsive. Journalist Samantha Power wrote that the president "did not convene a single meeting of his senior foreign policy advisors to discuss U.S. options for Rwanda." And later, the administration demanded the withdrawal of UN peacekeepers from the country.

With a choked voice, Clinton rose to address the assemblage, even as the engine of *Air Force One* continued rotating a few hundred yards away. "We in the United States and the world community did not do as much as we could have and should have done to try and limit what occurred in Rwanda in 1994. We must have global vigilance and never again must we be shy in the face of the evidence."

One of the genocide's survivors, Gloriosa Uwimpuhwe, seemed pleased with the president's empathetic display. She told reporter James Bennett that he "behaved as a real, real human being who felt what people were saying." Clinton inspired faith. "He said that he not only is sorry, but he's looking forward to taking positive options for the future," she said.

After the three-and-a-half-hour stay in Kigali, Clinton reboarded his plane for the remaining eight days of his trip. There would be ample time for taking in traditional song and dance. The Clintons enjoyed a two-day game safari in Botswana.

Most of the countries Clinton visited were already nearing—and in two of the six had already surpassed—adult HIV-infection rates of 20 percent. One in five adults, or significantly more, would be infected with a lethal virus.

Throughout the entire twelve-day tour, there was not one formal AIDS event. Barely a mention was made of the disease in a formal or public setting.

From her perch at UNAIDS, Sally Grooms Cowal was irate: "It's like one of those old movies when everyone goes on very nicely with their dinner party and there's this dead body under the table." Clinton was "going through the motions of these very lovely relationships at each of these stops, and there was this absolutely dead body under the table and nobody saw it."

The disease had clearly registered with Susan Rice. But, back then: "We saw it as the silent elephant in the living room, but not as the nuclear bomb that it seems today." In 1998, bombs were indeed exploding on the continent. In August, only months after the conclusion of the president's "good news" trip, a ringing telephone woke Rice at 4:15 A.M. in her Washington home. It was Johnny Carson, then ambassador to Kenya. He was calling with the devastating news that the U.S. embassies in Kenya and Tanzania had been attacked. Two hundred people were dead, including twelve Americans.

For the U.S. State Department, it was the capstone to a violent and tumultuous year. Conflict had broken out in the Congo, the beginning of violent multinational fighting that would take an estimated 3 million lives in the five years to follow. To the northeast, war had also erupted between Eritrea and Ethiopia.

At her swearing-in ceremony in October 1997, Rice had buoyantly declared, "There is now more reason for optimism about Africa's future than at any time in recent memory." It was a snapshot in time. Rice had positive news to report on economic growth and signs of democratization. The continent was in a period of relative stability. Rice was trying to seize the good news to woo investors and U.S. leaders to the continent. Still, it was a sharp miscalculation.

Under a microscope at State, the embassy attacks and the eruption of conflict threw the young assistant secretary directly in the line of fire. Crisis management became the order of the day. There were dire problems that demanded imminent attention.

"If you're living in the Congo, is AIDS a bigger problem than the conflict?" Rice asked. In the case of conflict, you have loud bullets coming at you, both as an African civilian and as a diplomat. AIDS was quieter; the problem wasn't going anywhere. The natural proclivity was to deal with the bullets first.

Even as immediate crises dominated her attention and agenda throughout 1998 and early 1999, a series of factors emerged during the same period that piqued Rice's interest in HIV/AIDS. The reports continued to come

in from embassies, and Rice's travels added visceral resonance to her intellectual comprehension. But once UNAIDS published its estimates and
media coverage picked up during 1999, the pandemic moved to the forefront of Rice's consciousness. "When the numbers became well documented and published widely," Rice said, "you could add up all the people
who died in conflicts in the last ten years and it would be millions, [yet]
they're still not going to add up to the same number of people who have
died of HIV/AIDS."

Rice also began to realize that the pandemic jeopardized the fulfillment
of her two main priorities—increasing economic ties with a vibrant and
prosperous Africa, and cooperation with the continent on transnational security issues. The disease was already poised to pummel Africa's economies
and undermine its stability.

Late in 1999, Susan Rice stood facing a packed conference room on the
seventh floor of the State Department Building. Using a PowerPoint presentation on a large screen, Rice spent the better part of an hour outlining
her budget request for the Africa bureau to roughly forty senior administration officials, including her boss, U.S. Secretary of State Madeleine Albright.

In the course of her presentation, Rice was about to unleash one of the
most ambitious ideas of her life. Jesse Helms and the Republican Congress
had left a searing mark on U.S. developmental assistance to Africa. Decreasing steadily over the preceding several years, the tally had fallen to
around $600 million by 1996, a 22 percent decline from 1995. With Al-
bright's support, Rice was able to inch up the figure in modest increments
thereafter. Congress's purse strings remained tight, though, and Rice wasn't
even able to obtain all the funding she had requested to help secure her
embassies, even after the bombings.

As she went through the usual items, Rice got to U.S. funding for AIDS
in Africa. The United States had just increased—moving the needle for
the first time in seven years—its aggregate funding for global AIDS from
$120 million to roughly $250 million for 2000. Rice was not content with
incremental progress though. She aimed to recalibrate the entire complexion of the U.S. effort in one swift stroke. Her budget request asked for
$1.5 billion in fiscal year 2000 for assistance and relief for AIDS in Africa.

The request "dwarfed everything else" in the budget. Most of her listeners were skeptical. Some were ecstatic. Almost all were taken aback by the size of Rice's request. She noticed Albright motion to her budget people to take note of the request, as if, Rice felt, she meant for it to be taken seriously.

In a sense, Rice was still the idealist who had organized a protest in her college days at Stanford, creating a fund in which the university's wealthy donors could withhold their contributions until either Stanford divested from companies doing business with South Africa or the country abolished apartheid. A scholar, she also had a keen sense of a larger historical context. She could place the pandemic as one of the most punishing catastrophes in world history. The lesson of Rwanda played heavily on the young stateswoman's mind: speak up and be counted for.

But she was also a pragmatist. Whether dealing with African despots or her own colleagues in Washington, Rice was a player in a tough world governed by crosscutting agendas, power grabs, and self-interest. Rice desperately wanted the funding. But with Jesse Helms presiding over the Senate Foreign Relations Committee and the issue's lack of profile, she estimated her chances at "not a snowball's hope in hell."

She submitted the proposal to Albright's office, where, together with all the other requests from the panoply of bureaus at the State Department, it would be parsed and shuttled to the secretary along with recommendations for the department's overall budget request.

Madeleine Albright had addressed global AIDS in a high-profile public forum as early as December 1, 1996, on World AIDS Day. Thereafter, she commissioned a State Department report on the pandemic. She incorporated a series of AIDS events into her travels to Africa. At one event in Botswana, both Albright and Rice embraced an HIV-positive woman. In the late 1990s, the gesture had significant symbolic import. Listening to Albright speak to a crowd in Botswana, as she departed from prepared remarks to tell her audience that as a mother and a grandmother she felt deeply for their suffering, no one could doubt her sympathy. She would speak with Rice about the pandemic intermittently throughout the waning years of the second Clinton administration.

But Albright had a full agenda. She had to deal with a host of important bilateral issues with China and Russia. Iraq and North Korea were grave security concerns and there was a great push to broker a peace settlement in the Middle East. There was European diplomacy, NATO, and international treaties and protocols to manage. The threat of terrorism was on the rise. Relations with the UN were poor.

Measured against the plethora of imminent challenges and other priorities, global AIDS never seemed to incite Albright's energies. "She didn't make it a very high priority," said Princeton Lyman, who served for part of her tenure as an assistant secretary of state. At Policy Planning, Stephen Morrison had no cause to doubt her sympathy, but "she didn't play on the issue."

Rice's funding request was dead on arrival. Albright had not made the issue a priority with her budget people. Her budget was tight, other crises were deemed more imminent, and this issue seemed like a political nonstarter. Rice's request never made it past Albright's office. To the best of Rice's knowledge, President Clinton was never made aware of it.

"The administration would have been laughed out of Dodge," Rice insisted, if Albright or anyone else in the administration had taken the proposal to Helms and the Congress. "He was hostile to everything," Rice believed. "It's not that the secretary or anybody else for that matter was arguing the importance of it. Everybody agreed it was important." But nobody was willing to fight for it.

--------◆◆--------

By 1999, Secretary of HHS Donna Shalala was becoming increasingly frustrated. The global death toll was mounting, infections were exploding, and U.S. funding for global AIDS had remained flat for seven years.

When she tried to prod her colleagues at State and USAID to ratchet up funding and leadership, she kept hearing one name: Jesse Helms. As long as Helms was running the Senate Foreign Relations Committee, they told her, funding wouldn't move. They didn't seem prepared to try.

A series of factors was emerging, though, that were emboldening Shalala on the issue. On the domestic side, U.S. infection and death rates had decreased steadily over the last several years. Domestic success amplified the failure of the international community to deal with the pandemic globally. The circulation of credible estimates highlighted the horrifying magnitude of the crisis. Inaction would no longer do. If Jesse Helms was the problem, as she kept on hearing, then Shalala had a solution.

Helms and the Congress had pummeled USAID throughout the mid- and late 1990s. The CDC, on the other hand, had been remarkably successful in attracting funds from Congress, often obtaining even more than the president proposed. The center's standing on the Hill was excellent. It was the inverse dynamic at work with USAID.

In 1986, the first U.S. funding for global AIDS was allocated to USAID, in part because everyone else was content to pass the buck. The issue continued to fly low on departments' and agencies' radar screens for the ensuing thirteen years. As the issue finally registered, in 1999, the dynamic would be thrown on its back. A leading department wanted in. There would now be, in fact, a bureaucratic turf war over the mandate to lead the U.S. response.

Shalala wanted HHS and CDC to assume primary responsibility for the U.S. effort. Like Rice, she had in mind not merely an incremental increase in funding, but a recalibration. Her domain housed the technical expertise and she felt she could attract the resources that USAID could not. It seemed a foolproof mechanism, a sensible structural adjustment in which bureaucracy would serve the solution, and not the other way around.

There was a hitch though. USAID administrator Brian Atwood had been housing the U.S. effort at his agency. Under perpetual assault from Congress, Atwood had grown conditioned to protecting what resources he could muster and fending off parries from all quarters.

As Shalala got increasingly serious about it in 1999, she perceived a stiff wall of resistance. "It's Atwood in particular," she said. "He just didn't want to weaken USAID or its role. . . . Atwood was extraordinary at protecting his turf. He was adamant." Atwood was close to Gore, and, "The White House supported him on this."

Atwood felt that HHS was a domestic department. USAID had the international mandate. USAID had very large missions on the ground and delivery mechanisms in place. "I think we were the right place to house the effort," Atwood said.

Shalala couldn't have disagreed more. HHS had technical expertise. With hundreds of millions or even billions more of funding, they could have built up their capacity. They could have outsourced through NGOs or financed local efforts where infrastructure and mechanisms were already in place. Most important, they could have attracted the funds. USAID's in-country capacity meant nothing if funding was going to remain at nominal levels.

"I would have given anything for more money on the international side," Shalala said. But she sensed that Atwood was not about to budge.

"The resistance was bureaucratic. USAID literally did not want to give up its portfolio."

For his part, Atwood recalled some discussion on the subject, but downplayed its import: "I don't recall any major effort on her part to make this—I don't think this ever became an issue. As a Cabinet secretary, if she ever wanted to take this up with the president she probably would have prevailed."

At a Cabinet meeting late in 1999, Shalala did just that. She turned to Madeleine Albright and told her that the health part of international aid should be put in the CDC budget, "because we can get it in the CDC budget," she argued. "And finally I said to the president, " 'This ought to go in the CDC budget. We can get it in the HHS budget. You've got no political clout on the State Department budget.' " According to Shalala "the president finally took notice."

But Clinton did not follow up with USAID. Shalala, perceiving the president's tepid posture and Atwood's intransigence, compounded by her sense that Gore would have sided with Atwood if it came to a full-blown showdown, relented on pressing the matter.

The tables had turned markedly from the dynamics that shaped the structural approach to the U.S. response. Some thirteen years later, instead of passing the buck, centers of the U.S. government—keenly aware of the magnitude of the pandemic—were now trying to stake their claim.

Still, no one could muster the political will or ingenuity to mend the gaping structural deficit. Elsewhere in the bureaucratic leviathan of the U.S. government, others would take their turns.

—∽∞∽—

TWELVE

A Foiled Plan,
"Too Little, Too Late"

On a simmering African day in the late fall of 1997, the van carrying Sandy Thurman and her small entourage pulled up to a dilapidated structure with rusting tin walls. Converted from an old abandoned army barracks, the orphanage sat nestled against a barren hill in the South African countryside. It was the last stop on Thurman's first trip to Africa. Appointed President Clinton's third and final AIDS czar six months earlier, Thurman, a forty-four-year-old divorcée (married, her ex-husband had claimed, to her work), was a striking blonde with a heavy Georgia accent. A seasoned domestic AIDS advocate, she had already seen, she estimated, several lifetimes' worth of suffering. But nothing could have prepared her for what she saw on that first trip to Africa. The sheer magnitude of death, the utter despair, shook Thurman to her core.

Stepping out into the arid terrain, she kicked up small plumes of dust as she made her way to the entrance. As she approached, she could hear wails growing louder. She steadied herself, took a deep breath, and entered. The old barracks was filled with thirty iron cribs, with two or three infants in each. The orphans were part of one of the world's fastest-growing populations: the 13 million children across the world who had lost a mother or both parents to AIDS. Most were infected themselves. Shaken, Thurman made her way around the orphanage. Her eyes gravitated toward one baby boy in particular. His tiny dark hands clasped the bars of his crib, as he precariously held himself upright.

The nurses told Thurman that out of love for her baby son, the infant's mother had defied the doctors' expectations, holding on for days, then weeks longer than anyone could have imagined. They had never met anyone so determined to stay alive. Unable to afford the drug treatment that might have extended her life through her son's childhood, she had died, emaciated to flesh and bones, shortly before Thurman's visit.

Thurman had spent a good portion of her life around destitute and sick children, and was particularly adept at making them smile. Despite her best effort, though, she couldn't get this baby to smile. He couldn't have been more than twelve months old, but it seemed to Thurman that his face wore a hundred years of suffering.

"This just should not be happening," she said to herself, "this is fundamentally wrong." It's an episode that remained seared in her conscience.

She arrived back in Washington late in 1997 "loaded for bear." The first thing she did was check into the details of the existing U.S. effort. In short order, Thurman discovered that global AIDS had remained flat-funded at $120 million for seven years in the face of a stratospheric increase in the global epidemic. Her reaction: "I hit the roof!"

In the months and years to follow Thurman would embark on a single-minded crusade to galvanize the U.S. response. No one would leave a larger imprint on U.S. global AIDS policy during Clinton's second term.

Thurman's newfound zeal was more than a little ironic. Only six months earlier, she had stiff-armed the White House in an attempt to avoid taking the job. At the time, she was still settling in to her new position as director of cultural and professional exchange programs at the U.S. Information Agency, or USIA. She had been there for all of three weeks when, in April 1997, the phone rang.

Thurman had received her plum post at USIA by way of a political appointment at the behest of President Bill Clinton. She had been a long-time political ally (and asset) and personal friend to the president. In 1992, her ex-boyfriend, James Carville, had summoned her to direct Clinton's primary campaign in Georgia. Following a defeat in New Hampshire, Thurman helped deliver an invaluable early win in the key southern state. She proved an asset again in Clinton's second presidential campaign in 1996.

A reward for her support, Thurman's plush corner office at USIA had huge windows that afforded her an expansive Washington view. She was delighting in her new post, though still fighting a miserable cold, when she picked up the phone.

It was Marsha Scott, from White House personnel, also a longtime friend of Thurman's. "Sandy, we are having trouble reaching consensus on the AIDS czar post, and we want you to consider it."

Thurman had been reared in a tradition of service and politics. Her mother, Marge Thurman, was a tall (six foot) and imposing woman, a pioneer who eventually became the first woman to head the Democratic National Party in Georgia. An only child, Sandy acquired a Southern lady's charms and wiles. Marge also raised her daughter to be tough, to survive and thrive in a world of "good old boy" politicians.

Mother and daughter worked side by side to lobby for the Equal Rights Amendment in the early 1970s. At the time the war in Vietnam was still raging, and a reporter from *The Washington Post* asked Marge, "Are you aware that if the ERA passes your daughter will be eligible for the draft?" Marge assured the reporter that she was, "and if that happens," she added, "all I can say is God help the enemy."

Coming of age, Thurman immersed herself in service. She found a cause of her own in the mid-1980s when the AIDS epidemic hit an ill-prepared Atlanta with impunity. She became executive director of AIDS Atlanta, an organization focused primarily on care. The patients piled in. Most had no homes, families, or money. In those days, a colleague said, "All we could do was make the sign of the cross, step over the dead body and keep on moving." At the apex of the crisis, Thurman found herself delivering an average of one eulogy per week—that's not attending one funeral per week, that's actually delivering the eulogy, one per week, for years.

She was exhausted by her experience in the AIDS community: the death, the thankless advocacy, the unending hours, the politics—the sheer emotional toll. Sitting at her new post, making grants to novel and fascinating cultural exchange programs, Thurman actually found herself flirting with serenity.

Previous AIDS czars, Thurman judged, were "very weak." The post "had no juice," it was a "lightning rod for the administration." It was exactly the sort of position she was trying to stay clear of. She looked around her new office at USIA, promptly thanked Marsha Scott, and declined the offer. As Scott prodded, Thurman got blunt: "There's no way. I am *not* going over there!"

Thurman may have been done with the issue, but it wasn't done with her. Scott and one of her associates called back about a week later. It was around Holy Week, and Thurman did a lot of praying. On a luminous spring day, cherry blossoms in full bloom, she went with a friend to the Holocaust museum. When she read the testimonials at the end of the tour—what people knew, and how they failed to act—she said to herself, "Holy shit, this is not good!" A day later Thurman called Scott to accept.

She agreed to do it on two conditions: first, that she would have access to the president; and second, that she could focus on *global* AIDS. Earlier work at the Carter Center had piqued her interest in international affairs, and she believed that the domestic AIDS community was robust and active, strong enough to wield a political voice with or without her undivided attention.

Scott and the White House responded on the spot: "Yeah, yeah, fine, fine," they told Thurman. The post's vacancy had become a political problem. They were relieved to fill it and didn't seem to pay much attention to Thurman's conditions.

The Office of National AIDS Policy, or ONAP, Thurman discovered upon assuming her post in April 1997, was little more than a shell of an office. It had a paltry budget, and a staff of only three or four.

Politically savvy, Thurman knew that access would be king. Her office, however, was located—in a telling sign reflecting White House priorities— by the McDonald's on Seventeenth Street, far from the corridors of power of the White House. "It's all about location, location, location," she said. "They don't lie to you when they tell you that."

She spent her first six months in office mired in bureaucratic and administrative wrangling, fighting for the very things she was promised upon accepting the job. Forced to employ all of her meager political capital in a push merely to get to the start line, she did not even try to accomplish anything on the policy front. Finally, by the fall of 1997 Thurman had managed to secure "prime property" in Lafayette Square and the Old Executive Office Building. The offices became the "bunker" out of which she could operate.

Situated and settled, Thurman left Washington in the late fall of 1997 for her trip to South Africa. On a spectacular morning, flowers in full bloom, she arrived at Rhodes University in Grahamstown. For Thurman, "it was love at first sight" with Africa. She was told that she was to give a brief lecture, and in the afternoon was brought to a small lecture hall that seated just over twenty. When she arrived, she found the room brimming with more than two hundred doctors, NGO workers, traditional healers, and HIV/AIDS patients.

They "had never had a common discussion, never had a common forum," Thurman realized to her horror. "They were desperate to get some help." She was overwhelmed and at a loss for what to say. She conceded to the group that she was still a novice, but pledged that she would come back with answers. "And I walked out of there, and felt like someone had hit me in the head with a bat."

Subsequent events and encounters on the trip—most notably that final visit to the orphanage—strengthened Thurman's resolve. Upon her return to Washington, Thurman assembled her team and began educating herself.

By March 1998 Thurman had drafted and submitted her first memo to the president. She recounted what she had seen in Africa and outlined the depth of the problem worldwide. The memo went on to take inventory of the feckless, almost nonexistent, U.S. response to date. "This is just unacceptable," was the primary theme of that first memo.

Generally, Clinton would get a stack of memos daily, take them up to his residential quarters, read them at night, and jot notes or questions in the margins before passing them back to the author. Thurman's memo came back replete with questions. He had underlined certain passages, including the estimated number of infections per day and the estimated number of orphans predicted one decade hence. The president wanted to know about the pandemic. More than that, he asked how it had gotten so bad, and why the U.S. response was so anemic.

It was the same pandemic he had spoken of in his first inaugural address in January 1993. Patsy Fleming and Donna Shalala had posted him on the global pandemic intermittently since then. During the government shutdown in 1995 he had spent hours reviewing the pandemic with Shalala and others and seemed to grasp the dimensions of what was brewing. But when Thurman entered the scene, the pandemic was "not even on the [White House's] radar screen," she said. "No one had a clue."

The White House "is an environment like no other," and "unless there is somebody in that building who can make the case," Thurman said, an issue will invariably fall off the screen. There was a retinue of officials who were concerned, but no one had made it a paramount priority. The president's senior health advisor, Chris Jennings, did not want to focus on it; Clinton's policy people never drove him on the issue; Shalala had an enormous agenda, and the two previous AIDS czars had prioritized domestic policy and never had considerable access. In Thurman's words, "There was not a real champion inside the White House on the issue."

With a strong AIDS community to carry the mantle on the domestic front, and against the backdrop of ARV treatment and waning domestic death rates, Thurman began spending as much as 70 percent of her time on the global dimension. She became the champion with access that had failed to emerge in those preceding years of quiescence.

The stakes were too important, and Thurman wasn't about to be deterred by Washington bureaucracy. "I tend to put my head down and work right through something," she explained. Moving U.S. policy, she concluded, would require tunnel vision; it's a style that's "sometimes good," but she conceded, presaging ominous turf battles that lay ahead: "It's sometimes bad."

Nevertheless, Thurman's memos to the president had framed and articulated the problem with a degree of lucidity and force that had not, until then, been directed toward the issue. So, upon receiving the president's response to her memo, in March 1998 she was left with the distinct impression that for Clinton, "it was a revelation."

It marked the beginning of a regular correspondence between Thurman and Clinton on the pandemic. There was, however, another matter of some import to the administration percolating in that spring of 1998.

———•◆•———

On January 21, 1998, the name Monica Lewinsky appeared for the first time in *The Washington Post*. It had been almost four years to the day since Janet Reno had named an independent counsel, with Clinton's consent, to investigate allegations of impropriety regarding real-estate dealings in Arkansas. The investigation took on a life of its own, moving from real estate to alleged sexual improprieties, eventually ending up with a young White House intern from Beverly Hills.

The media devoured the story. For eight months, the president denied the allegations. He waved his finger, looking sternly into television cameras, and asserted that he "did not have sexual relations with that woman." He wore a defiant look, as if to express disapproval with the media, legislators, and the public at large for allowing such dross to distract him from executing his responsibilities. Nimbly, the spin doctors spun: he was being unjustly besieged, but the president would continue, undaunted, to carry out the nation's business.

The intensity of the scandal kept mounting. A semen-stained dress, a thong flash, and a character named Linda Tripp and her taped phone calls became the stuff of national discourse. The press fervor sailed to vertiginous heights. A poll suggested that a month into the scandal, 80 percent of Americans considered the coverage "excessive." In the months to follow, pundits began assailing the president. At the crest of the media storm, 140 newspapers would call for the president's resignation. The Republican-controlled Congress seemed dead set on toppling Clinton.

As the accusations' veracity appeared increasingly likely, the war cries rose in pitch. On July 30, 1998, it was reported that Clinton had agreed to testify in front of a grand jury. He did so on August 17, 1998. Following his testimony, Clinton addressed the nation. Again, it was a defiant Bill Clinton, unwilling to utter the word that the nation seemed so poised to hear: sorry. His lackluster performance helped fuel the tempest that culminated with his impeachment in the House and finally the Senate's acquittal on February 13, 1999.

It was a year of scandal. The spin was that Clinton was focused on the nation's business all along. Surprisingly, it's a notion that those seeking to advance global AIDS policy support. Thurman noted a steady dialogue with Clinton during the year. He supported her trips to Africa and afforded her office greater political muscle than ever before. Similarly, Dr. Ken Bernard, Senior Advisor for International Health at the NSC, said that Clinton was engaged in correspondence on the issue. Clinton simply worked harder to get everything done, Bernard said. He encouraged all to move forward. He never subverted anyone's advocacy. He never encouraged anyone to pull back on the issue.

It is not what Clinton did, of course, that is of particular note, but what he failed to do. He would *correspond*, he would *discuss*, he would *agree*, and he would *encourage*. He was famous for doing all of these things, and leaving interlocuters feeling as though a great deal of progress had been made. Action, though, was another matter altogether.

The scandal had rocked Clinton to his core, and emasculated his ability to enact meaningful political change. Almost all emergent issues—particularly those long-term in nature—were consigned to the periphery of his agenda. Despite Thurman and Bernard's advocacy, Clinton did not move one inch on global AIDS in 1998. According to David Halberstam, in his detailed account of the period, *War in a Time of Peace*, "Despite the public denials . . . As soon as the story broke, the White House circled the wagons. All political risks were to be dropped. Coin was to be conserved for this massive winner-take-all political confrontation." He continued: "All of this meant that the middle of Clinton's second term, instead of being devoted to new initiatives . . . was devoted to hunkering down to fight off Special Prosecutor Kenneth Starr."

Clinton had been riding a wave of popularity and had all the moral authority of a two-term president. The economy was in the midst of a dizzying boom and the promise of years of surplus funds appeared likely. He was charismatic and distinctly adept at crafting a story and vision and selling it directly to the American public. Africa was riding a short wave of "good news" stories, and attention was at an all-time high in senior political circles, coinciding with the president's spring trip to Africa. With Thurman and Bernard's advocacy, and the support of senior players like Shalala on the rise, 1998 seemed the perfect year for Clinton to emerge on the issue, and to champion a recalibration in the U.S. response. A better backdrop for engaging a catastrophic global challenge seemed unimaginable. But it was not to be.

Scandal struck, generating a foreboding firestorm in which political capital needed to be conserved for survival. "By his conduct," Haynes Johnson wrote in *The Best of Times*, "Clinton weakened the office of the President . . . and wasted a critical year that might have been spent dealing with problems. Even worse, this neglect occurred at a time of unparalleled peace and prosperity when a second-term President had a rare historical opportunity to provide significant long-term leadership." He concluded: "That opportunity was squandered."

Years later, in July 2002, Bill Clinton took to the stage and received a frenzied welcome from a capacity stadium crowd at the International AIDS Conference in Barcelona. Speaking from a podium, he regretted that he was not able to do more during his presidency, but pledged that global AIDS would be one of the foremost priorities of his post-presidency.

In his trademark off-the-cuff style, Clinton shared a very simple plan. Developing nations should tabulate a bill for the drugs, care, and resources they need. They should designate all the funds they could muster to that end, and then, Clinton proposed, developed nations should foot the difference. The implied share for the United States would translate into billions of dollars in annual commitments. As the new millennium dawned, there was no greater challenge to humanity, Clinton exclaimed, to wild adulation from the crowd.

Activists who were not new to the issue looked on, some befuddled, others outraged. Even during the last two years of his presidency, once he had secured his acquittal and scandal had dissipated, Clinton had remained essentially inert on the issue. He supported Thurman's incremental advocacy, and he helped secure increases in funding for vaccine research and development, but he never lent the weight of his office to the issue.

"There is a staggering hypocrisy in Clinton's involvement as a shining knight in coming to rescue Africa and elsewhere from the pandemic," said one senior UN official. He had "tremendous opportunities when he was president, and chose to exercise none of them."

His defenders point out that the agenda in Clinton's last two years was a robust one. There were matters of great national security interest such as North Korea, relations with China and Russia, and the National Missile Defense debate. Clinton was trying mightily to secure a peace agreement in the Middle East. There were also formidable impediments, most notably, the Republican Congress led by Jesse Helms, who was opposed to global AIDS funding, and foreign aid at large. Against this robust agenda and unrelenting political opposition, Clinton did what he could.

The Office of Management and Budget would be the "no" men and women on global AIDS, rebuffing policy makers championing increases in funds. But the OMB takes its cues from, and ultimately works for, the president. Clinton made it clear that he supported the incremental increases in funding. But he never made it a major priority with OMB, and never pushed Thurman, the Congress, or anyone else to move funding into the billions—the solution he would prescribe in Barcelona, a mere fifteen months *after* relinquishing the reigns of power.

To be sure, there were impediments, and they mattered. But, on issues that Clinton made a priority he was remarkably deft, particularly when it came to funding, at weaving through those impediments. Clinton grew Head Start from $2.8 billion in 1993 to $6.3 billion in 2000. He grew child care supports from $4.5 billion to $12.6 billion and the Earned Income Tax Credit from $12.4 billion to $30.5 billion. "Even in 1998 and 1999," wrote Joe Klein, "with Washington allegedly paralyzed by the Lewinsky scandal and impeachment proceedings, Clinton continued his work, winning a few hundred million dollars here, a billion dollars there for programs he favored."

Global AIDS only drew his "favor" in the waning months of his presidency, if at all. He never employed his budget mastery to recalibrate the response to the levels he would prescribe only a year or so later. Ultimately, Bill Clinton was a champion in empathy, not in policy. The surplus was there, and the know-how was there, but the political will was not. Pressed to account for the president's record, Donna Shalala concluded, "He didn't see the politics in it, I guess."

Of his presidential record, champions and critics offered competing epithets: "Time ran out," say the former. "Too little, too late," say the latter.

———•◆•———

On September 3, 1998, just as scandal gripped Washington, Daniel Tarantola woke to terrible news in Geneva.

After his high-profile resignation from WHO's Global Program on AIDS, or GPA, in 1990, Jonathan Mann had left Geneva to launch the François-Xavier Bagnoud Center for Health and Human Rights at Harvard University. About a year later, Tarantola, an amiable Frenchman and Mann's former deputy at GPA, left Geneva and followed Mann to Harvard. Smarting from the debacle in Geneva, Mann resolved to make strides from his new perch at Harvard. With his knack for attracting funds, he was able to bring on other AIDS experts. The team at Harvard published two important books—AIDS in the World I and II—in 1993 and 1996, respectively. Mann continued to speak out publicly, still popular, charismatic, and well received.

He enjoyed certain parts of his new academic life, like the writing and the teaching. But he missed being in the field. He craved the action. Mostly, he yearned to be at the helm once again, formulating policy, commandeering the world's attention, and leading the global response. Unfulfilled, Mann grew increasingly despondent through the mid-1990s. He began writing less, and published almost nothing on AIDS in his final year at Harvard.

In January 1997, desperate to descend from Harvard's Ivory Tower, Mann resigned from the university to take a post at the Institute of Applied Health in Philadelphia. There he spent his days training paramedics in public health.

It was enough, though, to reignite Mann's passions. He wanted back into the fight. In the summer of 1998, he telephoned his old friend Tarantola, by that time back at WHO, under a new director general, Gro Harlem Brundtland. With his nemesis Nakajima since departed, Mann was interested in jumping back into global health. He scheduled a series of meetings, including one with his longtime colleague, Peter Piot, executive director of UNAIDS, for an upcoming trip to Geneva in early September.

Early in the morning of September 3, on the day of Mann's scheduled visit, Tarantola learned of the crash of Swiss Air Flight 111. Utter confusion ensued. He couldn't remember if Mann was flying out of New York or Washington. He had forgotten the time of departure. A secretary then shared an e-mail she had gotten from Mary Lou Clements, Mann's second wife, with whom he'd be traveling. The two were scheduled to be on a later flight, but at the last minute had changed their arrangement.

Tarantola rushed to the Crisis Management Center at the airport, where he waited for three hours to learn that Mann and his wife had been, as Tarantola had dreaded, on Flight 111. There were no survivors.

Mann had single-handedly revolutionized the global response to the pandemic. He had usurped the international spotlight and directed it onto the pandemic and its victims. He had done much to destigmatize the disease and to reconceptualize how it had to be fought. He had mobilized more than a hundred national programs—all to incalculable effect. With unshakable belief in his mission, he could at times appear egotistical and at other times messianic. He knew that to recalibrate the response, he would have to rattle the system.

Unlike so many others, Mann had not placed process or personal advancement above people. He had tendered his resignation from GPA in protest, becoming the first and last major player on the issue to do so, ceding his personal standing—and a career in international politics with boundless prospects—for a cause he deemed much greater.

On the afternoon of September 4, several hundred WHO and UN officials gathered in an auditorium at WHO headquarters in Geneva to remember Jonathan Mann. Gro Harlem Brundtland addressed the crowd, delivering an emotional eulogy, punctuated by fitful sobs from her audience. It was a short and dignified service. For Tarantola, Mann's longtime friend and comrade, the untimely loss brought untold grief. "It was very hard," he said, his voice still trembling with the pain of precious memories—and opportunity lost.

———•◆•———

A few weeks earlier, on a sweltering August morning in 1998, around the time of Clinton's grand jury testimony, Dr. Ken Bernard kissed his wife good-bye and left his home in the Virginia suburbs for his first day of work at the National Security Council. Forty-nine years old, the former physician's graying hair, soft monotone, and congenial manner gave every impression that he was not unlike the quintessential small-town doctor. How unlikely, then, that Bernard would find himself as a senior advisor at the NSC.

It was a position he had fought for. At the Department of Health and Human Services Bernard served a successful tour as the political officer to the U.S. mission to the UN in Geneva. After successfully completing his primary mission—ensuring that Director General Hiroshi Nakajima did not run for a third term—Bernard cashed in hard-won political capital with his boss, Donna Shalala, early in 1998, imploring her to lobby Sandy Berger, director of the NSC, to appoint him Senior Advisor for International Health. It was a position without precedent, to be created for him.

There were health issues, it seemed to Bernard, that had to be dealt with as national security issues. Two were of particular concern: bioterrorism and infectious disease. And there was no infectious disease as daunting, no health threat as perilous, Bernard believed, as the global AIDS pandemic.

Bernard had been on the ground in Southern Africa. He had seen the bodies pile up, dozens upon dozens. He had witnessed the suffering and despair. But Bernard pressed the argument further, positing that there would be seismic economic and even security implications as well. The pandemic was so prodigious, and so debilitating to civil society that it would help breed instability and disorder. In time, it would be a root cause of state failure and quite probably even conflict and war.

Bernard's new colleagues did not quite know what to make of the new senior advisor for global health. Even in the late 1990s, the NSC—created by the 1947 National Security Act, during the Truman administration—was still steeped in the Cold War mentality of its birth. Most at the NSC prided themselves on dealing with "hard" binational confrontational, politico-military issues. It was what they were trained to do, and the reason they got in the game in the first place.

Even with the dissolution of the Cold War, and with progressive thinkers like Anthony Lake and Sandy Berger at the helm, many in the national security machine were slow to adjust, and inherently skeptical of what seemed humanitarian or social—security speak for "soft" or "fluffy"— issues. In those halcyon days before 9/11, anthrax, and bioterror warnings, Bernard's colleagues agreed that health was important, but few bought into the notion of a health/security nexus.

Accordingly, Bernard would have a hard time getting taken seriously. Colleagues would say, "Hey, Doc, since you're over here, do you mind taking a look at my knee?" He actually had his secretary take the "MD" off of his White House business card, finding that he was taken more seriously as a traditional policy maker than as "a health guy."

Nevertheless, Bernard knew that if an issue was deemed of national security import, it attracted funds with a velocity that no other area of the U.S. government can match. He made it his mission to inject health, particularly global AIDS, into the national security agenda. If he could get key people to buy in, he knew, he could effect profound change. He became a door-to-door salesman, working the formidable high-ceilinged corridors of the Old Executive Office Building, knocking on the oversized, dense mahogany doors, selling his case to whoever would listen. The going was slow.

Pounding the hallways, Bernard began to hear from colleagues about a cerebral, if idiosyncratic, senior policy maker. At fifty-nine years of age, Leon Fuerth, Vice President Al Gore's longtime foreign policy advisor, could be disarmingly curt, but his fiercely independent intellect and his loyalty to the vice president won him the respect of colleagues and Gore's unequivocal confidence. Earmarked to be national security advisor in the event of a Gore win in 2000, Fuerth's abilities and the likely prospect of his ascension (most expected Gore to win) afforded him great influence in the foreign policy apparatus late in the Clinton administration.

As luck would have it, he was also a progressive thinker. For the 2000 election he crafted a foreign policy doctrine for Gore that he labeled "Forward Engagement." The doctrine called on the United States to consider and engage "nontraditional" security threats. They included: terrorism, transnational crime (e.g., weapons and arms proliferation, the drug trade), the environment, and health (including global AIDS). Though not as imminent as the "traditional" binational politico-military threats, Fuerth recognized that they were every bit as perilous, and that they would in fact lay the groundwork for the next epoch's wars. Fuerth wanted to engage these threats early. "The alternative," he wrote, "was to keep letting [them] wash over us again and again."

Bernard worked on Fuerth as much as he could, in passing in the halls, and in briefing sessions in Fuerth's office, where, to Bernard's distraction, Fuerth would munch incessantly on carrot sticks. He insisted that the pandemic would lay the groundwork for great instability and crisis. It was an argument that jibed with Fuerth's worldview. Well versed on the issue through his involvement in the binational commissions with Russia and South Africa, he hardly needed convincing. Both agreed the United States would have to start talking in billions, instead of millions. And they would have to start to think about an apposite structural response as well. Fuerth told Bernard that what was needed was a comprehensive national strategic plan—"like a battle plan as if we were going to war." "Finally!" Bernard thought.

They needed a strategy that outlined the objectives, the costs, and the tasks—who would do what when? Armed with that strategy, they could take it to the deputies (a collection of the deputy secretaries and directors of key U.S. departments and agencies), and then to the principals (secretaries and directors). With their recommendation and the president's approval, it would become U.S. national security policy. The funds and structural reform, they suspected, would follow.

To begin, Fuerth told Bernard, they should convene all the various players in the U.S. government with "equity" in the issue under an interagency working group. Bernard would be a co-chair. Sandy Thurman, it was decided, had to be a co-chair as well.

In late April 1999, Bernard, with even more bounce in his step than usual, strode through the marble-floored corridors of the Old Executive on his way to Room 208, the Cordell Hull Conference Room, for the first working group meeting.

He entered and took a seat at the head of a dark oval mahogany conference table. The room was elaborately decorated, with flowing velvet curtains and a baroque chandelier. Save for the table, it resembled a well-sized drawing room out of a Tolstoy novel. The meeting place added a sense of grandeur to the proceedings. Twenty chairs sat around the periphery of the conference table and another twenty around the edges of the wood-paneled walls.

Attendance exceeded expectations, and many had to stand. Leon Fuerth stopped by for a pep talk: "You are all undertaking a very important task," he told the group, providing the stamp of senior leadership. "I have the full confidence that you will be able to do this. And remember, all else being equal, this work just might get us into heaven." Bernard led the meeting, tasking out different assignments, with Thurman, as co-chair, interjecting intermittently. Leaving the meeting, Bernard had every reason to be optimistic.

About a month later, the second meeting convened. This time Sandy Thurman wasn't there. She had told Bernard that she had "another meeting, a prior engagement." She didn't send a deputy or anyone in her stead. And she hadn't submitted her comments to the working draft of the strategic plan memo.

Following that session, Bernard called on Thurman to engage in the process. Pushing the issue through the national security apparatus afforded them, Bernard argued, the best chance to recalibrate U.S. policy and enact a truly comprehensive U.S. national plan.

Thurman wasn't responsive. With her direct line of access to the president, Thurman had positioned herself as the foremost champion and spokesperson on the issue. She already had an advisory council, she told Bernard. They were formulating a plan of their own. She was reluctant to enfranchise others in the process. The national security realm was foreign to her. In part, she feared that such a group would be unwieldy and cumbersome, that it would impede her ability to "stick her head down" and advance the issue. In part, Thurman was being protective of her turf, her access.

Following that second meeting, the chemistry between Thurman and Bernard began to grow toxic. She would speak to him affectionately, calling him "love" and "dear." "Aren't we doing great work, dear?" she would say to Bernard when their paths crossed. But a senior administration official involved in the group remembered: "Frankly, Ken and Sandy couldn't stand each other, and they were always going in different directions." Much of the tension emanated from Thurman's obduracy. Stephen Morrison, then a State Department official recalled, "Sandy wouldn't even give him the time of day. She saw him as a threat."

The discord produced a comedy of mishaps. Intent on maintaining her direct line of communication with the president, Thurman would send Clinton memos without having shown them to Bernard or others in the group. Clinton's secretary would occasionally misdirect Thurman's memos, signed, "Sandy," and marked up with the president's comments, to NSC Director Sandy Berger, who would then pass them along to Bernard, who would, in turn, discover that he and the group had been cut out of the loop.

Thurman's unwillingness to cooperate became an impeding force in the group's effort. Support from key participants waned. Susan Rice could see the group "going not very far, very fast." Others agreed and stopped participating. They were slow to submit input and comments on the working draft of the "plan." Bernard and others found it impossible to achieve coordination and formulate an "integrative" U.S. government policy without the AIDS czar.

Pursuing her own distinct agenda, Thurman was having much greater success, winning her self-selected battle, even as the war was being lost.

At 7:15 on a brisk March morning in 1999, Sandy Thurman strode through the West Wing on her way to the Roosevelt Room. Months earlier Thurman had managed the unprecedented feat of injecting herself into the daily White House senior staff morning meetings. Elsewhere, Thurman had acquired a reputation for being boisterous, even outspoken. There was certainly much she wished to say, much she had to say. During the meetings, for months now, though, she had remained mute.

She was intimidated by the grandeur of the Roosevelt Room, and by the stature of the key players in the meetings: Robert Rubin, secretary of the Treasury; John Podesta, White House chief of staff; Gene Sperling, director of the National Economic Council; and the rest of Clinton's senior staff. They all knew each other and, unlike Thurman, represented the traditional power centers of the Executive. Thurman was a neophyte in the ways of high-stakes, closed-door senior policy making.

That spring morning would be different. Thurman had just returned from a presidential mission to Africa—her second visit and first comprehensive continental tour. Moving from hospital to hospital and orphanage to orphanage, Thurman's sense of outrage had been piqued and her resolve had solidified. She had crafted a passionate memo to the president, recounting the horrors she'd witnessed and pleading for resources and leadership. As ever, his response was supportive and encouraging. Emboldened by the president's tacit support, Thurman sought to win much-needed support from other senior colleagues. She would have to speak up.

Entering the Roosevelt Room, Thurman was, once again, intimidated by her milieu. As the meeting moved on, the principals went around the room. Each briefing was tendered seamlessly, without significant event— business as usual. Thurman remembered her grandfather, the former patriarch of the Thurman clan. He used to implore his granddaughter to live according to the Peter Principle: "When you arrive in heaven, that is, and meet St. Peter at the pearly gates, can you make your case?"

At approximately 8:00 A.M., Thurman stood up to make her case. "I've just gotten back from Africa," she told her colleagues, who were surprised to see Thurman take the floor. She forced the words out: "By the end of the decade we'll have forty million children orphaned. We have six thousand people dying a day. This epidemic is wiping out all the gains we've made in development in the last twenty years. Infant mortality is tripling. Child mortality is doubling. Life expectancy is dropping by twenty years or more."

She canvassed the room for reaction: silence. It was already 1999 and "they just didn't know. . . . People were looking at me like I had just come in there and had a seizure . . . they were just standing there staring and couldn't say a word."

Their reaction was indicative of the constraints and uphill battles that had already marked Thurman's mission to date. The pandemic was still mired in the stigma of early years. It was clear that AIDS still evoked notions of sexual promiscuity or deviancy, or drug use. Many simply preferred to dismiss the issue outright.

Finding little internal support in the government, Thurman was forced to look outside. "A very interesting thing about the White House [is that] you can't do it yourself," Thurman said. "You have to call outside and get your pressure cooks to call inside and then you go inside and say all these people are calling you, you've got to get this done." But, when Thurman looked to domestic constituencies she found a barren landscape. No one was interested. The AIDS community was still focused on the domestic front. The developmental community had yet to awaken to the gravity of the pandemic, and was still taken with its preexisting roster of issues. The African-American community was not yet interested. "There wasn't anyone for us to call on the international side," and it was an enormous impediment.

Thurman began to follow the money. And the money, she learned, was at USAID. Under administrator Brian Atwood's tenure, the division had been downgraded and had grown conditioned to its "hunker and bunker down" posture. The goal was not to build up the effort, but rather to maintain the effort and funding against the backdrop of an adversarial Congress, the balanced budget initiatives, and cuts in foreign assistance at large.

Thurman suspected that USAID would not be willing to reallocate existing funds to the detriment of their other programs, so she approached Duff Gillespie, a career USAID bureaucrat, and told him that she would work the White House and the Congress and try to secure additional funds for his agency. That way, nothing would have to get cut. Gillespie seemed pleased, but told her that USAID could accommodate only another $20 million. That was it, Gillespie said. At $20 million they would be at "absorptive capacity," bureaucratic speak for "their limit." Thurman was livid.

She responded, "You're sending out reports which complain [about underfunding and the pandemic's escalation] and how can you send me this information and when I respond to it, you can't respond to it! If that's true, then Jesse Helms is right; you need to be put out of business!" She would never get much proactive movement from USAID.

To add insult to injury, Thurman's interest in the global dimension had exposed her flank, leaving her vulnerable to criticism from the domestic AIDS community, who felt sold out and neglected. She considered the domestic constituency her base, and was stung by the criticism. Rifts developed with cherished old friends. As 1999 moved forward, the outlook for Thurman appeared bleak.

Then the tide began to turn.

The UNAIDS report providing the world with the first credible, consensus-based global estimates had been released late in the summer of 1998, and in the months thereafter the world was beginning to awaken and take notice. Increasingly, the media was taking note as well. Several of the major newspapers had allocated more print to the pandemic. With ARVs extending life in the United States, the global agenda was slowly gaining steam among an ever-broader base of U.S. activists. Members of the Congressional Black Caucus like Ron Dellums and Barbara Lee started trumpeting the need for a "Marshall Plan" for Africa. African leaders were also slowly awakening.

Thurman read the break of the waves and started paddling. In the spring and summer of 1999, she began conducting frequent trips to Africa, ushering delegations to the continent. They often included a colorful potpourri of policy makers and personalities. On one trip she traveled with philanthropists, members of Senator Ted Kennedy's staff, Congresswoman Nancy Pelosi's staff, Senator Jesse Helms's staff, ex-Mayor David Dinkins of New York, and a Methodist bishop from Washington.

Always bipartisan, Thurman would work on everyone and anyone to whom she was afforded access. Some derided her efforts, calling the trips "AIDS tourism," but she knew that if she could get policy makers to spend only thirty minutes on the ground in Africa, the sky would be the limit for U.S. funding and leadership. A gregarious "socialite" and "schmoozer," it was a strategy that played to Thurman's strengths. And it ultimately proved effective.

On July 19, 1999, the administration announced the LIFE (Leadership and Investment in Fighting an Epidemic) Initiative. It was to be Thurman's flagship effort, and she and her staff labored that summer to refine the features of the plan. She leaned heavily on the intellectual firepower and legislative wherewithal of Michael Iskowitz, a longtime Senator Ted Kennedy staffer, and one of her closest personal friends. Iskowitz was both openly gay and pointedly irreverent—he wore his long hair in a ponytail and sat behind a name placard on his desk that said "Jesse Helms."

By the fall of 1999, LIFE was ready to take to the Hill. The initiative called on Congress to increase U.S. funding. Importantly, it also invalidated USAID's sole claim to funds. LIFE would augment USAID's funding pot, but it would also allocate funds to HHS and CDC (as well as others in smaller slices), which enjoyed greater political support, clout, and technical expertise.

Their entry into the policy fold meant that the U.S. response would have a more robust and efficacious base from which to build. "It made USAID mad," Thurman said, but she didn't lose much sleep over it. The shift served the solution, if not bureaucratic agendas.

Thurman sat in the House chambers that fall of 1999, rustling papers, as policy makers debated LIFE. She had prepared comments roughly seven minutes in length. As she listened to the debate, she noticed that several of the supportive legislators had borrowed language directly from the proposal—a sure sign of success. She found herself whittling her comments further and further. When she was finally given her cue, Thurman delivered a two-and-a-half-minute presentation. LIFE passed comfortably, securing an additional $100 million in U.S. funding for 2000, bringing the U.S. total close to $250 million.

LIFE was Thurman's crowning achievement. After seven years of U.S. stasis and neglect, she had finally moved U.S. policy, and "no one," Ken Bernard said, "can take that away from her." The initiative also summoned U.S. leaders in all areas of government to make the issue a priority. In 2000, Thurman would help secure another turn in funding, so that by the time the administration departed early in 2001, that year's budget had allocated $450 million for global AIDS, a threefold increase in two years.

In the process, Thurman left more than a little scorched earth in her wake. "I just fight my way through it and write a thank-you note later," she said. "I do feel that in this instance, while it may not have won me the Miss Congeniality Prize, it got the work done." And it did. The achievement had Thurman's unique imprint all over it.

But it was also a choice that would exact an incalculable cost. Thurman's office was meek, almost feckless, which meant that she had to marshal all of her muscle, leverage all of her access, and spend all of her political capital to effect even incremental policy change. In the national security domain, by contrast, it was customary to speak of marshaling billions, not millions of dollars to engage threats. The national security crowd had the clout to tackle emergent problems with leaps, rather than in increments. It was also the one area of the government that could institute near-term, meaningful structural change to engage a problem. By rebuffing the "national security" effort, and choosing the go-it-alone option, Thurman had pried open an avenue, but in the process she had suffocated a major thoroughfare.

Otherwise occupied ushering delegations to Africa and on the LIFE Initiative throughout 1999, Thurman had opted out, almost entirely, of Bernard's Interagency Working Group process. Her absence and even circumvention were crippling his effort. The fall of 1999 was shaping up to be an inclement one for Ken Bernard.

Bernard expressed his reservations to Fuerth, his senior sponsor. Fuerth had little appetite for bureaucratic nonsense. He demanded that Bernard continue to press the effort forward. To generate momentum, Fuerth told Bernard that he would schedule a deputies meeting for that November where Bernard could present "the strategic plan."

Even as Fuerth pushed though, determined not to let the initiative die, he was unwilling to address the effort's fundamental Achilles' heel. Thurman was close to the president. Fuerth wasn't willing to take her on. He told Bernard that they would just have to do their best to engage her, and if she balked, they would just have to plow ahead without her.

But Thurman had come to speak for the White House on this issue, and Bernard could not, or would not, be so brazen as to unilaterally formulate a national strategic plan that did not cohere with White House policy. Furthermore, because the process had hit a wall, the other major departments and agencies were less than focused on formulating their own roles in the comprehensive strategy.

Putting together the war plan became an all-consuming obsession for Bernard. He persisted through late nights and obduracy from almost all quarters. But between Fuerth's relentless pushing, Thurman's circumvention, and the group's haplessness, Bernard found himself in between jagged rocks and in a very hard place indeed.

Laboring mightily during that October and November, Bernard found himself essentially alone, trying to do all he could to advance the effort. Progress was hard to come by. He found solace in his wife, who would welcome him when he got home at night, sometimes after midnight. As they talked about music, art, and other topics, she helped temper his anxiety. She assured him that it wasn't his fault. It didn't matter whose fault it was, Bernard explained to her. The effort would fail and the burden weighed heavily on his shoulders, and even more gravely on his conscience.

Around noon one late November 1999 day, Bernard made his way through the West Wing of the White House toward the Situation Room for the deputies meeting Fuerth had promised. It was the first deputies meeting of Bernard's career. Anxiously, he entered the room, carrying copies of the memo to be discussed at the meeting.

The oval mahogany conference table seated twelve, and the high-tech communications system, screens, panels, and sparse decor added a sense of gravity and foreboding to the moment. Bernard sat behind Jim Steinberg, deputy director at the National Security Council—a well-respected foreign policy expert—in a row of chairs lining the Situation Room's walls.

The meeting began on a disastrous note. Typically, Joe Gannon, director of the National Intelligence Council, or some other such top-level CIA figure, would begin the meetings by reading the "threat assessment" of whatever security issue was being addressed. Still trying to get her on board, Bernard had invited Sandy Thurman to present the threat assessment to the high-powered group.

Thurman did not speak the same language as her "security" colleagues. She spoke of humanitarian suffering, orphans, mother-to-child transmission. The security crowd leaned back, eyebrows bent cynically. They were skeptical of "nontraditional" issues to begin with, and Thurman's briefing seemed more a "public service think piece" than a threat assessment.

It set the tone for the rest of the meeting. Perusing the memo, it was clear to the deputies that it did not contain the hard, finite recommendations they favored. Instead, it seemed more like a briefing paper on the pandemic, and on the existing U.S. effort. The deputies only consider a meeting worthwhile if they are able to reach actionable conclusions. But "the plan" was inchoate.

The meeting became confused and disjointed. Jim Steinberg, chairing the meeting, deferred to Fuerth, the senior sponsor. It became more of a briefing session. Fuerth highlighted the problem and exclaimed that the United States needed a strategy, goals, and resources. He managed to pique some interest, and for most, the meeting was didactic. But deputies meetings are supposed to be conclusive, and for the most part it was "amateur hour," and provided ammunition to validate the skeptics' doubts.

After the meeting, Bernard got a tongue-lashing from his superiors. Fuerth told Bernard that the effort was too important to get mired in bureaucratic silliness, and that he was going to use his influence to get it moved forward. Fuerth was true to his word. He kept pushing Bernard. But again, he did not expend political coin or energy to fix the fundamental problem: Thurman's circumvention of the process and the working group's degeneration.

In the aftermath of the deputies meeting, Bernard tried to bring those who had participated in the working group back into the fold. He worked on Thurman, and labored on the draft of the plan, but all to little effect. Leon Fuerth continued to push. Fuerth could see the election looming, and calculated that he had a limited window of time in which to strike. He called another deputies meeting, despite Bernard's protestations.

Two nights before the late January meeting, Bernard went over to see Mara Rudman, chief of staff at the NSC, at her office in the West Wing. As he had tried to explain to Fuerth, the "plan" was nowhere near ready. Rudman received Bernard's appeal for counsel sternly. She was put off that Fuerth was pushing this issue—a disease, a security threat? She threw Bernard's memo on her coffee table and called in someone from the National Economic Council nearby to redraft it, apparently presuming that Bernard—a doctor after all—was inept. It was a grave insult, but he needed a miracle and didn't object.

The evening before the meeting was frigid. Outside the wind whistled and pounded relentlessly against the windows of Bernard's third-floor office in the Old Executive Office Building, no more than fifty yards from the West Wing of the White House.

For nine months the effort had summoned every ounce of Bernard's energy. He had spent countless late nights, working harder than he had since his days at medical school. Bosses and colleagues wondered: Could he deliver the plan? He would carry, he knew, the stamp of the outcome of the next day's meeting with him for the rest of his career in government.

Amidst the policy making, the strategic formulation, and the Washingtonian politicking, he made sure to remind himself of the human element—the millions of lives at stake. Above all, he was a physician.

Sitting at his desk, Bernard pored anxiously over the redrafted memo to be presented at the following day's meeting. The deputies would be expecting a comprehensive national plan, but the memo outlined only a disparate set of preliminary recommendations. It had gotten worse, not better. As the clock struck 10:00 P.M., fifteen hours before the meeting, it seemed to be tolling the effort's imminent failure.

For months the effort to formulate a viable U.S. strategy had been dying amidst internecine bureaucratic turf wars, scandal, politics, personal agendas, and egos. He had tried as best he could, but he could not save it, and now, he could not stop it. As the realization dawned, Bernard slapped the fifteen-page memo back on his desk, his hopes utterly dashed. He got up and walked toward his window looking out on the West Wing. Thinking about the opportunity that would be lost, tears of anger and frustration welled up and rolled down his cheeks.

Retracing his steps through the West Wing on his way to the Situation Room the next afternoon, Bernard carried a sinking feeling in his stomach. He took his seat, once again, behind Jim Steinberg, and waited with trepidation for the meeting to begin.

Thurman did not attend the second meeting, nor did she send anyone in her stead. She did not offer any comments or input into the working draft of the memo during the weeks it circulated. All the while, she continued to advance her own distinct agenda, pursuing incremental gains, and protecting her access to the president.

As the meeting commenced, Fuerth, once again, spoke passionately about the need for a comprehensive and ambitious national strategic plan. But the working group had not presented the deputies with a national strategy to approve. They became fed up, intemperate, and eventually—even worse—disengaged. The meeting was a debacle.

Following the meeting, Bernard tried, once again, to regroup, but his chance had come and gone. By late winter the election was heating up and attention was turning elsewhere. Most of the interested players had, in Bernard's estimation, "lost the stomach for battle, knowing that they wouldn't be there to complete it." Most predicted a Gore victory anyhow, and presumed that under Gore, Holbrooke, and Fuerth, the issue would be well taken care of.

Elsewhere, Bernard waged one final attempt to move policy; this time, though, through another angle. Richard Holbrooke's chief of staff, RP Eddy, had come up with a novel and innovative idea. It called on the president to appoint a special envoy for AIDS Cooperation. With Holbrooke's sponsorship, Eddy got Bernard on board. Brainstorming, the two envisioned a leading executive like Jack Welch, or a high-profile statesman like George Mitchell for the post. Reporting directly to the president, the new envoy would manage the U.S. response and champion a diplomatic agenda to summon national leaders to upgrade their countries' responses. As the two moved on the idea, they ran into only more bureaucratic resistance and red tape from the State Department and Sandy Thurman's office, both protective of their mandates and their turf. After much wrangling, Thurman was appointed the envoy with only months left in the administration, an empty symbolic gesture.

The Clinton administration's final days ebbed against the backdrop of an America giddy with unprecedented economic prosperity and a sense of immunity from the world's problems and cares. Bernard's final months in the NSC were relatively quiet. He had shifted gears, and spent most of his time on bioterrorism, which was beginning to garner increased attention.

Then, one August morning, a telegram arrived in Bernard's office inbox. It was a report from the ambassador from Swaziland, and outlined excerpts of a speech his king had just delivered in a local stadium brimming with tens of thousands of his countrymen. The king was furious at the plight of his people and at the world's seeming indifference. Bernard rightly read it as a rebuke to his own country. Ashamed, it scalded him deeply.

Hours after receiving the telegram, Bernard found himself in a senior staff NSC meeting in the Situation Room in the West Wing. Days earlier the Russian submarine Kursk had fallen to the depths of the Barents Sea, killing 118 crewmembers. The Kursk incident had dominated the news media for the past few days and the NSC staff was similarly abuzz. What would it mean for Putin, the Russian military, internal politics, the situation in Chechnya?

Bernard sat in the meeting listening as his colleagues could speak of little else. One hundred and eighteen military men died when the *Kursk* sank. Bernard knew that during the course of that very same day roughly eight thousand people would die of AIDS. As colleagues continued to talk about the *Kursk* and its implications, Bernard grew increasingly indignant. Finally, he could no longer resist.

He stood up, cleared his throat, and announced that he held a telegram from a speech the king of Swaziland had delivered to thousands of his countrymen. Bernard read from the telegram: "One quarter of you will die of AIDS. Nobody cares. The world is letting my country die."

There was not a word for ten seconds.

Finally, Gayle Smith, senior director for African Affairs, said that Bernard was right and that "we need to do more about this." With months left in the administration, everyone knew that her words would yield little of substance. Already leaning toward the door, folks were pleased that Smith had broken the uncomfortable silence. They seemed relieved to pile out and move on to other matters.

It was the only serious effort in U.S. history to devise a comprehensive *strategic* plan. It would take another three years until even the notion of a meaningfully upgraded U.S. effort would be taken up again. Nearly 9 *million* people would die in the interim, and roughly 15 *million* new infections would accrue. During those years, the pandemic would gain a menacing foothold in China and the former Soviet Union, and burgeon wildly in India.

It was one of the deadliest policy failures in the history of the U.S. government.

A Great Awakening?
(2001–2003)

THIRTEEN

—⚯—

A Bleak Outlook,
Finally—A Vehicle

A lmost immediately, the activists' worst fears seemed realized. After the closest and most contentious election in presidential history, George Walker Bush had been in office as the forty-third president of the United States for less than twenty days. In what he anticipated would be an entirely innocuous comment, the new White House chief of staff Andy Card mentioned to a *USA Today* reporter that the Bush II White House intended to dismantle the Office of National AIDS Policy.

To leading Beltway advocates like Terje Anderson, the comment seemed the fruition of a clear pattern of the new president's disinterest in global AIDS.

Years earlier, another Beltway advocate with conservative ties had won a meeting with then Texas Governor Bush's senior health advisor. "The one thing Bush is really uncomfortable dealing with is AIDS," the governor's advisor told the advocate. As governor, Bush still thought of the disease as a domestic phenomenon. He had little appetite for the issue for many of the same reasons as his conservative predecessors. It was sex. It was rowdy homosexual activists. Given his conservative political base, engaging the issue would have meant treading uncomfortable and precarious waters.

During the campaign, leading foreign policy figures like Leon Fuerth had picked up on a number of statements or comments that presaged that a Bush II administration would be disengaged on global AIDS. In the 2000 Republican National Platform, the section on foreign affairs entitled "Principled Leadership" took aim at Gore's foreign policy strategy. The platform

245

impugned the vice president's "new security agenda," which included items like disease. "If there is some limit to candidate Gore's new agenda for America as social worker, he has yet to define it," the platform read. "It is time for America to regain its focus," it went on. "A Republican president will identify and pursue vital American national interests."

It was a cardinal point of differentiation, the GOP argued. Gore and the Democrats were blurring the lines between "soft" humanitarian issues and "hard" traditional security issues. It would lead to costly overextensions in U.S. commitments and errant enterprises like nation building.

When asked how he would have addressed the genocide in Rwanda, Bush answered, "We should not send our troops to stop ethnic cleansing and genocide outside our strategic interests. . . . I would not send the United States troops into Rwanda." It was, in fact, one of the few points on which Bush would say of Clinton that he had done the right thing.

The implication was that the Democrats were conducting national security policy like adolescents. The Republicans were grown-ups and would put national security policy back into focus.

Throughout the course of the campaign, Bush offered further insights into how his administration might deal with global AIDS. On painfully unsure footing on foreign policy throughout the election, in an interview with Jim Lehrer in February 2000, Bush addressed Africa and its place in a new Bush II foreign policy matrix. Bush said, "While Africa may be important, it doesn't fit into the national strategic interests, as far as I can see them." With breathtaking economy—in twenty words—Bush had practically written off an entire continent's strategic relevance.

In the second of three presidential debates held in North Carolina about a month before the election, Jim Lehrer, this time as moderator, asked Bush about the role of the United States in intervening on the continent to prevent humanitarian catastrophe. "Africa is important . . . but there's got to be priorities," Bush said.

Because the election remained contested right up to the inauguration, Beltway advocates like Terje Anderson had little time to try and make inroads with the Bush camp. The Democrats had been in power for eight years. The activist community had few connections with the new administration. Bush's comments on Africa during the election, and the new administration's apparent lack of interest in reaching out, evoked memories of Bush's Republican predecessors.

Some of the activists who had particular insights into policy making were discouraged to learn that the office of senior advisor for international health at the National Security Council, previously occupied by Ken Bernard, was disbanded on the very first day of the administration. The new NSC director, Condoleezza Rice, had said that under Clinton the NSC had gotten turgid, too bloated to serve its function as honest broker and coordinator of other departments and agencies. It's not that global health was unimportant to Rice and the administration, just that it was better managed by HHS.

But to many it was emblematic of what the Clinton camp called "ABC"—"Anything But Clinton." It seemed an underpinning credo, a reaction to a predecessor who represented much of what the Bush camp reviled. Putting global health at the NSC seemed "another instance of woolly-headed Clinton thinking," said Stephen Morrison. And so they dismantled the post.

Many of the activists who had participated in the Gore protests began having doubts. Their target came to seem like their best friend. He had lost by only a few hundred votes in Florida, where tens of thousands of disenchanted Democrats had punched their chads for the countercandidate Ralph Nader. With such a slight margin, might the attacks made on Gore have made the difference? Even Jamie Love wondered. Could it have been a terrible mistake?

When Andy Card's announcement about ONAP came out in USA Today on Wednesday, February 7, 2001, it certainly seemed so. The office had scant resources and influence, but it held enormous symbolic import. It was literally the White House's interface with the activist community. Announcing its demolition less than three weeks into the new administration set off a firestorm.

Within hours, activists began pelting the White House with a barrage of phone calls, e-mails, and faxes. They put out a flurry of press releases. They got staffers and representatives on the Hill on the case. The Congressional Black Caucus, having gravitated toward the issue with increasing force, spoke out, as did Senator Tom Daschle and Congressman Dick Gephardt.

The protests launched a flurry of closed-door deliberations at 1600 Pennsylvania Avenue. Card had also announced that the Office of Race Relations was closing. Bush had won less than 10 percent of the African-American vote. It was clearly a demographic that he would have to win over, and a deep pool of potentially convertible votes. He filled three of his administration's most important seats with African-Americans, including two Cabinet posts.

Now, having announced that they were closing both the Office of National AIDS Policy and the Office of Race Relations, it appeared as if the new administration was not going to be friendly to a critical minority. It appeared as if it had carved the "compassion" out of compassionate conservatism. The infinitesimal election margin afforded little room for a debacle out of the gate. And the administration realized that it was in danger of casting itself in the very mold it had sought to avoid.

At a press conference the next afternoon, White House press secretary Ari Fleischer got to spinning. "A mistake was made," he said. Card had misspoken. Fleischer would not say whether or not the administration had been considering closing the two offices, but "there is nothing that is closing. That office is open." When pressed further, Fleischer said, "He made a mistake. It happens." The White House had recanted, assuring the AIDS community that ONAP would remain open. More than that, they pledged that they would increase funding for global AIDS.

"The White House chief of staff does not misspeak," said Terje Anderson. According to *The Washington Post*, the "confusion marked the first significant stumble of a White House that has basked in mostly favorable reviews for its smooth and disciplined performance." Concerned activists deemed it more than a coincidence that the administration's "first significant stumble" would involve AIDS.

However, in the aftermath of the July 2000 International AIDS Conference held in Durban, South Africa, critical mass had fomented among the domestic activist community, bringing the Beltway folks into the fold with the fringe ACT UP characters. Responding to the statistics and UNAIDS's advocacy, the increased media attention, the visibility of the Gore protests, and the constant escalation of the death and infection tolls, interest escalated sharply among the public health community, the African-American community, the developmental community, and—of particular importance to the administration—faith-based organizations.

It was an unlikely aggregation of players and voices, but together they generated a loud groundswell of noise. They made it clear that they were not going away and that they would demand more progress on U.S. policy.

For starters, the administration would have to demonstrate a measure of commitment by appointing a director to fill the vacant position at ONAP. They were in the market for an AIDS czar.

• • •

When Tommy Thompson was named Bush's secretary of Health and Human Services, Scott Evertz estimated that he would have a decent chance of obtaining a job in the new administration. Evertz had gotten to know Thompson, the former governor of Wisconsin, as a local figure in the not-for-profit community and as an advocate for AIDS programs. He had worked on one of Thompson's election campaigns, and later became one of the "Austin 12," the group of Log Cabin, or gay, Republicans to meet with the president during the election on gay issues.

After interviewing with some officials in the new administration, the president's personnel people were less than impressed with Evertz. Despite his affable demeanor, he had relatively little programmatic experience. He was passed over for a position.

Nearly two months later, the administration found itself in a quandary. Having assured the burgeoning U.S. AIDS community that it would be keeping the Office of National AIDS Policy intact, the director position at ONAP had remained vacant. A friend of Evertz's in presidential personnel threw out his name. He was loyal, both to the president and to the secretary. He had little experience, and so would not bring an aggressive agenda or get too far out on policy. He would become the first openly gay presidential appointee, which would translate into a political coup for the administration.

In mid-April 2001, Scott Evertz became the new director of ONAP. It was not a position he had applied for. His reaction upon learning that he would be the new AIDS czar: "I was horrified!"

When Evertz arrived at the White House he had the obligatory meetings with Bush's senior domestic political advisor, Margaret Spelling, and chief of staff, Andy Card. When a State Department official came to tell him that the king of Swaziland was arriving for a visit, and that Evertz would be the first U.S. official with whom he'd meet, it seemed emblematic of the surreal position he had been thrown into.

At first, Evertz found himself spending most of his time on the domestic front. He was also directed to develop recommendations for ways in which the administration should address the global pandemic. It was a loose mandate and he was given little guidance.

The broad-based activist community had become increasingly demanding on the global front, however, so Evertz had to get up to speed fast. Politically green, Evertz hadn't come on board with an agenda, or an interest in making particular progress in one area as Thurman had. Evertz tried to take on as much as he could, doing his best to please every constituency. Without a history of relationships or great political deftness, he found it hard to navigate the inclement waters.

Over the course of his relatively brief tenure, Evertz would meet with roughly forty-five national leaders. He would hobnob with celebrities like Elton John. He accompanied Secretary Thompson on a tour of Africa and made countless appearances and speeches.

It was an exhausting period for Evertz. The demands, the criticism, and the onus—"you've been asked to help solve a pandemic!" he said—weighed heavily. Evertz never had a clear sense of mission. Finally, fifteen months into his tenure he would find the administration's bounds, by unwittingly transgressing them.

———◆———

Just as Scott Evertz was settling into his new White House office in late April 2001, scores of senior national leaders flew to Abuja, the capital of Nigeria—Africa's most populous state—for the African Summit on HIV/AIDS, Tuberculosis and Other Infectious Diseases.

Colin Powell, the administration's secretary of state and the highest-ranking African-American in U.S. history, was scheduled to represent the United States. Powell had gotten the news that Libya's notorious leader, Moammar Khadafy, would be in attendance. Bill Clinton would come as well, citing a promise he was said to have made to Nigeria's leader, Olusegun Obasanjo. Powell wasn't interested in being at the same Conference as Khadafy, and the Bush II administration certainly wasn't interested in sending their secretary of state to Africa to be upstaged by Bill Clinton. Powell canceled at the last minute. His absence kept away prominent African leaders for whom the conference's main attraction was the opportunity to get an audience with the renowned African-American statesman.

Many of the continent's leaders were there, however. UN Secretary General Kofi Annan, originally from Ghana, had come to deliver the conference's keynote address. Also in attendance was a forty-six-year-old Harvard academic with a mop of brown hair and a deep baritone voice. His name was Jeffrey Sachs, and a few years earlier The New York Times Magazine had called him "probably the most important economist in the world."

Ebullient, Sachs had arrived two days early. He was a featured speaker. Mostly, he was eager to hear his good friend Kofi Annan's address. He anticipated that it would be an historic occasion.

On April 26, 2001, the final day of the conference, Kofi Annan rose to address the assemblage of attendees. Outside, people were moving about lethargically, negotiating the ninety-five-degree heat. Inside, Jeffrey Sachs was a study in bridled enthusiasm and concentration.

AIDS had become not only the continent's single greatest cause of death, Annan told his audience, but "our biggest development challenge" as well: "And that is why I have made the battle against it my personal priority."

Annan then outlined five key objectives for combating the disease. In addition to prevention, Annan threw unequivocal support behind treatment. It was feasible and necessary, he said. Back in Washington, the Bush administration was deeply skeptical.

The secretary general then turned to the means by which he hoped the global community could achieve the ends he had highlighted. He called for leadership, resources, commitment, openness. Profound change was necessary. "It sounds a lot, and it is a lot," Annan said. But Annan had something else up his sleeve. Sachs knew it and his pulse rose as Annan neared the denouement of his address.

"I propose the creation of a Global Fund, dedicated to the battle against HIV/AIDS and other infectious diseases," Annan announced. He would call for commitments of roughly $7 to $10 billion a year from the global community.

Sachs had to wait several hours for his turn, as the conference lagged behind schedule. Finally, at 4:59, forty minutes before his flight was scheduled to depart Abuja, Obasanjo summoned the American economist to the podium.

Leaning into the microphone, Sachs exhorted his audience: "If you call for a global fund there will be a response internationally. This is the chance finally—finally to mobilize resources," he bellowed. "I have every reason to believe this effort can be won. With the resources, think of what can be done."

It was the thought that had been consuming Sachs for the better part of the last six years, ever since a 1995 trip to Lusaka, Zambia.

In 1991, Jeffrey Sachs had been a thirty-six-year-old economist with

peerless international cachet. The son of a prominent Michigan labor lawyer who fought for the downtrodden, Sachs flew through Harvard, becoming one of the university's youngest tenured professors. During the 1980s
he had been the architect of audacious economic reform programs—later
dubbed "shock therapy"—that jolted foundering economies into free markets, almost overnight. His work invariably courted controversy. But in
1991, Sachs could point to Bolivia, Poland, and other economies as dramatic success stories.

And so, when the defining political and economic transition of the age
commenced, Jeffrey Sachs was called in, tasked with the historic assignment
of transforming the former Soviet empire into a western-style free market
economy. Though Sachs was the leading western economist managing
Russia's economic transition from 1991 to 1994, he had little success in getting the Bush I and Clinton administrations, the World Bank, and the IMF
to heed his recommendations. By any economic metric, Russia's transition
was a disaster. Wherever the culpability lay, it was clear that the endeavor
had been the biggest failure that Jeffrey Sachs had ever been associated with.

The Russian debacle would have ruined most economists, but not
Sachs. By 1995, he had taken over the reins of Harvard's Institute for
International Development. Having worked in depth in South America,
Eastern Europe, and Asia, the self-described natural "comparativist" recast
his sights on a continent in desperate need of development.

The Institute at Harvard had a project under way with the Finance Ministry and Central Bank in Zambia, a nation paralyzed by acute hyperinflation in its copper industry and plagued by general macroeconomic
instability. Sachs was keen to travel to Lusaka to see for himself what was
happening.

Almost immediately upon arriving in Lusaka in the fall of 1995, Sachs
was greeted with shocking news. Eight out of the thirty Zambian professional counterparts working on the project had died of AIDS. As he asked
questions to familiarize himself with the national economy and the project,
Sachs found the discussion constantly veering back toward AIDS and the
country's health catastrophes.

Sachs was seeing it, too. He had worked in places hard hit by economic
crisis, in which life expectancies had declined to sixty years. But, in sub-
Saharan Africa in many places life expectancy was approaching forty years.
Death was unavoidable. It meant that children were dying regularly of
disease. Adults would simply not show up for work one day, never to be

heard from again. Coffin makers seemed ubiquitous and stories of funerals and family disasters were the stuff of daily conversation. "When you work in hyperinflation," Sachs said, "everybody talks about money and price exchange rates. When you work in Africa, people talk about death." Sachs had found his new mission.

For the next three years, Sachs embarked on an intellectual traverse, tackling a "very steep learning curve." He got up to speed in the rudiments of public health and epidemiology. He began to postulate that health was not merely one of many issues impeding Africa's development, but that it lay at the very center of Africa's problems. Sachs charged himself with proving his postulation, and then devising an economic strategy to combat the crisis.

After two years of research and many visits to Africa, Sachs had come to a mind-bending conclusion: he had made a grievous error. "My mistake was to believe that you couldn't have an epidemic that could be completely ignored." But that is precisely what Sachs had found. Despite the speeches by national leaders professing active involvement and alleged international financial and developmental community engagement, around 1998, Sachs had come to realize that "this fulminant pandemic [had been] utterly and completely neglected by the rich countries."

Many of the afflicted African countries were allocating only $2 or $3 per person per year for health. Some had only the shells of national health systems. The international community had done little to help. An in-depth analysis revealed that the World Bank had made only "a pittance" in loans and aid and foreign assistance.

Sachs started speaking out. The journal articles, op-ed pieces, speeches, meetings, and conferences began to increase in frequency and intensity. He knew the data and had command of all of the figures. When he tried to appeal to national and international leaders, however, his words met a stiff wall of indifference.

In 1999, WHO Director General Gro Harlem Brundtland asked Sachs to chair a new task force at WHO entitled the Commission on Macroeconomics and Health. It was to be a two-year commission investigating the relationship between health and economic development, now—in part thanks to Sachs's advocacy—a high-profile issue. The appointment placed Sachs at the vanguard of both international health and international development, and made him the world's leading authority among those interested in understanding the nexus between the two. The position gave

Sachs a seat at the table. It also helped further solidify his relationship with leading international figures like UN Secretary General Kofi Annan.

The dynamics and aims governing Sachs's advocacy differed from those of his colleagues in international bureaucracy, national governments, or even in the nongovernmental sector. They were beholden to institutions, governments, bosses, crosscutting interests, agendas, and egos. Sachs, in contrast, was "not negotiating with them . . . I'm not a legislator. I'm not in the executive branch. I'm an academic. My job, I've always believed, is to tell the truth, as closely and as actively as I possibly can. . . . I just tell them that something needs to get done . . . and if you don't do it, you're going to leave millions of people dying and I'm going to do my best to make that clear to the world."

At the International AIDS Conference in Durban, South Africa, in mid-July 2000, Sachs would lend the force of his intellect and personality to a novel idea.

Addressing a capacity crowd of thousands, Sachs used a ten-page Power-Point presentation to outline his key points. He opened his remarks by explaining that health crises besieging the world's poorest countries had helped consign them to "a poverty trap" from which they did not have the resources to rescue themselves. The international donor community and international institutions had failed to meet the challenge.

What was needed, Sachs exclaimed—nine months before Annan's announcement at Abuja—was a "Global Fund." The fund had three basic architectural features.

It would be a *global* vehicle, comprising a pool of capital donated by the international donor community, public and private alike.

Proposals for projects would be originated at the local and national levels. Instead of a boilerplate approach, projects would be "sensitive to the ecological, epidemiological, and social context of each situation." This would also encourage self-sufficiency.

Finally, there would be an expert panel that would "review, monitor, and evaluate" incoming proposals for funding. Sachs hoped to reenfranchise the scientific community in the policy making process. An independent review board allocating a pool of resources would also help extricate national politics out of the disbursal process, helping to ensure that projects would be accepted based primarily on merit and need.

Sachs then went on to lambaste the international donor community. In light of the magnitude of the crisis, he exclaimed, "donor support for disease control [has been] shockingly small, and therefore in need of a substantial increase."

"Sub-Saharan Africa will require approximately $10 billion per year of donor support to mobilize an effective response," Sachs maintained. Based on its share of the global GDP, the implied U.S. contribution came out to roughly $3 billion. Total U.S. funding for global HIV/AIDS in 2001 had finally reached $450 million after having been flatlined for most of the 1990s. Now Sachs was calling for a sevenfold increase—immediately. Critics decried Sachs's proposal as unrealistic. Such lofty numbers would impugn their credibility. It couldn't be done.

Nonsense, Sachs answered back. He was calling for $3 billion per year from the wealthiest and mightiest power in world history. The commitment would mean that the United States would spend .04 percent of U.S. GDP. Measured against millions and millions of deaths per year, it was nothing. It was little more than $10 per American—less than the price of a movie ticket and popcorn.

No one had put it like that before. Former CDC director Bill Foege believed that Sachs's entry into the mix transformed the complexion of the advocacy effort: "He has gotten people thinking in a different league. Most of us have been willing to accept marginal increases in funding, and he says that isn't right."

Critics remained skeptical and resentful. It was easy to cast Sachs as a self-promoting academic, appointing himself as the leader of a crusade that others had started. Post-Russia, Sachs's star was in need of an image makeover, and speaking out on behalf of the world's most downtrodden and marginalized was the perfect way to do it.

Others like Foege and Harvard infectious-disease specialist Jim Yong Kim sensed that Sachs was beginning to orchestrate something extraordinary. By raising the bar of expectations, he was jump-starting the tectonic plates undergirding the world's response into motion.

"If we didn't have Jeff Sachs," Kim said, "we would have to invent him. Right now, he is among the most important people ever—historically—for the health of poor people."

Criticism was hardly foreign to Sachs. He was undeterred: "I know that some of these numbers start outlandishly high—but I've had the fortunate experience in my life to say things that people think are impossible and to see them come to fruition afterwards. . . . I've seen many times what is called the impossible become logical and inevitable."

---·◆·---

Jeffrey Sachs wasn't the only player to whom the idea of a fund to combat the pandemic had occurred.

In the waning months of the Clinton administration, Ken Bernard and a Nancy Pelosi staffer named Chris Collins had been working on a fund that would collect billions of donor dollars to create a market to encourage pharmaceutical companies to develop vaccines for HIV/AIDS, tuberculosis, and malaria. Similarly, Representative Barbara Lee was pushing the idea of a fund housed at the World Bank. Both efforts fizzled, but were not forgotten.

Shortly after Sachs's speech at Durban, Ken Bernard and other senior health officials from the world's wealthiest countries convened over a several-day period at Okinawa after the 2000 G8 Summit. The senior government officials agreed that a new global fund might be an effective vehicle to launch a multilateral assault on the pandemic. Okinawa brought the concept of a global fund from Sachs's pronouncement onto the desks of the world's leading officials.

As the idea dragged along through the summer, fall, and winter and through a contentious presidential election in the United States, Secretary General Kofi Annan was getting anxious. He was increasingly committed to the cause, and increasingly convinced that the UN system had to demonstrate leadership to jump-start the international response.

As chair of the WHO Commission on Macroeconomics and Health, Sachs was an official member of the UN system, and was becoming an important advisor to the secretary general. Together with Peter Piot, executive director of UNAIDS, RP Eddy, Annan's new senior advisor on AIDS, and senior UN officials like Louise Frechette, deputy secretary general and Mark Malloch Brown, administrator of the UN Development Program, or UNDP, Sachs worked diligently to add flesh to the idea of a global fund.

In March 2001, just one month before Abuja, Annan met with President Bush and broached the global fund idea. Bush later said that at that March meeting in the White House, he had agreed in concept to the creation of the fund, which the G8 had already been "discussing." Several of the G8 countries were not yet ready, and the global fund was still very much an abstraction, when Annan formally "proposed" the creation of the Global Fund in Abuja in April 2001.

The secretary general had presented the international donor community with a challenge and a vehicle. It needed institutional flesh and bones. Most of all it needed funding. All eyes turned to the United States.

If it appeared as if the new Bush administration was not particularly interested in global AIDS, a series of factors and events had led the administration to do an about-face on the issue. There was the February backlash from activists angry at the White House announcement that ONAP was closing.

Then, on June 7, 2001, Andrew Natsios, an international development veteran who had just been confirmed as the new USAID administrator, testified before the International Relations Committee of the House of Representatives on AIDS in Africa. He painted an abject portrait of Africa. Natsios hammered home the point that Africa had scant infrastructure and "capacity." He testified that even if drugs were made available, they would be hard to deliver and administer. In a point he would come to regret making, Natsios told Congress that administering the drug regiments would be a problem because many Africans "do not know what watches or clocks are."

Months later Natsios was scheduled to meet with Secretary General Kofi Annan at the United Nations. Annan, RP Eddy recalled, arrived forty-five minutes late to the meeting. "I'm sorry," the world's leading diplomat and Nobel winner feigned apology, "I've been having trouble telling time."

Many felt that the comments had a racial undertone. Several advocacy organizations and members of Congress, like Maxine Waters, called for Natsios's resignation. The episode was an embarrassment for the administration. It had become clear that AIDS would be one of the hot-button issues upon which Bush's merit as a "compassionate" conservative would be judged.

Early in 2001, Jeffrey Sachs requested a meeting with Condoleezza Rice, Bush's national security advisor. Rice, the former provost of Stanford University, was an old academic colleague Sachs had been acquainted with for years. The national security advisor, whose foreign policy speeches and essays showed little sign of suggesting that global AIDS was a prominent consideration, or much of a consideration at all, agreed to meet with Sachs.

"This is an emergency and there are ways to address it," Sachs told Rice at their White House meeting. "It is financially feasible to do, morally necessary to do, and politically smart to do," Sachs said of upgrading the U.S. response in dollars and to include treatment as well as prevention. Rice was "noncommittal," but listened closely and assured him that, "the president was interested."

Rice had enlisted her friend Jendayi Frazier as NSC Director for African Affairs. Frazier, also an African-American woman, and a former professor at the JFK School of Government at Harvard, was well attuned to the issue and sympathetic. Internally, she pushed Rice further along on the issue.

Then, shortly after Annan's announcement, prominent GOP senator from Tennessee and administration favorite Bill Frist made a trip to the White House to urge the president to assume leadership on the issue and specifically to support the Global Fund. There was also Annan's March 2001 White House meeting.

Interest and advocacy were percolating in a number of corners. Early stumbling had helped earmark global AIDS as one of the issues upon which the administration's moral leadership would be defined. And the president was digesting the magnitude of the crisis.

On the morning of May 11, 2001, in a special ceremony in the White House Rose Garden held in conjunction with a state visit from Nigerian President Olusegun Obasanjo, President Bush took to the lectern to address a crowd of reporters and senior government officials. With Bill Frist, Colin Powell, Tommy Thompson, and Obasanjo standing behind him, and Condoleezza Rice, Kofi Annan, and other senior dignitaries in the audience, the president lamented that the global AIDS crisis had reached a point "almost beyond comprehension. . . . We have the power to help," the president said.

The Global Fund was still merely a theory. It did not even have a bank account. Nevertheless, Bush announced that the United States would be the first to make a contribution, pledging $200 million. The pledge breathed life into the Global Fund.

The president called it a "beginning." Frist was publicly supportive, agreeing that the initial commitment constituted "a spark which will ignite a flame."

Still, it was billions per year short of what Sachs, Annan, and the rest of the fund's supporters were hoping for. To skeptical activists it seemed an empty maneuver, window dressing for an administration more concerned about its image than waging a battle against the pandemic. A group of roughly sixty protestors marched in a circle outside the gates of the White

House during the Rose Garden ceremony, chanting, "Tax cuts for billion-aires, nothing left for AIDS." Washington advocate Salih Booker agreed, telling John Donnelly, "Tomorrow's headlines ought to read, 'President Bush to Africa: Drop Dead.' "

Jeffrey Sachs's response was measured. He reportedly applauded the president's pledge as a "beginning" and the activists' exhortations for a greater commitment.

In the months following Bush's Rose Garden announcement, a series of factors and events helped stoke the expectations surrounding the Global Fund. The world-famous technology titan Bill Gates pledged an additional $100 million to the fund. With a stroke of the pen, Gates had pledged an amount equaling 50 percent of the U.S. government commitment.

In June 2001, the United Nations held a special session in the General Assembly on AIDS. It was the first special session of the UN General Assembly, or UNGASS, on one specific health threat. For three days the most high-profile forum in the world debated AIDS. National leaders came to address the pandemic and speak to their countries' commitment. There were roughly two thousand civil servants there. "For two to three weeks," UN official Ben Plumley said, "the GA and the UN itself was completely taken over by AIDS."

It was at the UNGASS session that African leaders began to emerge in a chorus, pleading for U.S. and international help in combating the pandemic. African leader after African leader rose to speak out on the horrors besieging their countries, and—even as they pledged to mobilize domestic resources and leadership—their sense of helplessness. The Global Fund became the vehicle they rallied behind.

Insiders from the UN system and national representatives were pleased about the momentum behind the fund. The attendant expectations, though, represented a daunting challenge. At a subsequent G8 meeting in Genoa, Italy, in July 2001, international donors made hundreds of millions of dollars in additional pledges. International enthusiasm was clearly percolating. Still, there was a problem: The Global Fund did not yet exist.

In the months following Annan's bold proposal at Abuja, senior UN officials and national representatives labored feverishly behind the scenes to give life to the concept. In August 2001, Annan named former Ugandan minister of health Crispus Kiyonga to run a Transitional Working Group to design and build consensus on the institutional and operational framework of the fund.

In its abstraction, the Global Fund had enjoyed popularity and lofty expectations. In short order, though, the idea was thrown into the more prob-
lematic realm of international policy making. UN officials and national
representatives gathered in several successions of three-to-four-day meetings to deliberate upon the details of the fund's institutional and operational design. Disagreement broke out immediately over where the fund's
secretariat would be based. Several European Union members wanted the
fund's home to be in Brussels. Others insisted that it be in Paris, or in
Geneva, closer to UNAIDS, WHO, and the rest of the UN system. Eventually, Geneva was named the fund's home.

Some, like Jeffrey Sachs, thought that the fund should be housed at
WHO. But the United States insisted that it be a separate, independent
entity, stressing the importance of "monitoring and evaluation." If the fund
was going to succeed in the long term, it needed to demonstrate efficacy.
Money needed to be well spent, and results had to be, as much as possible,
measured and proven.

By the Global Fund's first board meeting in January 2002, its basic archi-
tecture was in place. It would be an independent entity aimed at attracting
capital from international donors, both public and private, and disbursing
that money to fight HIV/AIDS, TB, and malaria. Sachs's three main features were fleshed out, refined, and incorporated.

First, project proposals would be originated at the national and local
levels. As Sachs had intended, projects would be customized and sensitive
to local needs. It also placed the initiative with the affected locales, a critical first step in promoting self-sufficiency and responsibility.

Second, its governing board had broad-based international representa-
tion, including representatives from the developed world and the nongovernmental sector. Grants were not subject to national strategic and
economic interests or relationships, or cultural or religious particularities.
This meant, for example, that if Cuba or North Korea submitted sound
grant proposals, those projects would go through, despite U.S. political
qualms. It also meant that the preference for abstinence-only initiatives,
distinct from those including condom distribution, often driven in part by
religious doctrine, would not override the fund's grant making. Of course,
national interests would factor in, but the fund had done its best to strip
politics and ideology out of the way, paving the way for a needs-based
grant-making capability.

Finally, the fund relied on an expert review panel to assess project proposals. The panel set a high bar for grant applications, aiming to ensure that those who applied were capable—had the resources, expertise, and credibility—of enacting their proposals, whether to provide ARVs to a local population, build hospitals and orphanages for care and treatment, or to promote prevention through condom distribution or awareness campaigns. The expert review panel would help ensure that corruption, mismanagement, and inefficiency—key U.S. concerns—were kept to a minimum. In addition, the fund enlisted private partners to perform disbursal, monitoring, and evaluation, helping further ensure that funds were being well spent.

What had been created was an international grant-making institution unlike anything that had ever existed. UN Special Envoy for HIV/AIDS Stephen Lewis remarked to senior fund advisor, Anil Soni, "The Global Fund is the most important thing that has happened to overseas developmental assistance since the creation of the World Bank, since the end of World War II." Not only was the Global Fund charged with leading the global fight against the AIDS pandemic, it had become a prototype for a new brand of international institution—independent, apolitical, results-and-performance-based, and sensitive to national and local particularities.

From January 2002, the Secretariat of the Global Fund moved at a frenetic pace to put its operational framework in place. Richard Feachem, a longtime British public health official with extensive academic and programmatic expertise, was selected as the fund's executive director in April and came on board formally in July. By then, the fund had already received four hundred project proposals for its first funding round. Without a permanent team of employees, the Secretariat scurried to institute the review panel to evaluate the incoming proposals.

When the dust had cleared, the review panel had approved just under sixty proposals valued at roughly $1.6 billion over five years. The board committed to two years of funding, which translated into about $600 million of actual commitments, with the rest conditional upon performance. By the time the fund entertained its second round in the summer of 2002, there were $5 billion in eligible requests. They expected their third round in the fall of 2003 to yield an even larger amount.

By its second round of funding, it was clear that the fund had upped the ante. National and local actors were responding. Paul Zeitz, formerly a USAID official, had since left Zambia to begin the Global AIDS Alliance, an activist organization mobilized to upgrade the world response. Very active in Washington, Zeitz was still in touch with friends and colleagues back in Zambia. After the fund's creation, he was noticing remarkable changes in-country: "On the recipient side . . . as the Global Fund requests for proposals went out to the country level, it was like real money was out on the table and it catalyzed innovation and catalyzed a response. I got calls from friends in Zambia, saying it was the first time we all sat together and worked on a common strategic plan."

However, the eligible project funding requested far dwarfed the amount the international donor community had pledged to the fund, which threatened to deplete the very momentum and credibility upon which the fund depended.

Predictably, bureaucratic and turf wars started to surface. Though many in the UN system had developed a fresh appreciation for the urgency and magnitude of the threat, "there is still territoriality and pride and all the other things that happen with human beings," one senior official at the fund said. "It's like a twenty-way tug of war." Competition and a lack of co-operation, most notably with the World Bank, slowed the fund's momentum. And while WHO and UNAIDS had been cooperative, many officials worried about their roles in the wake of the fund's emergence.

The challenges were monumental. But so was the opportunity. For the first time in the history of the pandemic, the world had a credible and independent global vehicle with which to battle the pandemic head-on. The fund had ignited the imagination of both African leaders and the international community. It was inchoate and unproven. But it was also ambitious and responsive.

As with the international institutions and vehicles that had come before, the fund's efficacy and vitality would be a function primarily of the commitment and will of its leading sponsors and donors. As it had each time before, the eyes of the international community turned to the United States.

———— ◆ ————

By the early summer of 2002, President Bush was keenly aware of the new Global Fund. When Scott Evertz was called in to the Oval Office to meet with the president, he anticipated that the meeting would be short and he would do most of the talking. Instead, the president launched into a revealing pep talk. "He explained how important this was to him," Evertz said, "how he recognized that it's not getting the attention it should, but that he was very committed to this and wanted to make sure that [the fund] would work." Evertz remembered the president's directive as something to the effect of: "There are a lot of loud voices around this issue, but you just remain focused and try to ignore all of it. . . . You help Secretary Thompson make sure it works, so we can do what I said we would do which is to commit more U.S. funds when this thing proves successful."

If the president had done a 180-degree turn on global AIDS a year and a half into his administration, no administration official had done more to affect the president's position than the venerated sixty-four-year-old general turned secretary of state, Colin Powell.

Powell was raised in the Bronx, New York, by immigrant parents from Jamaica. His ascent to the third highest-ranking position in the U.S. government constitutes one of America's all-time great success stories. With roughly thirty-five years of military experience, tours in Vietnam, and stints as Reagan's national security advisor and the first President Bush's chairman of the Joint Chiefs of Staff as well as commander of the U.S. military during the Persian Gulf War, no American leader had more stature in 2000 than Colin Powell.

Bush secured a boon for his presidential candidacy when Powell agreed to sign on as his future secretary of state. He brought experience and gravitas, assuaging concern among many in the electorate about the governor's shaky footing on foreign affairs.

In short order, though, Powell seemed more on the fringe of the administration's foreign policy deliberations than at its center. Bush had an unusually close relationship to his vice president, Dick Cheney, a hard-line neoconservative. It was widely reported that Cheney grew wary of his former colleague during Powell's first remarks as secretary in which he spoke mostly in the first person and made scant reference to the president. Cheney worried that Powell would be Powell first, and the president's man second. Bush's particularly close personal and professional relationship with Condoleezza Rice—whose office was just down the hall from the Oval Office and who shuttled in and out of his office many times per day—further pressed Powell to the margin.

Powerful leadership from Secretary of Defense Donald Rumsfeld and the unilateral, neoconservative proclivities of his deputy Paul Wolfowitz had a big impact, further diluting Powell's influence. Powell's worldview stood in marked distinction from neocons like Cheney, Rumsfeld, and Wolfowitz. He was an internationalist, strongly favoring multilateral approaches when possible. He believed that modernity and globalization meant that every corner of the globe held strategic significance for the United States and that as the world's greatest power, the United States had to be active and engaged.

Driven in part by his sense of U.S. priorities, the secretary spent a significant portion of his time during the transition seeking briefings on Africa. He had visited the continent a few years earlier, and its problems and challenges had made a big impression. Powell had acknowledged that his roots were in Africa, and he held the continent in special regard. There was also the matter of Bush's unfortunate comments during the presidential election in which he awkwardly managed to downgrade Africa, suggesting it did not fit in the bounds of the U.S. national strategic interest. Powell would have some diplomatic fence-mending to do.

Cheney, Rumsfeld, and Rice—the three other loud voices on foreign policy—showed little interest in the continent. Powell was not prepared to allow Africa to drift into the nether regions of obscurity on the U.S. agenda.

The new secretary of state was aware of the AIDS situation in Africa prior to his briefings, but when the State Department's senior official on Global AIDS, Jack Chow, briefed the secretary, the magnitude of the crisis in Africa was brought into even greater focus. Powell had spent much of his time out of government during the 1990s chairing a not-for-profit devoted to the advancement and well-being of America's youth. Estimates of up to 14 million AIDS orphans did not sit well with the former general.

By 2001, global AIDS had been injected onto the media radar screen. Though it struggled for attention and priority amidst a long list of favored crises, conflicts, and news items, the issue would not disappear again. And so, during Powell's first televised interview as secretary of state on February 4, 2001, on ABC's This Week with Sam Donaldson and Cokie Roberts, Roberts asked the new secretary if he shared his predecessor's view that global AIDS was in fact a "national security problem."

Without missing a beat Powell responded, "AIDS is a national security problem; it's an economic problem; it is a devastating problem, especially in Africa. . . . It is a pandemic and it requires our attention." In an interview on the Jim Lehrer NewsHour two months later, Powell was asked the same question, and gave almost the same exact answer.

At the State Department, Powell upgraded the issue in priority almost immediately. He promoted Jack Chow to ambassador status and built out his office. "I was a one-man show and now I have a fully operational office," Chow explained, shortly after the promotion. The secretary spoke of global AIDS often at his daily 8:30 morning meetings at State. He highlighted the issue for his new assistant secretary of state for African Affairs, Walter Kansteiner—a former NSC official who had also been a businessman with industrial connections in Africa—as one of his top five priorities for the region.

During a twenty-minute telephone conversation with Powell in early 2001, it was clear to Jeffrey Sachs that the secretary was "sympathetic." Powell wanted to do his part. But he had proposed a relatively modest 10 percent increase in funding in the State budget. He was skeptical of how far the issue would move in the administration. When Sachs spoke of the need for billions of new dollars, he remembered Powell saying, "It's going to be very hard to get that amount of money."

While Powell publicly called for a global "full-scale assault" on the pandemic, he did not launch his own "full-scale assault" back in Washington. Powell, it appeared, was straddling the fine line between the loyal soldier serving "at the pleasure of the president"—a refrain he would repeat often—and advocate for a worthy cause.

Then in late May 2001, Powell left for a four-country tour of Africa. As it had for so many key players before—Thurman, Holbrooke, and Sachs—the trip would have a profound impact on him.

From the outset, it was clear that this was not the run-of-the-mill diplomatic tour. On the flight from Washington to Mali, Powell confided to journalists on board that he felt "an emotional twinge" when he thought about venturing to Africa.

Upon arriving on the continent and throughout his trip, Powell was given a hero's welcome. "As [the secretary] traveled from site to site, local people told him of the pride they felt in him, and the hope he brought as a black leader," recalled journalist Ben Barber.

The secretary had made sure to schedule AIDS events in each of the countries he visited. In Nairobi, the capital of Kenya, Powell and his wife, Alma, attended an AIDS awareness demonstration at a clinic at the edge of the notorious Kibera slums. Powell was greeted by a beautiful young child bearing bright flowers. The child, Powell was told, had AIDS. The Powells watched as young girls "act[ed] out ways to resist having unprotected sex."

Later at that same event, Powell and his wife shared an encounter with a forty-nine-year-old woman who explained that she had been HIV-positive for nine years. She had lost her husband and her six-year-old son. "It was difficult to see the young boy die," she wept. "Instead of giving my children life, I gave them HIV. I live with the guilt that I infected my own child."

On that same trip at a clinic in the remote hills and valleys of the infamous Soweto Township in South Africa, Powell spoke with AIDS orphans. In Soweto, the secretary also met an HIV-positive woman named Florence. Her child, also HIV-positive, had been placed in her in-laws' care. After her child died of AIDS, her in-laws refused to inform her of her own child's death. When they finally told her, they castigated her and insisted that she did not even deserve to go to the funeral.

"I see you as a role model," she told Powell. "You have come to show us the light even though you have not brought us anything. Your visit means a lot to us." To the proud and empathetic military man, the words must have stung: "even though you have not brought us anything." Months earlier Powell had told a congressional committee: "I can assure you that Africa will not be a photo-op foreign policy matter for this administration."

The pandemic came alive for Powell during the course of his African tour. During the trip, the secretary of state proffered the strongest public statements of any sitting senior U.S. leader: "Even though there are wars in other parts of the world, even though there's a crisis in the Middle East, even though people are dying in these conflicts around the world, there's no war more serious, there's no war causing more death or destruction, there's no war on the face of this earth that is more grave than the war we see here in sub-Saharan Africa against HIV/AIDS."

The secretary echoed a familiar refrain: "You don't really get a full appreciation until you see the people who are stricken. I hope I can convey the passion of what I've seen." Powell pledged that he would "go back and make a case in Washington of the need for more resources."

At the UNGASS session on global AIDS in June 2001 in New York, Powell's remarks demonstrated that his pronouncements in Africa were not just sentimental. He declared: there is "no enemy in war more insidious than AIDS."

• • •

On September 10, 2001, *Time* magazine ran a cover story entitled "Odd Man Out." With a barrage of comments and quotes from key insiders and luminaries in the foreign policy establishment, the extended piece portrayed Powell on the fringe of the administration's foreign policy team. The story detailed the schism in worldview and policy between the State Department and the Pentagon and listed the travails that had beset Powell during the first two hundred days of the administration. But "Powell has certainly had his successes," the article allowed. "The White House lets him run free on Africa and AIDS." He was carrying the administration's water, true to his pledge in Africa.

The issue had picked up a surprising degree of traction in the administration's first two hundred days. The Office of National AIDS Policy had been salvaged and the administration had appointed Scott Evertz director. The USTR pledged that it would not rescind Clinton's executive order not to pursue punitive measures against developing countries pursuing affordable AIDS drugs. U.S. funding had increased by several hundred million dollars. The administration had played a key role in endorsing, establishing, and sponsoring the new Global Fund. And now, those pressing the issue could count the administration's most publicly venerated official an ally.

Most activists, like Paul Zeitz, who were pessimistic in the early days of the administration, were buoyed by the positive developments. "We thought we were riding a momentum wave," Zeitz said. Advocate Terje Anderson similarly recalled some of the positive developments. The issue was gaining momentum, "but then 9/11 happened and everything froze."

Terrorists had hijacked four American commercial aircrafts, turning, in one staggering sweep of madness, America's bearings in the world on its head. As the smoldering rubble was cleared from Ground Zero in lower Manhattan, the United States faced a new world of grave peril and profound uncertainty. With a serious economic recession, a prodigious tax cut, an ambitious war on terrorism, and two impending wars, the prognosis for "peripheral" or "long-term" issues like global AIDS suddenly seemed dire.

That's not the way Colin Powell saw it, though. Less than a week after 9/11, still processing the catastrophic attack and struggling to devise a path forward, Powell carved time out of his day to meet with his ambassador on global AIDS and the Global Fund's new temporary director. He wanted an update on the Global Fund. He also had a message for Jack Chow and Crispus Kiyonga: "Regardless of what happened last week, you guys have to drive ahead and create this Global Fund."

Unaware of Powell's behind-the-scenes advocacy, the activist community grew despondent, assuming that the crises would consign global AIDS to a subaltern position on the administration's agenda. Almost no one imagined, in those dark days, that they would have the very opposite effect.

—⁓—

FOURTEEN

Righting the Response, Getting Religion

In the tumultuous months following September 11, the Bush administration became consumed with ridding Afghanistan of the Taliban and implanting a new stable regime in its place. The task of restructuring much of the U.S. federal government to enhance domestic security, a demanding diplomatic agenda, an economic recession, and escalating concern over Iraq, Iran, and North Korea also helped saturate the new administration's agenda in the aftermath of the attacks.

For many, the attacks triggered an impulse to pull back from American commitments abroad, to erect walls and barriers. For others, they demonstrated that America's fate could not be extricated from even the most remote corner of the globe. The attacks summoned America to wake from the insularity and slumber of the 1990s to consider the world anew.

The final death toll for 9/11 came out at around 3,000 lives. It was one of the deadliest days in the republic's history. It struck some that at the same time global AIDS was taking roughly 8,000 lives—nearly three times 9/11's death toll—every day. They were not prepared to let that catastrophe drift off the policy screen, the critical demands of the moment notwithstanding.

In the year following the attacks on America, a remarkable cast of players and an unlikely series of events generated a powerful groundswell of interest in the pandemic.

At a luncheon on February 20, 2002, roughly five months after 9/11, Jesse Helms, the powerful senator from North Carolina who was entering the thirtieth and final year of his career in the U.S. Senate, addressed a crowd of hundreds of Christian AIDS activists at the Prescription for Hope conference organized by Franklin Graham, the son of the evangelist Reverend Billy Graham. In the preceding years and months, Graham's leading faith-based organization Samaritan's Purse had become increasingly committed to mobilizing U.S. engagement in global AIDS. Missionaries were coming back from Africa with wrenching descriptions of a holocaust. Leading voices and core faith-based communities had gravitated toward the issue. Their faith demanded that they help.

These were Helms's people. They spoke the same language—both religious and political. Helms's words at the conference were among the most startling and powerful in the history of the U.S. response.

"I'm so ashamed I've done so little," Helms said of his record on global AIDS. "I will do better than I have done in the past and I will work together with you." It was a decidedly unexpected mea culpa from a perennial adversary of U.S. funding for global AIDS. Helms's remarks were big stories in *The Washington Post* and *The New York Times*.

On March 24, 2002, Helms wrote an op-ed piece published by *The Washington Post*, "We Cannot Turn Away." The article called for an additional U.S. commitment of $500 million to "eliminate, or nearly eliminate" mother-to-child transmission, still the safest area of focus for Helms. "In the end," Helms concluded in the op-ed, "our conscience is answerable to God. Perhaps, in my eighty-first year, I am too mindful of soon meeting Him, but I know, like the Samaritan traveling from Jerusalem to Jericho, we cannot turn away when we see our fellow man in need."

Many were skeptical. Some were enthused. Almost all were shocked, and wondered just what—or who—had brought about Helms's volte-face.

The senator attributed his awakening to three people. The first was his "dearest" friend Franklin Graham, who had framed the necessity for assistance in moralistic Christian terms. The second was Secretary General Kofi Annan, who in the course of private conversations had stressed the macabre impact that the disease was having on the already struggling African continent. There was one more, though, and he was a little different. He was an Irish rock star and his name was Bono.

In 1984, an erstwhile little known Irish band named U2 released an album entitled *The Joshua Tree*. The album was a mega-hit, and it catapulted the band to superstardom. For the band's lead singer, a young man from Dublin named Paul Hewson, though better known as Bono, music had always been a window into, and a mouthpiece with which to express, the social condition. When Irish punk rock star Bob Geldof asked the band to come and perform at Live Aid, a concert bringing together stars to raise money to combat famine in Ethiopia, the band eagerly accepted. After the concert, Bono and his wife, Allison Stewart, ventured to Ethiopia for about a month to volunteer, and to see for themselves what was happening.

In the decade and a half to follow, the charismatic front man and his band became one of the most popular groups in the history of rock and roll, releasing a string of hit albums in which they were able to refashion their sound time and again, all the while remaining popular and relevant.

In the summer of 1998, Jamie Drummond, an Irishman who had been working for years on a debt relief campaign for countries in the developing world, was looking for a public face for his campaign. Drummond got in touch with Mark Marot, who worked at Bono's music label, and Chris Blackwell, an Englishman who had signed U2. His contacts told him they would try, but they couldn't promise anything.

In the late summer of 1998, when the global markets were in a tailspin, Drummond's phone rang. "Hello, Jamie. This is Bono," the voice on the other end said. "I suppose your debt relief campaign is not going to do well because of the crisis in Southeast Asia," the voice continued.

"I thought it was the guy from downstairs trying to take the mickey out of me," Drummond said later. Then he realized that it was Bono and that he was asking a pertinent question. And he was very serious.

Vast wealth and fame now afforded the singer a chance to engage in the social issues in which he had long demonstrated an interest. Bono and his new compatriots on the debt relief campaign—known as Jubilee 2000—recognized that it was imperative to bring the United States to the table. Bono called Bobby Shriver, a record-producing Kennedy scion who had vast connections in the political and financial worlds. The two agreed to partner up to force political movement on U.S. debt relief.

Bono was not interested in being yet another celebrity activist making self-righteous, sanctimonious speeches. He decided that if he was going to get involved, he wanted to learn about the issues in depth, to be well informed on the nuances of policy.

The rock star was in the market for a teacher. There just happened to be an economics professor in Cambridge, Massachusetts, who had long been speaking out on debt relief and development. With an entree from

Shriver, Bono called Jeffrey Sachs. He requested a meeting and further asked that Sachs invite a conservative colleague, so that he might hear the other side of the argument. It was the beginning of a personal friendship as well as a humanitarian odyssey. The tale might be entitled, "The Education of a Rock Star," or perhaps "The Miseducation of a Harvard Professor."

Delivering the Class Day Address to Harvard's graduating class of 2001, Bono reminisced: "Jeffrey Sachs not only let me into his office, he let me into his Rolodex, his head, and his life for the past few years. So, in a sense he let me into your life here at Harvard. A student again."

Armed with a first-rate education and access to the world's best minds, Bono set his sights on Washington. All told, he and his partner Shriver made fourteen visits to Washington through the end of 2000, pounding the halls of Congress and the Clinton White House. Bono's activism helped press rich countries to agree to waive $20–30 billion in poor country debt. On the back end of Jubilee 2000, Sachs—who was doing much thinking about the issue as chair of the WHO Commission on Macroeconomics and Health—began pointing Bono toward AIDS. Late in 2000, Bono, Shriver, and Drummond founded DATA, a new advocacy organization promoting debt relief, aid for Africa, trade reform—and AIDS.

In March 2001, Bono met with the new secretary of state, Colin Powell. He presented the secretary with a signed note from one of Powell's heroes, former Secretary of State George Marshall. Just as his hero had mobilized a multibillion-dollar effort to save Europe after the war, this was Powell's chance, Bono lobbied, to initiate a Powell Plan for Africa.

Just months before his meeting with Powell, U2 released an album entitled *All That You Can't Leave Behind*. It was the most heralded album of the year. It received eight Grammy nominations and won the award for best rock album. Bono's public star had never shone brighter. He parlayed his celebrity into access. He became a fixture at international events like the World Economic Forum. He could be found sharing a table or even a dais with the likes of Bill Clinton, Bill Gates, or George Soros.

In the midst of their strategic deliberations, Bono, Shriver, and Drummond had gleaned a critical insight into U.S. political advocacy for the developing world. It was usually the conservatives who were opposed to funding for international aid or global AIDS, they knew. Yet faith and religion played a very strong role in most conservatives' thinking. "Pointing out that discrepancy and appealing to that religious conviction and then the religious right is a way to change things more than just appealing to the usual base of liberal Democrats who care about these issues," said Drummond.

Bono "is also a Christian and serious about it, without being tedious about it. . . . That means he can appeal to something which is not very European, but is very American." The team was armed not only with Bono's cachet and celebrity, but with what Drummond called the "greatest marketing book" of all time: the Bible.

Jesse Helms was not a big U2 fan. In fact, he had never heard of the band. Bono and Shriver estimated that if they could appeal to Helms, the sky would be the limit. In the summer of 2001, Helms met with Bono. The meeting went on for two hours. Helms was floored by his unusual visitor. During the meeting at the senator's office, Helms said later, in his February 2002 luncheon speech, "Bono told me there were 2002 verses in the Bible instructing us to help our fellow man."

In June 2001, Helms hosted a lunch for Bono at the Senate Foreign Relations reception room in the Capitol. With Bill Frist, Pat Leahy, and other senators looking on, Helms welcomed Bono. "You'll never be an outsider. You'll always be a friend here," Helms said, shaking the singer's hand.

The U2 front man called Helms "a brave and bold man" for inviting him to the lunch. "It's an extraordinary thing, I will admit, to have Jesse Helms throw a lunch for you," Bono said. "You know," he added with a grin, "it's a bad thing for both of our images."

Helms seemed to relish the new attachment to the star as well as the kudos for the reversal of his stand that would come in February 2002. Clearly, Helms was thinking about his legacy as well as his own mortality. But if image and political considerations were part of the equation, Helms's expression of remorse over his position and his willingness to up his commitment were real. After attending a U2 concert with his grandkids, Helms conceded that his grandchildren seemed to be enjoying the music more than he. He wasn't necessarily a big fan of Bono as a musician, he said, but he was a big fan of Bono as a man.

Helms's newfound interest in the issue translated into legislative initiative in the spring of 2002 with the proposal of his co-sponsored $500 million Supplemental Bill for reducing mother-to-child transmission. Of even greater importance, perhaps, was the symbolic value from Helms's high profile and vehement reversal. With Helms, the biggest and most obstinate domino had fallen. Others would follow.

• • •

On March 4, 2002, the cover of *Time* magazine featured a picture of Bono wearing his trademark tinted sunglasses and pulling open his jacket to show its American flag lining. The cover read: "Can Bono Save the World? Don't laugh—the globe's biggest rock star is on a mission to make a difference." A few months earlier U2 had performed at the Super Bowl, playing songs from *All That You Can't Leave Behind*. The CD's evocative hit single "Walk On" became something of an anthem for a country still grieving after the attacks on 9/11. At forty-one he was at the crest of his fame and influence.

Three months later, in July 2001 at the G8 Summit in Genoa, Italy, Bono met with Condoleezza Rice, the president's national security advisor. A concert-level pianist, Rice was also relatively close to Bono in age and decidedly hipper than the retiring senator from North Carolina. Rice's specialty was the former Soviet Union and Russia. She saw the world primarily through the lens of Great Power conflict and a "hard" "politico-military" U.S. national interest calculus—at least before 9/11.

In an essay in *Foreign Affairs* during the presidential campaign in 2000, Rice chided those who she thought fatuously co-joined "humanitarian interests" with the "national interest." "To be sure," she wrote, "there is nothing wrong with doing something that benefits all humanity, but that is, in a sense, a second-order effect." She wished to refocus the country on a taut interest-based foreign policy. Things like nation-building and humanitarian intervention diverted the United States from a more focused national mission.

By the time she met with Bono in Genoa, 9/11 had helped expand Rice's conception of the national interest. Terrorists had secured harbor and autonomy in Afghanistan, demonstrating that state weakness, in a monumental historical shift, was now a greater threat to U.S. security than state strength. Bono argued that U.S. assistance was critical in providing stability in the developing world.

The entreaty came at a propitious time. Rice and her colleagues in the White House and the State Department were interested in doing something to bolster the U.S. image abroad. In March 2002, the president would travel to Monterrey, Mexico, to discuss global poverty with other world leaders. Rice foresaw that the United States was due for another lashing just as had happened at Seattle, Genoa, and other recent international conferences on trade and/or development.

Bono enjoyed considerable access to Rice leading up to the Monterrey Summit. Before Monterrey, he was called in to meet with the president in the Oval Office. He spoke about debt relief, aid, and AIDS.

In a *New Yorker* piece on Karl Rove, Nicholas Lemann asked the political mastermind behind the Bush machine to delineate the difference between who is a Republican and who is a Democrat. Rove's answer was revealing: "First of all, there is a huge gap among people of faith. You saw it in the 2000 exit polling, where people who went to church on a frequent and regular basis voted overwhelmingly for Bush. They form an important part of the Republican base."

Bono and his people were very much attuned. During his meeting with the president he laid out all the arguments he had crafted with Sachs and Shriver and honed in sessions with Helms, Rice, and others. He quoted scriptures to the president. The two spoke for an hour. By the end of the meeting, the president and his guest were in sync. Bush told Bono that the pandemic was tantamount to "genocide."

Each had reason to be wary, though. Clinton had basked in the company of celebrities. The Bush camp, on the other hand, looked down upon the glitterati and the idea of the celebrity spokesman. For his part, Bono constantly had to worry about being used. It would be all too easy for politicians to offer empty promises, pose for a photo op, cash in politically on the tacit endorsement, and then to do nothing concrete.

Skepticism quickly faded, though. Bush took pride in disarming those who underestimated his abilities. He delighted in Bono's own disarming acumen and substance. For his part, Bono came to trust Bush and deemed him a man of his word.

On March 14, 2002, at an event at the Inter-American Development Bank in Washington, D.C., standing behind a podium flanked by long flags, and with World Bank president James Wolfensohn, the Archbishop of Washington, Cardinal McCarrick, and Bono seated behind him on stage, Bush announced a new initiative he called the Millennium Challenge Account, or MCA. The MCA promised to raise U.S. international assistance by 50 percent over the next three years. It aimed to provide assistance to good governments who were willing to demonstrate accountability and an interest in demonstrable results. The announcement was made just a week before the president's trip to Monterrey.

"As you can see," Bush said toward the beginning of his address, "I'm traveling in some pretty good company today: Bono." The crowd laughed and then applauded. "We just had a great visit in the Oval Office. Here's what I know about him: first, he's a good musician; secondly, he's willing to use his position in a responsible way. He is willing to lead to achieve what his heart tells him, and that is nobody, nobody should be living in poverty and hopelessness in the world.

"Bono, I appreciate your heart," the president said, "and to tell you what an influence you've had, Dick Cheney walked into the Oval Office [and] said, 'Jesse Helms wants us to listen to Bono's ideas.' "

The administration had just banked some political coin: Bono on the stage with the president. There would also be handshakes in the Rose Garden. Not since Elvis Presley visited Richard Nixon had there been such a "lopsided transfer of cool in Washington," wrote one journalist. Bono was helping the White House put the "compassion" back in "compassionate conservatism." And in MCA, Bono had gotten a significant portion of what he had hoped for.

However, he and his comrades had asked for more. In the weeks leading up to Monterrey, in addition to a boost in foreign assistance at large, the group had pushed for an historic AIDS initiative. They called for leadership and billions in funding per year. Drummond recalled: "We were not happy that AIDS was not included as a strategically connected initiative to the MCA. We thought it would be and said it very carefully. We [felt] like we extracted a political promise from them that they would deliver an historic AIDS initiative."

Bono was not finished. He started traveling to Africa, making frequent trips as a tour guide for a broad, diverse group of people. On his most high-profile trip in May 2002, Bono brought along actor Chris Tucker and did a documentary for MTV. Top billing on the tour, though, was shared between Bono and Treasury Secretary Paul O'Neill. The press dubbed it the "Odd Couple" tour. The two traveled to four countries in ten days. They were photographed in traditional tribal garb in Ghana and spent much time at AIDS clinics and orphanages in Uganda and elsewhere. "I think Paul O'Neill is going to be a very different person going out of this trip than he was coming in," Bono predicted.

By the summer of 2002, Bono's hopes were piquing. He was also becoming more anxious. Every White House meeting, every press appearance, and every award nomination drew him closer to the inside, to the establishment. His celebrity had become a political commodity. His advocacy, though, was an outgrowth of a strong desire to serve the suffering, not politicians. He was walking a tightrope, and he knew it.

Still, Bono thought of himself as a rebel. He admitted as much to Harvard's graduating class of 2001: "If I am honest," he said, "I'm rebelling against my own indifference. I am rebelling against the idea that the world is the way it is and there's not a damn thing I can do about it. So, I'm trying to do a damn thing."

The AIDS crisis was a "holocaust," Bono exclaimed, an "unsustainable problem for Africa . . . an unsustainable problem for the world." Still, the United States and the rest of the developed world had managed to turn away.

Bono had his own explanation: "It's hard to make this a popular cause. It's hard to make it pop, you know? And I guess that's what my job is."

————•◆•————

On January 19, 2000, the last day of the Clinton administration, Ken Bernard headed to a farewell gathering in the West Wing. He figured that he was due a free drink. As Bernard ambled into the party, he bumped into Donna Shalala on her way out. "What are you going to do now?" Shalala asked Bernard, who had served under her while at HHS.

Bernard explained that his position at the NSC was being dismantled and that he was planning on going back to HHS. "I might have something for you," Shalala said. It was a position with a senator from Tennessee working in international health. "I can make it happen today, but not tomorrow. You've got three hours," Shalala told him.

Bernard had had some contact with the senator, and, of course, he knew him by reputation. He had thought well of him. He had never worked in the Senate. It couldn't hurt to align himself with a rising star in the GOP. After thinking it over for a few hours, Bernard accepted. He would go to work for Bill Frist, then still the junior senator from Tennessee. In short order, he became both a trusted senior advisor and an enthusiastic acolyte.

Not yet fifty, Frist had been a senator for all of six years when Bernard showed up for his first day of work. Brandishing a lustrous and unusual résumé, Frist had already secured himself a place in the firmament of the upper echelons of the Republican party. He had graduated cum laude from Princeton, a certified pilot at age sixteen. After receiving his medical degree from Harvard, Frist went on to a storied career as a cardiothoracic surgeon. In his spare time, he ran marathons and did pro bono surgery in Africa.

Just as Frist's father had been a doctor turned businessman, Frist—whose nickname in high school was "Mr. President"—was intent on a career change and wanted to throw his hat in the political arena. His conservative agenda, his telegenic appearance, his credentials as a healer, his personal fortune, and his sheer desire had all enabled him to unseat a popular three-time incumbent.

In Washington, Frist won the admiration of his colleagues for his tireless work ethic, his cordial desk-side manner, and his sharp policy acumen. By the time George W. Bush arrived at the White House, Frist's star had jumped several notches. He was a longtime friend of the city's new power broker and the president's political eyes and ears, Karl Rove. An "administration darling" from the outset, Frist cemented his status by running his reelection campaign in tandem with Bush's. The tactic helped deliver Tennessee, Vice President Gore's home state, to Bush—not an insignificant favor.

When Bernard made his first office call to his fellow doctor, Frist welcomed him in and told him he really wanted to make a difference in his second term. As his new director of international health, Bernard was directed to identify and focus on several key priorities. As it turned out, they were interested in the same issue: global AIDS.

The senator had spent a good deal of time in Africa and was also chairman of the decidedly unglamorous African affairs subcommittee. As a doctor, he was well aware that the pandemic constituted the most pernicious health crisis of modern times. Trumpeting the alarm, Frist declared: "History is going to record what we do when we face the terrible waste of life and hope that is the global AIDS epidemic today. Our grandchildren will ask us what we did to fight it."

Shortly after Kofi Annan announced his proposal for the Global Fund, Frist grabbed Bernard for a trip to 1600 Pennsylvania Avenue. They met with Rice and others at the White House, and Frist was vehement in advocating U.S. support for the Global Fund. "I'm convinced . . . without question it was because of Bill Frist," Bernard said of Bush's pledge to support the Global Fund in the Rose Garden in May 2001.

Frist was becoming a fixture at all sorts of administration meetings, appearances, and ceremonies. At meetings in the White House and on trips on Air Force One, Frist used his access to the president to advocate for an upgraded U.S. policy on the pandemic.

Throughout much of 2001 and 2002, the senator joined forces with Massachusetts Senator John Kerry, to promulgate legislation to increase U.S. funding and commitment. In March 2002, Frist found an unexpected ally on his side of the aisle in an awakened old senator from North Carolina. Together, Frist and Jesse Helms co-sponsored an Emergency Supplemental Bill, which called for an additional $500 million with which to fight mother-to-child transmission.

There was a political opportunity. But Frist was also a doctor. The senator's nameplate was emblazoned with "Bill Frist, MD." He kept a medical bag in his office at all times. The bag came in handy on several occasions in treating his ailing 100-year-old colleague Strom Thurmond and perhaps most notably during an infamous shooting at the Capitol where Frist raced to the scene to try and resuscitate the lone gunman and a police officer the gunman had fatally wounded after bursting into the building. Each incident added to Frist's legend and, of course, his political sheen.

Less heralded were his frequent visits to Africa, including his trip in January 2002 to the Kenyatta National Hospital in Nairobi, Kenya, where one in seven mothers tested positive for HIV. During his visit he was briefed about the hospital's mother-to-child initiatives and their desperate need for assistance. "Our actions will show the world America's commitment to fighting the AIDS crisis and demonstrate our continued resolve to be a compassionate nation which refuses to simply look the other way," Frist said.

The $500 million Emergency Supplemental Bill that Frist co-sponsored became known as the Helms Legacy Amendment. It would have "had to have been a $20 billion amendment to make up for all the crimes that Helms had committed, $500 million was not quite adequate," said activist Paul Zeitz. Frist certainly agreed that the amount was inadequate: $500 million wasn't going to be enough. But, Helms's reversal afforded a window of opportunity and he wanted to seize it.

During the early summer, Helms fell ill. Frist's strong comments about the need for an upgraded U.S. response to the pandemic and Helms's subsequent health problems meant that he had become the face behind the proposed Supplemental Bill.

Meanwhile, at 1600 Pennsylvania Avenue, a core group of officials representing disparate White House offices had already been working for months, formulating a mother-to-child initiative. The Bush administration was hoping to lead on the issue. The plan's details and its level of funding remained up in the air. Yet they wanted a Bush plan, not a co-sponsored initiative from the Senate. The predicament pitted the Bush White House against one of their favorite senators.

One of the White House officials working on the inchoate Bush plan foresaw a grave political problem. He sent an e-mail to other senior colleagues working on the Bush effort reminding them that Frist was a friend of the administration. He acknowledged the importance of keeping the effort closely held, but noted that the Frist camp was playing a blind game and was going to do something that wouldn't be good for the administration and could be potentially embarrassing for Frist. The e-mail exhorted the White House to talk to Frist and to bring him in the loop.

In early June 2002, Andy Card reportedly called Frist to let him in on the White House initiative. In subsequent meetings and telephone calls, the president requested Frist's cooperation. He asked his good friend in the Senate, in what would be a familiar White House entreaty over the ensuing seven months, "to be patient." "Things are going to work out the way that you want them to," the president assured Frist, according to a senior White House aide.

It was a defining political moment for Bill Frist. He could stick with his own initiative and defy the president, thereby imperiling his standing with the administration and perhaps his political future. Or he could relent and trust in the president's assurance that the short-term damage would be minimal, and the long-term payoff enormous.

Frist acquiesced to the president's request. He pulled the amendment. The Frist camp was not in a position to share any of the details of the president's assurances with the media or activists, who had a pronounced skepticism about pledges and admonitions about "being patient." To many, the move seemed to confirm suspicions about a possible dark side to Bill Frist, the man some called "Doc Politic." When forced to decide between a principle and political advancement, it seemed, Frist had selected the latter; he had chosen to shelve his initiative in order to cement his "darling" status with the administration.

The backlash was furious and immediate. The activist community—with whom the Frist camp had tried to cultivate a relationship—besieged the senator's office with angry telephone calls and e-mails. There were protests outside of his house. Most painfully, Frist was castigated by a *Washington Post* editorial printed on June 12, 2002, entitled, "Senator Frist Backs Down." The editorial explained that Frist had cut the $500 million proposal by 60 percent down to $200 million "just hours before the measure was due to go to a vote."

There were several possible reasons why. One possible explanation, the editorial suggested, was "that the administration didn't want to spend the money, and that Mr. Frist put his relationship with Mr. Bush ahead of his commitment to the promised $500 million. . . . Mr. Frist should not walk away from his promises on AIDS," the editorial chided.

It was not the sort of press Frist had grown accustomed to expect, particularly on an issue on which he considered himself a national leader. "I was furious when I saw that editorial," said Ken Bernard, who had moved back to HHS following 9/11. Frist cared deeply about the issue. He had made very strong statements about the need for U.S. engagement and staked part of his reputation behind championing policy movement. "I know Bill Frist, and he did not want to lower funding on AIDS," Bernard said. "I think he was just trying to be helpful to the White House to meet their needs without diminishing the amount of support for the funding. . . . He was strategizing. He was waiting for the right time."

Frist had taken one on the chin for the administration, hoping that it would reap long-term dividends. Little more than a week later, the president announced his own $500 million mother-to-child initiative at a Rose Garden ceremony. With $200 million already approved by Congress, and the remaining $300 million spread out over two years, it was a meager effort, a retreat rather than a forward charge, in the words of Senator John Kerry.

The meager proposal invited a host of criticism from all quarters. *The New York Times* editorialized: "The White House is taking the wrong approach. . . . Although Mr. Bush and members of his Cabinet speak as if they understand the catastrophic impact of AIDS worldwide, their willingness to help apparently stops at the point where it could cross key financial supporters or require real money." Prominent Democrats like John Kerry, Dick Durbin, Patrick Leahy, and others assailed the President's shallow effort.

The activists were not pleased either. The evening after the Rose Garden ceremony, the president, Frist, and several other Republican leaders arrived at a dinner at the Mayflower Hotel in downtown Washington, D.C., honoring the head of GlaxoSmithKline, a multinational pharmaceutical company, attempting to raise millions for the GOP.

A group of roughly twenty activists assembled, including Paul Zeitz from the Global AIDS Alliance, some of the usual suspects from ACT UP, and others. The activists were ready to chain themselves to the building. It was the day that a small plane had been flown into the White House complex, though, and the activists sensed that the Secret Service and the eighty or so policemen on guard were on edge. And so, in a rare display of restraint, they opted for a more traditional picket-style protest.

Frist had met Paul Zeitz before. Following the senator's acquiescence, Zeitz had been speaking out strongly against the senator in the press. As Frist walked to the entrance of the hotel he recognized Zeitz and said, "Hello." Zeitz was flushed. He had been calling him a traitor in the press "and so was not winning Frist's good graces," the activist recalled. Frist had two words for Zeitz: "Be patient."

———◆———

July 9, 2002, was a stifling day in Barcelona, Spain. Secretary of Health and Human Services Tommy Thompson was getting ready to address an audience of several hundred in a theater-sized complex at the Thirteenth International AIDS Conference. It had been a dozen years since Louis Sullivan, the last HHS Secretary to attend an international AIDS conference, had been booed and heckled at San Francisco. "No other Secretary [of Health] has had the courage to come back since then," Thompson later remarked.

Thompson had attracted more attention than most of his predecessors at HHS. In the aftermath of 9/11, concerns about bioterrorism, anthrax, and smallpox were front and center on the national security agenda. It seemed that the health-security nexus had a newfound resonance. Thompson was charged with leading the U.S. response.

A former governor of Wisconsin, Thompson had overseen one of the country's most progressive state-level AIDS initiatives. The secretary was well attuned to the global dimension of the disease and had demonstrated a strong interest in increasing HHS's role in demanding more funding and in assuming the reins of leadership in the U.S. response.

Thompson was not the only Cabinet secretary, however, who wanted to lead the U.S. response. It was also a foreign policy issue, and Colin Powell wanted the U.S. response centered at the State Department.

In an attempt to delegate authority to both Cabinet members and their departments and to appease hostile activists who demanded policy movement, the administration announced a joint commission Cabinet-level task force, to be co-chaired by Powell and Thompson. It was, in the words of Ken Thomas, deputy director at ONAP, an attempt to achieve "better coordination . . . to see to it that [the issue] was no longer treated in a stovepipe manner." With both departments jostling for the lead, it was an attempt to bring them together under the aegis of a senior-level convening body. With a plethora of fragmented efforts still scattered throughout the government's departments, agencies, and centers, it was also an effort intended in concept to provide a measure of structural and institutional coherence.

The Cabinet task force met for the first time in the spring of 2001. It was a run-of-the-mill inaugural meeting. Anthony Fauci, the longtime director of the National Institute of Allergy and Infectious Diseases and other experts were called in to deliver presentations about the state of the pandemic and the status of the U.S. response. Suggestions were made and pep talks were given. When asked what the task force accomplished, a senior HHS official smiled and made a zero with his hand. The spring of 2001 session would be the task force's first and only meeting.

Thompson would deputize a young HHS official named Bill Steiger to take the lead from his side, and Ambassador Jack Chow would run with the ball for State. The two had worked together to help design and create the Global Fund. They were also in regular contact on U.S. global AIDS policy at large. In the wake of 9/11, though, as both Powell's and Thompson's agendas swelled, neither would muster the time to convene another meeting, rendering the task force all but defunct.

For the next two years, the Cabinet task force remained the ostensible coordinating body of the U.S. government's policy on global AIDS. In reality, though, the U.S. response remained governed by the same haplessness and structural deficiency that had plagued it from its inception.

With Powell's focus fixed on the war on terror, Afghanistan and later Iraq, and other pressing diplomatic matters, and the task force having been rendered a shell of a body, Thompson had a wide opening to take the lead on the U.S. response. Whereas before, at international events like UNGASS, Powell appeared to speak for the United States on the matter, Thompson emerged the representative voice at Barcelona.

Only three months prior to his arrival in Spain, Thompson had ventured to Africa for a seven-day, four-country tour of the continent. He had gone to learn more about the pandemic's grip on the continent and the possibility for further U.S. assistance. Visits to orphanages and AIDS clinics and hospitals—as they had for so many others—had a profound personal impact on the secretary and he resolved to get out in front on the issue.

Now, as Thompson rose to the podium to deliver his address, he did not foresee the scene that was to soon unfold. Before he could even begin his speech, dozens of activists, primarily from ACT UP, stormed the stage chanting "Shame, shame," and "No more lies." Placards read: "Bush and Thompson Wanted: For the murder and neglect of PWAs." Security surrounded Thompson forming a human barrier as he stood on the stage while the protestors continued chanting for fifteen minutes.

Thompson finally steadied himself and began to deliver his speech. The chanting continued, though, and scores of others in the audience were hollering and blowing whistles that had been distributed prior to the speech. The secretary was clearly caught unprepared. He had never experienced anything like it. He struggled to finish his ten-minute speech, most of which was rendered inaudible by the din.

The assault seemed excessive even to some leading advocates in the audience like Terje Anderson, who had expected the audience to blow on their whistles intermittently throughout the secretary's speech. "People thought when he'd say something offensive, we'd whistle," Anderson said. "That's what I expected would happen. Most people did. It took on a dynamic entirely its own when it got there."

True to form, Jeffrey Sachs, also in attendance, did not mince words: "Secretary Thompson probably was surprised by his reception, but he should not be surprised. It is a reflection of the utter confusion in the U.S. government of what they are actually doing. . . . They pick numbers out of thin air from week to week . . . they have not done their homework."

Thompson was livid. He considered himself a vigorous advocate. Meeting with reporters backstage, he touted the president's recent "$500 million" mother-to-child initiative. Thompson was the key senior champion behind the initiative. In addition, under President Bush, the U.S. had pledged roughly $500 million to the Global Fund, hundreds of millions more than any other country. "We will meet the objectives of the protestors, but not the way they want," he said.

Later that afternoon, Thompson consented to a side-room conversation with a handful of leading advocates. Throughout the first half of the Bush administration, contact between the community and the administration had been scant and desultory, and advocates like Terje Anderson were eager to gain an audience with the Cabinet member. Sitting with the secretary, the activists' enthusiasm quickly waned. Thompson was furious. He had taken the demonstration very personally, and was irascible for the first twenty minutes of the meeting.

Luckily, Anthony Fauci, for whom the secretary had a great deal of respect, was there. Fauci was a senior government veteran who had been on the receiving end of similar protests. He told the secretary that ten years earlier, activists had called him a "murderer, too, and now some of them are my best friends. It's not about you personally, it's about the passion they have for these issues." Fauci helped diffuse the tension, establishing a dynamic in which the two groups could speak constructively.

As the secretary's anger tapered, the activists outlined their four major issues with the administration. Three were domestic issues. The activists were surprised to find that the secretary was in agreement on all three points.

The fourth issue was the administration's policy on global AIDS. The activists expressed concern about the administration's request that Frist pull his amendment. They were also now trumpeting Jeffrey Sachs–like levels of funding for the issue, in the billions not hundreds of millions. As soon as they broached the issue, though, the secretary re-ignited and became angry and defensive. The Bush administration had practically tripled funding over the Clinton administration, he pointed out. He was irate at being accused of not doing enough. To Terje Anderson, "It was very clear that he had a personal investment in this; that he believed that this was a program that he wanted to leave his mark on."

Thompson seemed to be conveying the message that the administration had been "generous," but that it was not practical to do more. To several of the activists, the implication was that limitations in African infrastructure meant that pouring more money into the problem was not going to do any more good.

It was a rare and revealing window into the thinking of one of the administration's senior-most—and sympathetic—officials. It was July 2002, and the prognosis for a recalibrated U.S. effort was not good.

Back in Washington the right wing of the Republican party was speaking out. Outraged by the activists lashing out at the secretary, a group of twelve congressmen wrote a letter addressed to Secretary Thompson dated July 17, 2002, in which they expressed their displeasure. They called on the department to launch an investigation into the groups and to disclose whether or not they received U.S. federal funding.

It was a shot across the bow from the socially conservative side of the party. They generally frowned upon many of the U.S. activist or not-for-profit groups, often comprising significant numbers of homosexual members or employees. The far right opposed condom distribution and other "risqué" or unacceptable methods of prevention that most groups endorsed.

Many social conservatives had become supportive of U.S. efforts to combat the pandemic. The bedrock of their prevention strategy, however, was the promotion of abstinence-only solutions, at home and abroad. They pointed to religious institutions or faith-based groups as playing a leading role in implementation.

The conservative elements were ardent in their views. As the U.S. commitment ramped up and more and more taxpayer dollars were being spent on global AIDS, they were also becoming increasingly vigilant and vocal. Activists, moderate policy makers, and public health experts alike worried about the impact that social or religious doctrine might play in the U.S. effort. An effective prevention program had to be informed by sound science and health, not politics or dogma.

In June 2002, AIDS Czar Scott Evertz was feeling the heat from conservative factions both in Congress and at HHS. Evertz felt that some people had never really gotten over the fact that he was a gay man. It was a point of further difficulty for some to have an openly gay man as their boss.

Of course, Evertz had never been told precisely what he could or could not say. There was still no manual for the job. He would soon receive a lesson about Washington hardball, though. "One thing that I learned is that you don't have to ruffle many people's feathers, but if you ruffle the wrong ones you get into trouble."

Evertz knew that he represented the White House, but he also felt it important to speak his mind. He was asked about a program called StopAIDS that focused on prevention campaigns in San Francisco. Some of the group's marketing literature contained relatively provocative messages. To the dismay of some conservatives, who found the material thoroughly disagreeable, the group was also receiving federal funds. When asked about it, Evertz said that he supported the group. Their marketing was targeted at a certain demographic, and he estimated that their work was effective.

Evertz's answer didn't wash with a select group in Congress. Similar answers and positions had gotten members of the right increasingly agitated. Federal funds were not to be spent on lewd material.

Several congressmen voiced their vehement disapproval to Karl Rove, the president's political handyman and the primary interface with the far-right wing of the party. With stealth precision, Rove orchestrated Evertz's transfer to HHS, where he would help work on the creation of the Global Fund.

The elephants, it appeared, did not have short memories. Rove, Card, and others well remembered the reception that they had received when they announced that ONAP would be dismantled. They knew that they would have to fill Evertz's post, and name a new AIDS czar. Shaken by the secretary's reception at Barcelona, driven by the president's own political, moral, and spiritual convictions, a growing groundswell of voices—Sachs and Bono as well as the activist and faith-based communities—and advocacy from Powell, Thompson, and Frist, the administration had grown determined to make global AIDS one of its flagship issues.

First, the president would need someone to lead.

—⚊—

FIFTEEN

Behind Closed Doors, Coalescence

In mid-July 2002, the president hosted a new administration official in the Oval Office for what was supposed to be a standard ten-minute "meet and greet" session. The new official was Dr. Joe O'Neill, Scott Evertz's replacement as the new director of the Office of National AIDS Policy. Like his predecessor, the new ONAP director was openly gay. Some activists, disappointed with Evertz's appointment and naturally skeptical of the administration, assumed that O'Neill's appointment heralded business as usual. They had underestimated the new AIDS czar.

O'Neill was a graduate of the University of California at San Francisco's School of Medicine. He was board certified in internal medicine and held a faculty appointment at the Johns Hopkins School of Medicine. From 1997 to 2001, he directed the Ryan White Comprehensive AIDS Resources Emergency, or CARE, program. Under O'Neill's stewardship, CARE provided medical care and treatment, social services, and drug treatments to people living with HIV/AIDS throughout the United States.

Running CARE, O'Neill had overseen an annual budget of $1.7 billion and a staff that served more than 500,000 people a year. He was a straight-shooting, no-nonsense operative. He was a good communicator and had a proven record as an administrator and a wealth of medical and health expertise as a clinical and a palliative care physician.

O'Neill was the most experienced and qualified AIDS czar yet. And while some in the AIDS community were skeptical, his appointment was a reflection of the administration's strengthened position on global AIDS policy.

In the weeks leading up to the June 2002 White House announcement of the president's $500 million mother-to-child initiative, a series of key players from disparate centers of government, primarily from the White House, had already begun thinking beyond the impending initiative.

There had been discussion and position papers written since the beginning of the administration that made global AIDS an important foreign policy issue for the president. "It had gotten sidetracked after 9/11. It never went away. It shuffled around for a year, and then we picked it back up again," said deputy director of ONAP, Ken Thomas, a former Goldman Sachs banker who focused on the office's global AIDS efforts. Well aware of the skeptics, Thomas said, "I don't know if they'll ever believe it, but it was going on."

Many issues, however, receive similar measures of preliminary consideration. In this case, as in most others, the initial attention did not equal a firm mandate for a recalibrated initiative.

By the summer of 2002, as the administration began to focus on the mother-to-child initiative, the president was becoming more politically and personally attuned, and as relatively senior administration officials were delegated to focus on the issue, the genesis for a truly upgraded U.S. effort began to emerge.

In May 2002, Thomas said, in the course of mapping out the administration's mother-to-child initiative with Dr. Anthony Fauci, "we did a blue sky, which is if we were going to do something, what would we do in terms of a really big bilateral effort."

Then, in June 2002, Fauci, who had taken the lead on drafting the administration's mother-to-child initiative, walked senior administration officials through the proposal. All of the key players were there: Colin Powell, Tommy Thompson, Andy Card, Karl Rove, and the president. Sitting in the Hamilton Room in the White House, everyone offered enthusiastic approval. "I like it. It's a go, let's go," said the president. As the crowd got up and milled about the room, the president made his way over to White House Deputy Chief of Staff Josh Bolton, and said, "This is a great start, but it's not enough. We really need to do something more, something that has a broader impact on many more people."

Bolton, a former financier and a highly respected figure in the White House, called Fauci the next day. "OK, we're going to go for this now," he said. Bolton then assembled a core group of senior White House insiders to examine the possibilities for a recalibrated U.S. effort. The group came to include Josh Bolton, the group's interface with the president; Robin Cleveland, head of national security and international affairs at OMB; Gary Edson, deputy national security advisor; Jay Lefkowitz, deputy assistant to the president for domestic policy; and Anthony Fauci.

In that same month, scores of activists descended upon the White House to protest the administration's mother-to-child initiative, calling it disgraceful and anemic. A flurry of negative editorials and coverage followed in the news media. Then, in early July, Thompson's gruesome reception at Barcelona further shook the administration.

By mid-July, the administration was looking for an experienced, credible, and loyal operative to help lead the core team's efforts to formulate an upgraded U.S. initiative. Joe O'Neill became the clear candidate, and after considerable deliberation, he accepted.

When O'Neill walked into the Oval Office to meet the president, he introduced himself and began to outline the details of the pandemic. Moments into O'Neill's tutorial the president interrupted: "Just stop right there. I know it's bad. The money is not going to be a problem. I want you to figure out how we do it."

The ten-minute "meet and greet" reportedly turned into a forty-five-minute session. The president wanted to get a read on O'Neill. He asked him about the AIDS community, their expectations, and the protests at Barcelona. He was well versed in the statistics and the current U.S. response. The president expressed a firm intent to recalibrate the level of U.S. engagement. But he wasn't interested in throwing U.S. taxpayers' money away. O'Neill's job, Bush explained, was to examine what was viable and how to do it. The will, the president assured him, was there.

"Apparently," said the U.S. ambassador for global AIDS, Jack Chow, "the president had made a commitment by the time of O'Neill's appointment to do something big. It was [just] a matter of shaping it and structuring it."

O'Neill, Bolton, and the rest of the team working on designing the president's new global AIDS initiative were handed a blank slate. They didn't know how much funding they would get, or over how many years it would be spread out. They didn't know who would get it, or how it would be disbursed. They had yet to reach a consensus on its breadth; that is, would the plan be primarily prevention, or would treatment and/or care make up a major part?

The president had another directive: the details and nature of the team's deliberations—in fact, its very existence—were to be kept a secret.

The president and his key advisors had seen the politics, the emotion, and the noise attending the issue. He wanted to do something big, but he wanted to do it on his own terms and according to his own timetable. What ensued was a clandestine, behind-closed-doors effort. The mission: to reset the bar with respect to U.S. policy on the issue George W. Bush was steadily coming to think of as the defining humanitarian catastrophe of our time.

———◆———

Through the late summer and early fall, Washington was abuzz with speculation about what seemed like an impending war with Iraq. With the hawks in the administration pressing for U.S. action and key figures at the State Department pressing for Bush to pursue a multilateral approach, on September 12, 2002, the president went to the United Nations in New York to proclaim that the United States would chart its course along with the UN. The president made clear, though, that his country would set the direction of that course, and would be willing to proceed with or without UN support.

The president's speech was widely acclaimed. It seemed a victory for Colin Powell and the significantly more multilateralist inclined State Department. A war, U.S. relations with Europe, stability in the Middle East, and the very fabric of the U.S. relationship with the rest of the world seemed in the balance.

At the same time, under the world's radar screen, a core team of insiders was holding meetings all over the White House complex. Stealthily, they would assemble in the Situation Room, the Old Executive Office Building, Senior Policy Advisor Margaret Spelling's office in the West Wing, offices at the NSC, or "wherever we could find an empty room and not get interrupted."

From the beginning of the administration, the president and his key advisors had expressed skepticism about the viability of providing treatment in Africa and the developing world. The mention of phrases like "absorptive capacity" and "lack of infrastructure" had theretofore been sufficient to quell discussion about a serious effort to provide treatment. When Jeffrey Sachs met with administration officials early on and insisted that treatment on a wide scale was possible, it seemed, he said, as though "they thought I was crazy."

The advent of a drug called nevirapine and its proven efficacy in reducing the odds of the virus's transmission from pregnant mothers to their children helped breathe life into the June 2002 mother-to-child initiative. Finding itself committed to reducing mother-to-child transmission, the question naturally followed: What would happen to the rest of the family—the mother, the father, and the future orphan?

The dilemma caused the group to confront the question of the viability of treatment with renewed vigor. It was further becoming clear that, as experts had been arguing since at least the Durban Conference in the summer of 2000, without the potential for treatment, there was little incentive for people to get tested. Lack of treatment was keeping the virus underground, where it spread most effectively, and in turn it was crippling prevention efforts. The group came to understand that treatment was not separate, but rather an integral element of a comprehensive prevention campaign.

Still, senior officials who controlled the administration's purse strings, like Josh Bolton and Robin Cleveland, needed assurance that the provision of treatment was viable. The president had made clear that he was not interested in simply spending funds. The plan would need to be buttressed by evidence that a wide-scale treatment effort would work.

Surreptitiously, the group began requesting information and data from groups like the Elizabeth Glaser Pediatric AIDS Foundation and the Global Health Council. They solicited views and research from experts at institutions like Harvard and Columbia. Fauci and O'Neill directed the group to the world's most notable success story, Uganda, in which a comprehensive and aggressive national campaign helped reduce the country's level of infection by several times.

Bush was scheduled to travel to Africa in January 2003 on a multicountry, several-day tour of the continent. The trip had been scheduled to demonstrate that Africa, despite Bush's campaign comments, was of strategic relevance to the United States. By the end of the decade, it was now expected, Africa would provide the United States with 25 percent of its imported oil. With problems in the Middle East, Africa's importance as a major oil exporter gained it increased status. Several African countries had become key military partners in the war on terror, and the U.S. military presence on the continent picked up markedly. In addition, with the Iraq war approaching it was good diplomacy to show the international community that the United States cared about Africa. It was also, the president's advisors hoped, good politics with the African-American electorate.

The upcoming trip crystallized the importance of the core team's efforts and the need to move quickly to design a plan so that the president would not go to Africa and face its greatest crisis empty-handed. Still very much inchoate, the AIDS plan was to be the president's big deliverable. Moving into November, the pace of the team's meetings and the intensity of deliberations accelerated.

On November 13, 2002, the core team assembled an array of leading experts with extensive medical, public health, and clinical experience. Meeting in Room 248 of the Old Executive Office Building, the core team of six—Joe O'Neill, Josh Bolton, Anthony Fauci, Robin Cleveland, Gary Edson, and Jay Lefkowitz—spent three hours consulting with the outside experts. The specialists who participated in the meeting recalled months later that there was strong impetus to put forth an upgraded effort. In addition, they sensed that the administration was on the verge of making a watershed change in exploring the provision of treatment. One of the key questions put to the experts was "whether there was enough medical infrastructure in place for the program to be successful.

Fortunately, the invited specialists were the right group to take the questions head-on. Nils Daulaire was a seasoned and well-respected global health expert. Dr. Eric Goosby had spent much time in Rwanda working on AIDS. Dr. Paul Farmer and Dr. Jean William Pape were renowned international clinical physicians who had both been working for years treating HIV/AIDS patients in Haiti. All of the experts assured the team that with resources and drugs, there was no question that treatment could be successfully provided.

In addition, to better understand the Uganda model, the core team had invited Dr. Peter Mugyenyi, director of the Joint Clinical Research Center in Uganda. Five thousand HIV/AIDS patients were being treated successfully throughout Mugyenyi's network of clinics. They could treat many more people. "Our biggest problem," he explained, "is lack of funds, which has not allowed us to scale up."

Over the preceding months, the core team had gathered the data points from U.S. NGOs. It had summoned testimonials and input from leading experts around the globe. Treatment was possible and infrastructure was sorely inadequate, but with some will and ingenuity, millions more could be treated.

In addition, the pharmaceutical companies had finally lowered drug prices. If the president was willing to support the procurement of generic drugs, the drugs would cost only several hundred dollars per person per year—a huge decline.

After months of deliberations the group determined that drugs were now affordable and treatment was viable. Experts had been shouting as much for years, but it had finally registered for the pertinent political players. "If in fact what we've said is true," Ken Thomas recalled, "then we have a moral obligation to provide integrated care, treatment and prevention."

As the president's January trip neared, it appeared increasingly likely that treatment for the general infected population was going to be a part of the new initiative. Still, the big questions remained unanswered: How many dollars would the United States spend? How would it spend them? Who would get them?

Champions for an upgraded response were becoming increasingly anxious. U.S. Ambassador for Global AIDS Jack Chow ran an office at the State Department and reported directly to Secretary of State Colin Powell. The core team's efforts had been held so close to the vest that Chow, the senior-most official to focus exclusively on global AIDS in the U.S. government, was actually unaware of the effort.

Attending planning sessions in preparation for the president's Africa trip in November and December, Chow was disconsolate. At one meeting, called by Jendayi Frazier, the director of African Affairs at the NSC, at the Old Executive Office Building, Frazier walked the attendees through the events planned in each of the countries, soliciting feedback and input from the officials present. Dismayed, Chow proclaimed to the eclectic group: "Look, this is all great and I'm happy to do this, but the president ought to have a much bigger deliverable than this. It ought to be a multibillion-dollar initiative."

Frazier, who as a White House insider was one of the very few non-core team members to know about and participate in the planning, was purposefully oblique. "Well, we'll consider it," she told Chow. "We're basically here to focus on the planning." Chow thought that a golden opportunity for moving U.S. policy was slipping away.

Chow persisted, though, and tried to convene the president's Cabinet task force on AIDS for a second meeting. Chow thought the president's upcoming trip might enable him to galvanize the players. He had trouble getting movement, though. He solicited support from AIDS czar Joe O'Neill. The two had gone to UCSF Medical School together and were good friends. Chow called his old friend to try and fire up the task force meeting. "The time is not right," O'Neill replied vaguely, frustrating his old classmate enormously.

In the course of Chow's and O'Neill's regular phone conversations, Chow would express his dismay. "How can the president go to Africa and not do more?" Tight-lipped to the end, O'Neill tried to calm his friend. "Jack, don't worry. I can't say anything, but help is coming."

It was O'Neill's trademark refrain through the fall of 2002. As AIDS czar, O'Neill was the mouthpiece of the administration on AIDS. Yet, compared to his predecessor Sandy Thurman, he managed to cut a remarkably inconspicuous figure. He made comparatively few public appearances, was guarded and reticent to grant interviews. When speaking with colleagues, activists, or others with whom he had relationships, the line was almost always the same: "Be patient. Help is on the way."

Some sensed that O'Neill and Bush were both men of their word. Slowly, rumors began to trickle out. The history of the U.S. response, though, was littered with discarded pledges and half-truths. The administration's clandestine modus operandi did little to instill faith.

Meanwhile, global AIDS was gaining ever more traction with the media as well as with prominent thinkers and public personalities. The groundswell of interest put pressure on the core team and the president to deliver.

In the summer of 2002, *The New York Times*, the *San Francisco Chronicle*, and other publications ran stories or editorials on the burgeoning AIDS crisis in Russia. By 2002, Russia had the world's fastest-growing rate of HIV infection, and the U.S. media was starting to notice. The country was officially reporting two hundred thousand infections, but experts put the number at closer to five times that, or quite possibly more. The World Bank estimated that by 2020, as many as 15 million Russians would be infected with HIV.

Yet even as the epidemic advanced, Russia's response remained mired in stigma and discrimination. Few Russians understood how the disease was transmitted. Many doctors still refused to treat patients, and orphanages refused to house HIV-infected infants. Later in the summer of 2002, one of Russia's neighbors started to capture headlines as well.

In late August 2002, China's most prominent AIDS activist, Wan Yanhai, a former official in the Chinese Health Ministry, was reported missing. In the previous months, the activist had incurred a great deal of wrath from the Chinese government for publicizing the epidemic's growth in the Henan province. Yanhai, whose activist group, the AIDS Action Project, banned by the government a month earlier, had achieved international prominence and acclaim for trying to alert the world to the disease's hold on certain regions of the country.

It soon became apparent that Yanhai had been arrested and placed under government detention. The news released a flood of condemnation by international human rights and activist organizations. It seemed emblematic, as Elisabeth Rosenthal of *The New York Times* wrote, of "China's deep official ambivalence about becoming more open about AIDS." The incident helped shine a light on AIDS in China in articles and pieces like "China's Looming Catastrophe," printed in *The New York Times* on September 16, 2002.

The growing U.S. media interest served as a flush backdrop for the release of a groundbreaking National Intelligence Council report at the end of September 2002 entitled, "The Next Wave of HIV/AIDS: Nigeria, Ethiopia, Russia, India and China." The NIC singled out those countries for several reasons: they were among some of the world's most populous states—comprising roughly 40 percent of the world's population; they were all "of strategic importance to the United States"; they were all in the "early to mid-stages" of the epidemic; and they were all "led by governments that have not yet given the issue the sustained high priority that has been key to stemming the tide of the disease in other countries."

The report projected numbers for the next-wave countries out to decade's end. The figures were staggering. Infections in the five countries would grow from current levels of around 14 to 23 million to an estimated 50 to 75 million by 2010. The next-wave countries would soon "eclipse" central and southern Africa—projected to host 30 to 35 million infections— as the pandemic's epicenter. Combining the next-wave countries and central and southern Africa, even excluding the rest of the world, brought the 2010 NIC estimate to between 80 and 110 million infections.

Each of the next-wave countries had been woefully deficient in addressing and combating the disease. The levels of response and the factors governing them varied in each case, but the litany was familiar: lack of resources, lack of political will, taboo, denial, other public health issues, other pressing geopolitical, economic, or political matters.

The report conferred a sense of gravity on this emerging dimension of the crisis. "The rise of HIV/AIDS in the next-wave countries is likely to have significant economic, social, political, and military implications," the report argued. All of the five "next-wave" countries were either key U.S. strategic partners or strategic competitors. The disease was poised to extract a prodigious toll in human life, and be sufficiently destabilizing as to factor into U.S. strategic plans.

Estimates in Russia of HIV infection tallied between 1 and 2 million. By 2010, the report predicted, the figure would climb to between 5 and 8 million. HIV infection levels in China were estimated to range between 1 and 2 million. By 2010, the report predicted, the virus would infect between 10 and 15 million people. None of the three nuclear powers and Great Power states profiled in the report was positioned as precariously as India. Experts put India's infection level at between 5 and 8 million. By 2010, the report projected, India would far surpass South Africa as the most infected country in the world with between 20 and 25 million infections.

The year 2010 was hardly the endpoint. Rather, the forward estimates implied that the virus would have been introduced into each nation's mainstream population, making it even harder to contain thereafter. For the "next-wave" countries, the 2010 estimates were only the beginning.

The NIC report was widely covered and cited. *New York Times* health and science journalist Lawrence Altman profiled the report's findings in an October 1, 2002, piece entitled, "AIDS in 5 Nations Called Security Threat." Later in the month, Sebastian Mallaby of *The Washington Post* wrote an emotive editorial entitled, "An Optional Catastrophe."

Mallaby opened the editorial: "This isn't going to be a clever column. It's going to say something blindingly obvious. But sometimes the obvious needs stating, because it is taken for granted and then quietly ignored. A century from now, when historians write about our era, one question will dwarf all others, and it won't be about finance or politics or even terrorism. The question will be, simply, how could our rich and civilized society allow a known and beatable enemy to kill millions of people?"

The day Mallaby's editorial appeared, Kofi Annan was bestowed with an honorary doctorate from Zhejiang University in the eastern Chinese city of Hangzhou. Addressing thousands of faculty and students in a majestic auditorium, Annan, donning an academic gown, pointedly addressed the AIDS crisis: "China is facing a decisive moment," he proclaimed. The country stood "on the brink of an explosive AIDS epidemic. . . . There is no time to lose if China is to prevent a massive further spread of HIV/AIDS." Annan's comments stirred attention worldwide.

He was not the only person with international cachet to confer his energies on the "next-wave" countries during the fall of 2002.

———•◆•———

Sitting on a multibillion-dollar fortune that had made him the richest man in the world, Bill Gates had been deeply interested in embarking on an ambitious philanthropic program for years. Reading a magazine article in 1998, the Microsoft mogul came across a statistic that staggered him: developing countries were carrying 90 percent of the world's disease burden, yet they had only 10 percent of the world's health resources.

Gates's father, a prominent local figure in his own right, and chairman of the Bill and Melinda Gates Foundation, Gates's philanthropic vehicle founded in 1994, recalled to journalist Geoffrey Cowley, "Trey [Gates's boyhood nickname] sent me [the] article. . . . And he said, 'Dad, maybe we could do something about this.' " It was the beginning of what was to become one of the largest and most remarkable individual philanthropic ventures in human history.

Developing world health became the number one priority for the Bill and Melinda Gates Foundation, endowed less than a decade after its creation with roughly $24 billion. Tax law required the foundation to distribute in excess of $1 billion a year. By 2002, the foundation had already pledged billions. It doled out smaller chunks to efforts such as a special task force on global AIDS co-chaired by senators Frist and Kerrey at the prestigious Washington, D.C., Center for Strategic and International Studies. In June 2001 the foundation cut a $100 million check to the Global Fund in its fledgling days, helping to provide the fund with critical early momentum. Gates funded an HBO documentary entitled *Pandemic*, produced by Rory Kennedy, Bobby Kennedy's youngest daughter. It was hard to find a private, or even public, sector initiative focused on developing world health or global AIDS without a check signed by the Gates Foundation in its bank account.

In November 2002, Gates made a journey to India to pledge $100 million to help curb the tide of the epidemic. He felt a particular personal and professional kinship with India due in part to its burgeoning technology industry. In a November 2002 editorial in *The New York Times* entitled "Slowing the Spread of AIDS in India," Gates explained that India was on its way to becoming a global economic superpower, and that the country's purchasing power was the fourth largest in the world. "Much of this progress will be threatened by AIDS," he cautioned. Gates proclaimed elsewhere that his $100 million donation marked the beginning of his commitment to India.

In addition to funds, Gates wrote op-eds, appeared at international conferences like the World Economic Forum, and made sure to speak about the disease on programs like *Charlie Rose*, even though he came on to speak about developments at Microsoft. By the late fall of 2002, Kofi Annan and Bill Gates had come to round out a most remarkable assortment of personalities publicly committed to fight the pandemic.

At the Waldorf Astoria in midtown Manhattan before a session at the World Economic Forum in late January 2002, Bill Clinton arrived for a meeting with Bill Gates and a few other leaders from the not-for-profit world. It was the first time that Clinton and Gates would meet since the Justice Department's high-profile case against Microsoft's alleged monopolist practices. At first, participants could feel the tension between Gates and Clinton. Then the conversation veered toward global AIDS. The two leaders got engaged. Clinton mentioned that he had met with Bono the previous night. Everyone laughed. As the spirit warmed, Clinton chimed, "Maybe an impeached president, a monopolist, and an aging rock star can do something about this."

The quip spoke volumes about the motley crew that had emerged to fight the disease. Membership now included: Bill Gates, the world's richest man; Kofi Annan, one of the world's most prominent diplomats; ex-President Bill Clinton, who worked through his foundation to transform the South African response, to enhance Southern African and Caribbean health care systems, and to broker landmark deals to make AIDS drugs more affordable; Jeffrey Sachs, one of the world's leading economists; Ambassador Richard Holbrooke, who founded the Global Business Coalition on HIV/AIDS, an alliance of leading companies spearheading the business fight against the disease; Secretary of State Colin Powell; and Bono, one of the most popular rock stars in the world.

To varying extents they had all proclaimed publicly that at the dawn of the new millennium there was no challenge more pressing, no problem more daunting than the global AIDS pandemic. They all pledged their personal commitment to do their part to upgrade the world's response. While they collaborated with one another on occasion, they were an unofficial crew; each wielded his own distinct voice. Collectively, the remarkable assemblage of personalities was becoming impossible to ignore.

The motley crew's involvement helped further drive press coverage and public interest in the issue. At the same time, leading thinkers and publications were providing the pandemic greater degrees of attention and profile.

The November/December issue of the prestigious foreign policy journal *Foreign Affairs* featured global AIDS as its leading cover story for the first time in the pandemic's twenty-year history. The extensive article by Nick Eberstadt, entitled, "The Future of AIDS: Grim Toll in Russia, China and India," profiled the three most prominent "next-wave" countries, further helping to extend U.S. perceptions of the scope of the pandemic beyond Africa's shores.

Hazarding predictions over an even longer timeline than the NIC report, Eberstadt's article estimated that from 2000 to 2025 under three scenarios—mild, intermediate, or severe epidemics—the three Eurasian powers would incur 66 million, 193 million, or 259 million new infections, respectively. According to Eberstadt's numbers, the possibility of hundreds of millions of cumulative global infections by 2025 was very real.

He then explored what that might mean for the countries' long-term economic futures. In the "intermediate epidemic" scenario, Russia would incur 13 million new infections from 2000 to 2025. Already beset by severe economic and demographic challenges, AIDS would send Russia's economy into a 40 percent decline from 2000 to 2025.

In the same scenario, China would incur 70 million new infections in the twenty-five-year period. AIDS would cut into China's economic growth over the time period by well in excess of 33 percent. Eberstadt forecasted 110 million new infections for India under the "intermediate epidemic" scenario; in which case AIDS would lower the emerging power's economic growth by roughly 40 percent.

The disease would have a profound economic and geopolitical influence on the stability of the region and its relationship to the United States and the world. Eberstadt likened the pandemic's explosion in the region to a gathering tempest. Yet Moscow, New Delhi, and Beijing continued to regard the crisis with "a curious detachment. . . . When they come to their senses," Eberstadt cautioned, "the tempest will be even nearer than it is and they may discover that their ability to navigate out of harm's way is more limited than they would have supposed."

———•◆•———

Even as the gale swirled through Eurasia, quietly picking up force, the storm clouds of war were descending upon the Middle East and Washington, D.C.

Proceeding in stealth, the core team had been continuing to consult with outside specialists attempting to flesh out the contours of the president's new global AIDS initiative. They were making a reasonable amount of progress, but the details of the plan were still far from finalized.

The new initiative was to be the president's key deliverable for his upcoming trip in January 2003 to Africa. With the probability of war very high, and the White House walking a diplomatic tightrope, several insiders wondered if the trip would go forward. "International and domestic" considerations and—though not publicly acknowledged—concerns about the president's safety led the White House on Saturday, December 21, to announce that in fact the president would *not* make the planned January trip.

The White House insisted that the trip would be postponed, not canceled. Skeptics outside the administration interpreted it as a lack of will and interest in Africa. Even insiders who were aware of the administration's interest in Africa wondered about the probability of a future trip with war looming on the horizon.

The cancellation of the trip seemed to bode very poorly for the prospects of a recalibrated U.S. global AIDS initiative. The war on terror, an economic recession, the prodigious tax cut and the resultant deficit further dampened the prognosis. On top of it all, the imminence of another war that would cost at least tens of billions and bring peril and uncertainty seemed to many—both inside and outside the administration—to drain all the promise of a bold initiative on an issue that had long been perceived as "long-term" and "humanitarian" in nature.

Jeffrey Sachs had another take. For some time Sachs had been an intermittent contributor for *The Economist*, writing about globalization, development, and international economics. In an article printed in the magazine in late October 2002, Sachs reiterated a point he had been expressing in various guises for years. "One of the reasons why the Bush administration is losing the battle for the world's hearts and minds is precisely that it fights only the war on terror, while turning a cold and steely eye away from millions dying of hunger and disease."

An administration with an abiding faith in American righteousness had presided over a precipitous decline in America's image throughout the world. Pursuing a preemptive war with Iraq despite widespread international dissent, and U.S. willingness to shun international opinion and go it alone—even after attempting to work through the UN system—alienated much of Europe, Asia, and the developing world.

America, it seemed to many, was all force. The time was ripe to inject some "compassion" into U.S. foreign policy. Sachs's article—which he was told was widely read, particularly by Condoleezza Rice and others in the White House—spoke to the deficit of compassion: "If George Bush spent more time and money on mobilizing Weapons of Mass Salvation, in addition to combating Weapons of Mass Destruction, we might actually get somewhere in making this planet a safer and more hospitable home."

Most presumed that war with Iraq would squeeze global AIDS off the administration's agenda. Few, if any, imagined that it would in fact help catapult it to an unprecedented level of priority.

Yet there was a historical consistency to the president's approach. In the war planning for America's earlier incursion into Afghanistan to topple the Taliban, it was the president, according to journalist Bob Woodward's account, who insisted that even as fighter planes dropped bombs on Kabul and other regions of the country, other planes drop food aid. It was not an easy thing to do, but the president's approach coupled mass humanitarian assistance with the prosecution of war. Bush was willing to flex American muscle, but wanted to demonstrate American generosity and humanity at the same time.

There seemed to Stephen Morrison, directing the CSIS task force on global AIDS, among others, four big reasons driving the Bush administration's willingness to pursue a global AIDS plan of immense proportions: "Iraq, Iraq, Iraq, Iraq." There was a keen desire, Morrison said, in the weeks leading up to the war "to do something to demonstrate that it was not all Iraq all the time."

In late November, several hundred activists marched in front of the White House protesting funding for both domestic and global AIDS. Several carried mock body bags reading: "Bush: Stop AIDS Deaths." Others waved cardboard skulls as the group marched from McPherson Square at Fifteenth Street NW to Lafayette Square, right across from the White House. At 1:45 P.M., thirty-one protestors, who had chained themselves together, lay down right outside the gate of the White House. They were promptly arrested.

Days later, on December 1, World AIDS Day, Colin Powell and Tommy Thompson gave a strong address to scores of foreign diplomats highlighting the urgency of combating the pandemic and upgrading the global response. *The New York Times* published a lengthy op-ed written by William Jefferson Clinton that dominated the editorial page. Under the title "AIDS Is Not a Death Sentence," Clinton called on the United States and the rest of the world to provide treatment for the 95 percent of the HIV-positive population in the world who did not have access to the drugs. While the administration may have welcomed a robust discourse on the pandemic, they may have been less enthusiastic about Clinton's attempt to cast himself as a global leader on the issue.

Also on World AIDS Day, Bono launched an advocacy campaign dubbed the Heart of America Tour, enlisting a cadre of celebrities like Chris Tucker and Ashley Judd to tour the American Midwest. Traveling to ports of call like Iowa, Illinois, and Nebraska, Bono, Shriver, and Drummond had purposefully targeted constituencies for key members of Congress. Going directly to churches and larger venues, they were also probing the very core of Bush's political constituency.

Bono had Warren Buffett, the wealthy investor, and Lance Armstrong, the indefatigable cyclist and Tour de France champion, join him at certain events, ensuring that he had enlisted personalities that would appeal to every possible demographic. Medical and health experts from Harvard and leading not-for-profits rounded out the touring company, along with a young HIV-positive woman from Uganda who told her personal story. She told of giving AIDS to her child and watching both her child and her husband perish from the disease. If America's heartland couldn't go to Africa, then Bono would bring Africa to them.

The tour generated a good deal of publicity and launched a shot directly across the bow of Bush's political base. It inspired thousands of letters and telephone calls to the White House and the Congress requesting U.S. aid for the crisis. It was an important and timely effort, "which we know had an impact," said Jamie Drummond.

In mid-December, at a birthday celebration for one-hundred-year-old Senator Strom Thurmond, the Senate majority leader, Trent Lott from Mis-

sissippi made an offhand comment suggesting that the country would be better off if Thurmond—a well-noted former segregationist—had won the presidency decades back. The comment went little noticed for a day or so. Then
Lott's comment began spreading on the Internet and in no time the mainstream media picked up on it, opening up the floodgates to a storm of media
coverage and a crisis for Karl Rove and the Republican party.

Lott's comments, whether serious or not, touched a highly sensitive
nerve. They reflected everything that Rove, Bush, and their team had tried
to steer clear of in remaking the image of their party. Picking up more than
the 9 percent of the African-American vote that Bush won in 2000 was a
key political priority from the outset. Lott's comments put the administration in an awkward situation and heightened the impetus to reach out to
African-Americans in Congress as well as to the African-American public
at large. Supporting Bill Frist's emergence as majority speaker, and his
ascent as the new face of the party in the Senate, was one way to do that.
Demonstrating that the president cared about the death of millions of
Africans a year was yet another.

In mid- to late December 2002, the administration and the core team
working on the AIDS initiative faced a critical question: Should they
shelve the announcement of the president's global AIDS initiative—still
very much under construction—for Bush's future trip to Africa, or should it
be announced at the upcoming State of the Union Address in late January
2003? At some point in the weeks to follow, it was decided that the announcement would be made at the State of the Union.

Three days before Christmas, on December 22, 2002, a story appeared in
The New York Times Magazine entitled "What Will Become of Africa's
AIDS Orphans?" It was an extensive piece that touched on the dimensions
of the orphan crisis, but was primarily a human-interest piece exploring the
author's own adoption of an AIDS orphan. The title of the piece appeared
on the cover of the magazine, but was second-feature to a story on college
athletics.

On the following day, December 23, a lengthy *Washington Post* editorial
entitled "Denial Here at Home" suggested that the global AIDS pandemic was "probably the most underestimated enemy of all time." Having
gotten wind that something was stirring at 1600 Pennsylvania Avenue, the
editorial ended: "The Bush administration is preparing a strategy on AIDS;
it was to be released in time for the president's trip to Africa next month.
Now that trip has been postponed; once again, Africa is taking a back seat

in policymaking. There can be no similar postponement of an American commitment on AIDS," the editorial insisted: "This is a big moment for the Bush presidency . . . Mr. Bush needs to be bold."

The following week, on December 29, Kofi Annan submitted an editorial to *The New York Times* entitled "In Africa, AIDS Has a Woman's Face." Annan explained that women comprise more than half of Africa's infected population. The secretary general spoke to this critical dimension of the catastrophe and of the pandemic as an elemental force in "threatening the backbone of Africa—the women who keep African societies going."

In an unusually lengthy editorial printed in *The Washington Post* one day before the State of the Union entitled "Mr. President, Africa Needs Us," Bono wrote: "When President Bush delivers his State of the Union address tomorrow, he will focus on the military threats to national security. . . . But I hope for a few minutes the president will talk about the global AIDS crisis—and define a historic American response." Bono went on to say that when he met with Bush the year before, "he promised despite the deficit, if we could show him effective programs, these efforts would not go without funding. We can."

Then Bono repeated a refrain promulgated by his good friend and tutor Jeffrey Sachs, but this time in his own words: "It's a chance to show what America is for, not just what it is against." The line had pop.

Bono's editorial was an attempt to hold the administration to its pledge. Inside the White House, though, unbeknownst to all but a very few select insiders, the gauntlet had already been dropped.

A small group of upper-level administration officials had gathered in the White House only days before the Tuesday State of the Union address. The agenda was the president's new AIDS plan. Colin Powell had heard a lot of numbers floating around over the preceding weeks. Up until the final days, in fact, the group had been considering three options for its five-year plan: $5 billion, $10 billion, and $15 billion; or the Chevrolet, Oldsmobile, and Cadillac versions, respectively, according to Anthony Fauci.

"I must admit," Powell said months later, "I was kind of on the low end of the range knowing the demands and the pressures on our federal budget."

The president was sitting in the Oval Office on the other end of the range. "It's going to be $15 billion," the president announced to Powell's astonishment.

"You want to say that again, Boss?"

"Fifteen billion dollars," the president said.

———•◆•———

At 9:01 P.M. EST on January 28, 2003, President George W. Bush walked to the podium in the Capitol Building with a confident but somber gait. The president's demeanor reflected the mood of the chamber and the country he was about to address on the state of the American union. For months, the United States had been dissatisfied with the Iraqi government's response to UN weapons inspectors' demands, and much of the international community's calls for more time.

Few now doubted that war was imminent.

As the applause that greeted him drew into silence, the president looked grave but resolute. "This year, we gather in this chamber deeply aware of decisive days that lie ahead. You and I serve our country in a time of great consequence. We have a duty to reform domestic programs vital to our country; we have the opportunity to save millions of lives abroad from a terrible disease."

For the next several pages of his address, the president outlined the state of, and his plans for, the economy, health care, the environment, and the importance of mentoring and volunteerism as a civic pillar of American society. He then delivered a few lines about America's commitment to Afghanistan, the Middle East, and alleviating hunger worldwide.

"As our nation moves troops and builds alliances to make our world safer, we must also remember our calling as a blessed country is to make this world better. Today, on the continent of Africa, nearly 30 million people have the AIDS virus—including 3 million children under the age of fifteen. There are whole countries in Africa where more than one-third of the adult population carries the infection. More than 4 million require immediate drug treatment. Yet across the continent, only 50,000 AIDS victims—only 50,000—are receiving the medicine they need.

"A doctor in rural South Africa describes his frustration," Bush continued. "He says, 'We have no medicines. Many hospitals tell people, you've got AIDS, we can't help you. Go home and die.' In an age of miraculous medicines, no person should hear those words."

Both sides of the political aisle burst into applause. The television cameras panned to the chamber's balcony. They pulled focus on first lady Laura Bush, and the president's guest of honor, sitting to the first lady's right,

Dr. Peter Mugyenyi, the physician from Uganda who had consulted with the core team and played a central role in their efforts. The first lady was flanked on her other side by a uniformed military servicewoman. It was the desired snapshot: to one side the stick and on the other the carrot, American might and beneficence, both on display.

"AIDS can be prevented," the president went on. The cost of AIDS drugs had fallen from $12,000 a year to under $300 a year, he said, in a seemingly implicit endorsement of generic drugs—to many, a staggering feature of the plan Bush was beginning to outline on this most high-profile of occasions.

"Ladies and gentlemen, seldom has history offered a greater opportunity to do so much for so many," the president said, delivering the words with dramatic effect. "And to meet a severe and urgent crisis abroad, tonight I propose the Emergency Plan for AIDS Relief—a work of mercy beyond all current international efforts to help the people of Africa."

The plan would aim to provide treatment for 2 million people, prevent 7 million new infections, and care for millions of infected and orphaned. The chamber erupted in applause, setting the stage for the denouement.

"I ask the Congress to commit $15 billion over the next five years, including $10 billion in new money, to turn the tide against AIDS in the most afflicted nations in Africa and the Caribbean." Both sides of the aisle sprang to their feet and unleashed a clamor of approval. The panning television cameras managed to catch senators and congress members, some nodding their heads in shock, others wearing cynical smirks even as they joined in the applause.

Bush devoted roughly seven paragraphs of his historic address to set up and outline his Emergency Plan for AIDS Relief. His pledge meant a tripling of current U.S. funding, which was already more than double Clinton administration funding. Moreover, the president seemed to meet the AIDS community's demand of $3 billion a year in U.S. funding.

With one dramatic and unexpected stroke, President Bush had punctured the bubble of U.S. abdication and inaction that had engulfed the country throughout the twenty-year history of the pandemic's flight.

Historians rightly caution against the mono-causal explanation. History and the leaders who make it are almost always driven by multiple forces and motivations. A panoply of causative factors helped set the stage for an upgraded U.S. policy. Still, the contours and magnitude of the initiative remained to be decided by one man, the ultimate arbiter. If a "genocide" of unprecedented proportions was sweeping through a continent almost unabated and it was well within U.S. means and competency to prevent millions of deaths, then the president's sense of religious and moral duty prescribed action.

President Bush ended his historic speech asserting, "We Americans have faith in ourselves, but not in ourselves alone. We do not know—we do not claim to know all the ways of Providence, yet we can trust in them, placing our confidence in the loving God behind all of life, and all of history. May He guide us now."

Speaking to members of the AIDS Support Organization Center in Entebbe, Uganda, during his July 2003 trip to Africa—indeed postponed, not canceled—the president exclaimed: "You know, I believe God has called us into action. I believe we have a responsibility. My country has a great responsibility."

————•◆•————

10:00 P.M. EST, January 28, 2003.

Eric Sawyer was walking his dog in Morningside Park near the Columbia University campus in New York City. The longtime activist had heard mumblings about an upcoming announcement at the State of the Union. Sawyer had heard similar discussion for years. He assumed that it was the administration sending up "trial balloons," and he remained skeptical.

Sawyer's cell phone rang. It was Heidi Ostertag, one of the co-producers on a film entitled A Closer Walk, a poignant account of the pandemic narrated by Glenn Close and Will Smith, which Sawyer was also co-producing and had been laboring on extensively for months. Ostertag told Sawyer about the president's initiative. His reaction: "Holy fucking shit."

Sawyer's head was spinning. He thought back to his opening remarks at the Vancouver Conference in the summer of 1996 when he had called on drug companies to drop their prices and for a multibillion-dollar response. Sawyer began dialing some trusted friends, the ones who through his thirty-plus arrests, the degradation and tumult, had thought he was crazy, but had stuck by him anyway.

In succeeding months, as the details of the actual legislation trickled out, Sawyer once again turned skeptical. The administration's pledge of $15 billion seemed to suggest that the United States would now spend $3 billion in each of the five years going forward. And though the president had never specified how the aggregate plan would be weighted, Sawyer was dismayed that the administration pledged only $2.1 billion, instead of $3 billion, in its 2004 budget. He further learned that the legislation merely *authorized* the government to spend up to $15 billion. The legislation was replete with outs, and there was no guarantee that the dollars would be there.

Burned out, Sawyer remained in the thick of things, but he had tried to calm the pace and intensity of his activities. He awoke early, though, the morning after the State of the Union, to grab a copy of *The New York Times* for a full transcript of the president's remarks. He wanted to parse through the president's language to see how he could use it "to keep the pressure up [and] to make sure that it wasn't just more false rhetoric and [yet] another good public relations statement that didn't materialize."

A few blocks south, Jeffrey Sachs was watching television in his new home near Columbia. Sachs had just moved to New York to run a new institute at the university. Having heard to expect something, Sachs telephoned his wife and kids back in Massachusetts to make sure that they were watching, too.

He was displeased with the Bush II administration on several fronts. He was against a preemptive war in Iraq and felt that the administration was being deceptive. He also had serious qualms with the administration's fiscal policies. On global AIDS, he was skeptical of their assurances. "Be patient" did little to instill confidence.

His friend Bono believed that something big was in the works. During calls to Sachs, he insisted, "It's going to happen."

Sachs was elated to hear the dollar amounts announced. They were identical to those he had first proposed two and a half years earlier in Durban, South Africa, and had been vigorously promoting since. Even more than the figures, though, Sachs was thrilled with the "bluntness" of the president's insistence that people should not be sent home to die. What pleased him most was that the president had now stuck out his neck politically. He was accountable, and it seemed to Sachs, "things could never be put back in the box the way they were."

The next morning, Sachs called Bono and for a moment the tutor became the pupil. "You were right," Sachs told him. "I was losing heart. [You were] right—they actually did something."

Later that day Sachs took a briefing call from the White House and in the course of subsequent inquiry learned something disturbing. Out of the $10 billion in "new" money the administration pledged, only $1 billion, or 10 percent, would go to the new Global Fund. The rest would be administered directly by the United States in a bilateral capacity. For Sachs, the decision was "preposterous."

While it may not have been a nostrum, the Global Fund promised to be one of the most effective vehicles for generating global financial and political support and disbursing funds effectively to those who needed help most. While there was certainly room for bilateral activity, particularly as the fund continued to scale up, a predominantly bilateral approach, as it had before, threatened to beget duplication, fragmentation, and inevitably national politics; and quite possibly religious dogma would seep in. In bypassing the Global Fund, Sachs worried, the United States would forego the best leverage it had for coaxing other nations to join in what very much needed to be a global effort.

John Donnelly, the *Boston Globe* journalist, was sitting at home on his couch in Chevy Chase, Maryland. He had also heard that the administration had something in the works. Listening to the address, Donnelly was stunned at the magnitude of the president's pledge. Donnelly turned to his wife and exclaimed, "Amazing." Then he said, "I've got to write about this."

He followed the rest of Bush's comments on AIDS. Then he jumped to his feet and got on the phone with his paper's news desk. He insisted that they make space for him. In thirty minutes he pounded out a short piece and sent it off. Then the journalist took a moment to reflect on the occasion.

It seemed to Donnelly that the announcement had heralded a turning point. Donnelly predicted that finally, even if fitfully, rich countries would begin to "start addressing this with the seriousness with which it deserves."

Only a few days before, Donnelly had joined a group of six or seven journalists for a session with Colin Powell on the seventh floor at the State Department. A congenial group, they met beforehand to discuss the questions that each would ask. Donnelly said that he would ask about global AIDS. No one argued, but the looks Donnelly received were all too familiar. His colleagues' expressions seemed to be saying, "That's nice, but why do you want to ask about that?"

He had been one of only a very few foreign policy journalists to cover the issue on a consistent and continual basis. For Donnelly, the president's announcement was satisfying both personally and professionally. Looking forward, he anticipated that the new plan would also mark a turning point in the depth and breadth of the media's coverage of the pandemic and the world's response. In the months following the announcement, he was still waiting.

Ken Bernard was logging yet another late night at the Old Executive Office Building. After 9/11, Bernard had left HHS to join the Office—not yet Department—of Homeland Security, functioning effectively as the president's special assistant for Bio-Defense. Walking the halls, Bernard stopped by a colleague's office. The television was on, and Bush was front and center delivering his State of the Union. Bernard sat and watched.

White House "operational security" on the announcement was "extremely good." The core team and the handful of others who knew kept the plan "very, very, very close hold." Bernard only learned about the plan when he saw a copy of the speech on a senior colleague's desk the day before the address. He was both shocked and ecstatic.

Listening to Bush's words on the pandemic meet wild applause, Bernard felt gratified. The announcement evoked memories of desperate late nights in the Old Executive, of internecine turf battles with Sandy Thurman, and of the primary impetus for Bernard's interest in coming to the National Security Council as its first Senior Advisor for International Health back in August 1998: to get the U.S. government to deal with global health and global AIDS in particular as a threat to "U.S. national security."

To be sure, some of the administration's leading policy makers, including Secretary of State Colin Powell, had acknowledged the health-security nexus. But in characteristic fashion, the administration had not reached a consensus on the issue. In the State of the Union, Bush defined his plan as a "a work of mercy." And so, even as the disease was at work destroying Southern African states, creating breeding grounds for conflict and terrorists, and burgeoning in the "next-wave" countries, where it would have destabilizing effects of untold proportions, the U.S. approach remained humanitarian, without the urgency, priority, or scale of traditional "national security" threats.

Dr. Joe McCormick, the old virus hunter, was sitting on the couch in his living room with his wife in his hacienda-style home in Brownsville, Texas.

After years of living overseas, the itinerant public health expert had settled down to start a school of public health, the first of its kind in South Texas. With Mexico five minutes, by foot, from the door of his office, McCormick's gaze continued to extend beyond America's borders.

The president's AIDS initiative caught McCormick entirely unaware. He had been focusing on lassa fever and other matters, and had no inkling that something monumental was in the works. It was a pleasant surprise. Immediately, McCormick began thinking about precisely how the money would be spent. If it was spent well, the administration was capable of achieving enormous progress; if not, it could all just trickle "down the tubes."

Thrilled that Africa would receive billions in U.S. funding, McCormick was still deeply exasperated. It was almost exactly twenty years earlier that he had first determined that the disease was present in Africa. "This is great," McCormick thought, "but it's about ten years too late." He couldn't help but notice that the U.S. funding would be directed toward fourteen countries—twelve in Africa and two in the Caribbean. The rest of the world, including the "next-wave" countries, had been excluded. "Africa ten years or so ago was more or less where these countries are today." In the first wave of the pandemic, "We waited until the horse was out of the barn and several pastures away until we did anything significant."

At the State Department, Colin Powell and his former ambassador for global AIDS had done much to press the "next-wave" countries and others to mobilize their societies to combat the disease. U.S. economic and security interests were at stake, and so were tens of millions of lives. But without deeply intensified presidential and cabinet-level diplomatic engagement, and without the carrot of vastly upgraded financial and technical assistance, these states appeared likely to remain mired in the plethora of obstacles that had underpinned African leaders' abdication for so long. History, it is said, does not repeat itself; rather, statesmen keep making the same mistakes.

Through it all, not a day had gone by in which McCormick had not thought about his dear old friend Jonathan Mann. The pioneer had passed, but his legacy still brimmed with resonance.

Mann had been the first, and really the only person, in the history of the global response to devise and attempt to implement a comprehensive global strategy to combat the pandemic. Two months before the State of the Union, the longtime senator from Vermont, Patrick Leahy, took to the floor of the Senate. "What we lack, even after all these years," Leahy said, "is a global plan. This administration, like the one before it and the one before that, has no plan for how to mount a global campaign to effectively combat the most deadly virus the world has ever faced."

The president's initiative heralded a recalibration in U.S. policy. Focused on only fourteen countries in Africa and the Caribbean, lacking a sufficiently aggressive diplomatic plan of attack, assuming a bilateral approach, and conceptualized as a humanitarian "work of mercy," it was not a comprehensive global strategy. The Emergency Relief Plan aimed to prevent 7 million infections and treat 2 million people. The initiative was historic. Yet measured against the potentiality of a world likely to host hundreds of millions of HIV infections in the decades to follow, the effort remained woefully inadequate.

In Leahy's view much was at stake: "When future generations look back at this time and place, I believe they will judge us, more than anything, on how we responded to AIDS. It is the most urgent, the most compelling, moral issue of our time."

That had been the way Jonathan Mann saw it. "The disease is trying to teach us," Mann would say. Denial, obfuscation, timidity, agendas, egos, and quiescence would all lead to failure. Vision, will, tolerance, sacrifice, cooperation, and humanity were the ingredients of a successful response. In meeting the pandemic's challenge, the United States would do more than save tens of millions of lives and help provide peace, prosperity, and stability. The world's greatest power would embrace a worthy national mission that would unleash its better and nobler angels. It would take one giant step closer to realizing its potential as that shining city upon a hill, a beacon for mankind and what man might be.

The great Renaissance artist Michelangelo once remarked: "The greater danger for most of us is not that our aim is too high and we miss it, but that it is too low and we reach it."

At the dawn of the new millennium, humanity faced no challenge more daunting, no crisis more lethal than the global AIDS pandemic. In all of its resplendent power and potential, the United States knew of no cause more worthy of its aspirations.

A Note on Sources

Introducing myself to interviewees for this book, I would explain that I was writing a book on the U.S. response to the global AIDS pandemic. At least four or five responded, "It should be a short book." The details and insights gathered from more than two hundred interviews with roughly one hundred policy makers and thinkers form the better part of this book. I interviewed many multiple times—two, three, four, or even five times—in sessions lasting anywhere from thirty minutes to three hours.

Without the following core list of interviewees (listed in alphabetical order), whose accounts were particularly central, it would have been a very short book indeed: Terje Anderson, Brian Atwood, Kenneth Bart, Seth Berkley, Ken Bernard, Paul Boneberg, Kate Carr, Ambassador Jack Chow, Jon Cohen, Ambassador Sally Grooms Cowal, Chester Crocker, Nils Daulaire, Paul Davis, Paul DeLay, John Donnelly, Jamie Drummond, Nick Eberstadt, RP Eddy, Scott Evertz, Anthony Fauci, Patsy Fleming, Leon Fuerth, Laurie Garrett, Helene Gayle, Bart Gellman, David Gordon, Jeffrey Harris, Ambassador Richard Holbrooke, Walter Kansteiner, Rory Kennedy, C. Everett Koop, Brad Langmade, Ambassador Stephen Lewis, Jamie Love, Ambassador Princeton Lyman, Joe McCormick, Mora McLean, Congressman Jim McDermott, Michael Merson, Sheila Mitchell, Stephen Morrison, Trevor Neilson, Bob Orr, Peter Piot, Ben Plumley, Susan Rice, Eugene Rivers, Jeffrey Sachs, Eric Sawyer, Mark Schneider, Bernhard Schwartlander, Donna Shalala, Kenneth Shine, Bobby Shriver, Gayle Smith, Shepherd Smith, Anil Soni, Ambassador Dan Spiegel, Karen Stanecki, William Steiger, Steve Sternberg, Todd Summers, Daniel Tarantola, Ken Thomas, Sandy Thurman, Anne Van Dusen, Paul Zeitz.

I have not mentioned several who, though no less helpful, I spoke to on condition of anonymity. I conducted the interviews myself from January 2002 to December 2003. Quoted material comes from these interviews, unless otherwise attributed.

Laurie Garrett's seminal book *The Coming Plague* was an indispensable source in the first section of this book. Garrett's account of policy making in the U.S. and international science and public health arenas throughout the 1980s was particularly valuable. Also, Bart Gellman's *Washington Post* article, "The Belated Global Response to AIDS in Africa," provided valuable material, and first unearthed several of the themes that were explored here. Interviews with both authors, who were particularly gracious and supportive, helped complement their written work.

The following articles and books were critical sources in the specified chapters. **Chapter One:** Joe McCormick and Susan Fisher-Hochs, *Level 4: Virus Hunters of the CDC*; Laurie Garrett, *The Coming Plague*; Randy Shilts, *And the Band Played On.* **Chapter Two:** Laurie Garrett, *The Coming Plague* and *Betrayal of Trust*; Alan Brandt, *No Magic Bullet*; Bart Gellman, "The Belated Global Response to AIDS in Africa." **Chapter Three:** Laurie Garrett, *The Coming Plague*; Bart Gellman, "The Belated Global Response." **Chapter Four:** Princeton Lyman, *A Partner to History*; Bart Gellman, "The Belated Global Response." **Chapter Five:** Haynes Johnson, *The Best of Times.* **Chapter Six:** David Halberstam, *War in a Time of Peace*; Joe Klein, *The Natural*; Bart Gellman, "The Belated Global Response." **Chapter Eight:** Bob Davis, "Gore Hopes New AIDS Pact Will Help Shake Protestors"; Bart Gellman, "A Conflict of Health and Profit." **Chapter Ten:** Kurt Schilinger, "AIDS and the African: Denial"; Samantha Power, "The AIDS Rebel." **Chapter Thirteen:** John Donnelly, "The New Crusade." **Chapter Fourteen:** Josh Tyrangiel, "Bono's Mission"; David Grann, "The Ascent of Bill Frist: The Price of Power." **Chapter Fifteen:** John Donnelly, "Big Spending on AIDS Seen as Go-It-Alone Plan"; Nicholas Eberstadt, "The Future of AIDS: Grim Toll in Russia, China and India."

Hundreds of other sources, as listed in the Notes that follow, provided invaluable information and insights. Detailed bibliographic information accompanies the sources, as first listed in notes.

Notes

PREFACE

xi "Every day, 8,000 people": The most recent death toll available for the World Trade Center was 2,752 according to Dan Barry, "A New Account of September 11 Loss, With 40 Fewer Souls to Mourn," *The New York Times*, October 29, 2003. An additional 189 at the Pentagon and 40 on the plane that crashed in Pennsylvania bring the total number of 9/11 deaths to 2,981, not including the 19 hijackers.

xi "Since the first century": William Eckhardt, "War-Related Deaths Since 3000 B.C.," *Bulletin of Peace Proposals*, December 1991.

xi "There will be as many": In his "intermediate" and "severe" scenarios Nick Eberstadt estimates there may be as many as 193 million and 259 million new infections in Russia, India, and China alone from 2000 to 2025. There will be tens of millions of additional infections from Africa, Southeast Asia, Eastern Europe, and elsewhere. Nicholas Eberstadt, "The Future of AIDS: Grim Toll in Russia, China and India," *Foreign Affairs*, Volume 81, Number 6, November/December 2002.

xi "By 2010, several African countries": "The AIDS Pandemic in the 21st Century: The Demographic Impact on Developing Countries," Released by USAID, and conducted by Karen Stanecki of the U.S. Census Bureau, July 2000.

xii "By 2010, Africa will be host": "UNAIDS/UNICEF Fact Sheet: Children Orphaned by AIDS in Sub-Saharan Africa," October 23, 2003.

xii "Within several generations": "The Long-Run Economic Costs of AIDS: Theory and an Application to South Africa," The World Bank, July 2003.

xii "as high as 50 percent": Interview: Alex de Waal.

xii "Southern Africa is": Interview: Stephen Lewis.

xii "By 2025, one expert estimates": Nicholas Eberstadt, "The Future of AIDS: Grim Toll in Russia, China and India." Under the "intermediate" scenario, Eberstadt projects Russia's economic output will decrease by 40 percent; India's output is projected to decline off of its baseline growth by 40 percent, and China's output is projected to decline off of its baseline growth by "much" more than 33 percent.

xii "Russia faces the additional": Jon Tedstrom, "Russia Must Tackle AIDS Without Delay," editorial in *The Financial Times*, September 17, 2003. Also 8 million figure is high range in National Intelligence Council, prepared under auspices of David F. Gordon, "The Next Wave of HIV/AIDS: Nigeria, Ethiopia, Russia, India, and China" Intelligence Community Assessment, September 2002.

xiv "Months earlier, a *Washington Post*": Editorial entitled, "Denial Here at Home," in *The Washington Post*, December 23, 2002.

xiv "Throughout the pandemic's": Of course, the disease originated well beyond the early 1980s. It was during the early 1980s, however, when the U.S. confirmed and processed that the disease had international dimensions. That is why I speak of a twenty-year response.

A Feeble Beginning (1983–1990)

CHAPTER ONE. A CONTENTIOUS START, BUCK PASSING

3 "A few minutes into": Interview: Joe McCormick.

4 "Yambuku, McCormick would learn": McCormick gives primary credit to Karl Johnson for naming the virus. Interview: Joe McCormick.

5 "He felt, he would later tell friends": Joe McCormick and Susan Fisher-Hoch, *Level 4: Virus Hunters of the CDC* (New York: Barnes & Noble Books, 1996), pp. 14, 16–18. The details of McCormick's experiences in both Yambuku and Nzara come primarily from this account.

6 "These microscopic cells function": Laurie Garrett, *The Coming Plague* (New York: Penguin Books, 1994), p. 292.

6 "Through 1981 and '82": The CDC reported roughly 900 cases by the end of 1982. Randy Shilts, *And the Band Played On* (New York: St. Martin's Press, 1987), p. 214.

6 "By year's end a seven-year-old": Laurie Garrett, *The Coming Plague*, p. 309.

6 "To health and science journalist": Ibid., p. 296.

6 "In February 1983, the CDC": Randy Shilts, *And the Band Played On*, p. 233.

7 "As a consequence": There was, of course, a good deal of thought given to the Haitian cases. But the Caribbean was generally considered an extension of the North American continent. The Haitian cases were of interest to the scientific establishment or the media, early on, mostly in terms of how they related to what was emerging in the United States. They were not particularly concerned about what was happening in Haiti, or elsewhere, and were not concerned, by and large, with the global dimension.

7 "He was a family man": Randy Shilts, *And the Band Played On*, p. 70.

8 "Piot, it turned out": He had in fact requested a grant from Curran for his own Africa trip in the early spring of 1983, months before McCormick's request. Reportedly, Curran was "noncommittal." Laurie Garrett, *The Coming Plague*, p. 345.

8 "Dr. Tshibasu, a tall man": McCormick and Fisher-Hoch, *Level 4: Virus Hunters*, pp. 165–67. Account of devaluation and dinner at Greek restaurant also from here.

8 "He would be happy to cooperate": Ibid., p. 166.

9 "He clung to the one pillar": Ibid., pp. 167, 168, 171–73. Detail on Yema and McCormick's experience at Mama Yemo come primarily from this account.

10 "When the results came back": Interview: Joe McCormick.

10 "To the team's outrage": Laurie Garrett, *The Coming Plague*, p. 347.

10 "He cautioned the scientific community": Ibid., p. 324.

12 " 'What we saw with the disease' ": McCormick and Fisher-Hoch, *Level 4*, pp. 175–76. The details of McCormick's interaction with Foege and the call with Brandt come in part from this account. Details also come from interview: Joe McCormick.

12 "It was, for McCormick": Interview: Joe McCormick.

12 "approximately forty thousand lives": UNAIDS data, provided by Karen Stanecki, March 13, 2003. Unless otherwise noted, this is the source for all of book's historical estimates on infections and deaths. A revised schedule on infections, made available in December 2003, decreased historical estimates on people living with HIV/AIDS. The decrease was relatively slight. As of December 2003, the corresponding schedule for deaths was not yet available. As such it was not possible to estimate historical cumulative global infections based on the more recent December estimates. Thus, the March 2003 estimates were the most recent comprehensive set of historical estimates available.

13 "Those who rose to positions": The inability of scientists and public health leaders to succeed at political advocacy is a leitmotif in Laurie Garrett's section exploring the history, and the state of, the U.S. public health system in *Betrayal of Trust* (New York: Hyperion, 2000).

13 "McCormick would later assert": McCormick, Fisher-Hoch, *Level 4*, p. 176.

13 "Gallo, the director of the eminent": Gallo and his team had in fact been in a highly contested, and contentious, and (later) much publicized—perhaps most compellingly documented in Randy Shilts's seminal book *And the Band Played On*—with a French team of scientists from the In-

stitut Pasteur. The competing scientific agendas, jostling, and prodigious egos detracted from the dire mission at hand.

14 "She suggested that the discovery": Heckler said, "We hope to have such a vaccine ready for testing in approximately two years." Transcript, "Targeting AIDS," *The NewsHour with Jim Lehrer,* June 27, 2001.

14 "An internal 1983 WHO memorandum": Anil Soni, "From GPA to UNAIDS: Examining the Evolution of the UN Response to AIDS," undergraduate thesis, Harvard University, 1998, p. 26.

14 "It would attract approximately two thousand": Laurie Garrett, *The Coming Plague,* p. 352.

15 "Robert Biggar of the U.S. National Cancer Institute": Ibid., p. 352.

15 "The African scientists were aghast": Interview: Peter Piot. Also from Laurie Garrett, *The Coming Plague,* p. 353.

15 "Piot was utterly dejected": Laurie Garrett, *The Coming Plague,* p. 354.

16 " 'African AIDS reports are' ": Ibid., p. 354.

17 "Almost 4 million had": UNAIDS data, provided by Karen Stanecki, March 13, 2003.

17 "The total U.S. appropriation": Institute of Medicine, *Confronting AIDS: Directions for Public Health, Health Care and Research* (Washington, D.C.: National Academy Press, 1986), p. 274.

18 "In the late 1980s, the Soviet Union": Interview: Chester Crocker.

18 "State wasn't opposed to U.S.": Interview: Jeffrey Harris. Leading USAID's global AIDS effort through the mid- and late 1980s, Harris was well-positioned to opine on the State Department's level of activity and interest.

18 "From 1981 to 1983 Reagan": Laurie Garrett, *Betrayal of Trust,* p. 384.

21 "Enlisting USAID to tackle": Interview: RP Eddy.

CHAPTER TWO.
THE PRISM OF THE U.S. EXPERIENCE, ABSENCE OF LEADERSHIP

24 " 'Well, we want you to do that' ": Interview: Jeffrey Harris.

24 " 'We are fighting a war here' ": Laurie Garrett, *The Coming Plague,* p. 506.

25 "On July 8, 1982, the CDC": CDC, "Cases Reported to the CDC as of July 8, 1982."

25 "By decade's end there were almost": CDC, "HIV/AIDS Surveillance Report," Year-End Edition. Issued January 1990. Diagnosed cases tallies do not include cases reported from Guam, Pacific Islands, Puerto Rico, and Virgin Islands, as specified by CDC reports. Death tallies may include these areas; however, they are relatively small. This same methodology is used whenever domestic figures for cumulative diagnosed cases and death totals appear throughout the book.

25 "By the end of 1995, roughly 500,000": CDC, "HIV/AIDS Surveillance Report," Year-End Edition; Vol. 7, No. 2, December 1995.

25 "A group of miscreant arsonists": "Robert Ray, One of 3 Hemophiliac AIDS Brothers, Dies at 22," CNN.com, October 20, 2000.

25 "Harvard University public health expert": Alan Brandt, *No Magic Bullet* (New York: Oxford University Press, 1987), p. 5.

26 "Nineteen percent of those polled": National Center for Health Statistics, "AIDS Knowledge and Attitudes for May and June 1988," from Laurie Garrett, *Betrayal of Trust,* pp. 404, 405.

26 " 'We can all learn and grow' ": Bruce Hilton, "AIDSWEEK: Reagan—Better Late Than Never," *San Francisco Sunday Examiner and Chronicle,* February 4, 1990.

26 " 'It's a virus like measles?' ": Edmund Morris, *Dutch* (New York: Modern Library, 1995), pp. 457–58.

27 "Reagan's handlers had systematically": Interview: C. Everett Koop.

27 "Reagan aide Patrick Buchanan": Alan Brandt, *No Magic Bullet,* p. 193.

27 "Ronald Godwin, director of the Moral Majority": Laurie Garrett, *The Coming Plague,* p. 470.

28 "AIDS was affecting marginalized": Interview: C. Everett Koop.

28 "He did not speak": Ibid. Much of the detail from the "Meeting on the Potomac" comes from Joseph McCormick and Susan Fisher-Hoch, *Level 4: Virus Hunters of the CDC.* Much also comes from interview: Joe McCormick.

28 "Reagan called for abstinence": Laurie Garrett, *The Coming Plague,* p. 470.

28 "No one responded": Edmund Morris, *Dutch*, p. 624. The proposition was considered "too draconian" and dismissed.

28 "If we're not going to worry": Interview: C. Everett Koop.

29 "Hundereds of scientists, in an impromptu": Laurie Garrett, *The Coming Plague*, pp. 470–71.

29 "Pat Robertson brought the issue:" Ibid., pp. 469–70.

30 "There were not that many combatants": Bart Gellman, "The Belated Global Response to AIDS in Africa," *The Washington Post*, July 5, 2000.

30 "By the end of 2000 there were": UNAIDS data, provided by Karen Stanecki, March 13, 2003.

30 "The reaction, according to the principal author": Bart Gellman, "The Belated Global Response . . ."

31 " 'So, there was very little' ": Interview: Princeton Lyman.

31 "Though by marginal increments": "U.S. International Response to HIV/AIDS, 1999," Department of State publication, January 1999, p. 24.

32 "And by the end of the decade": UNAIDS data, provided by Karen Stanecki, March 13, 2003.

32 "His hosts showed little concern": Interview: Jim McDermott.

32 "That rate of infection": Laurie Garrett, *The Coming Plague*, pp. 697, 698. Source: Thai Ministry of Public Health.

32 "Thai policemen told journalist": Ibid., p. 496.

37 "Many of these problems would have": Harris claimed that under his leadership, his division did in fact approach Bill Griggs at the CDC about playing a role in prevention. "They talked about it and thought about it and the answer was no," Harris recollected. "They just didn't feel like they could mobilize the human resources to do it." Interview: Jeffrey Harris.

38 "A landmark August 1993 USAID report": "HIV/AIDS: The Evolution of the Pandemic, The Evolution of the Response," U.S. Agency for International Development, Program for Prevention and Control of HIV Infection, August, 1993, p. 2.

CHAPTER THREE. A MAVERICK GOES TO GENEVA, TURF WARS

42 " 'There's no question,' he exclaimed": Interview: Joe McCormick.

42 "On his first day, Mann arrived": Laurie Garrett, *The Coming Plague*, p. 462.

43 "Two factors would turn him around": Interview: Daniel Tarantola.

43 "Tarantola remembered Mahler telling him": Ibid.

43 "The former skeptic proclaimed": Comes from Bart Gellman, "The Belated Global Response . . ."

44 "Dated 1986, and adopted by the WHA": Interview: Daniel Tarantola.

44 "There could be anywhere from": Ibid.

44 "Mann would later write": Laurie Garrett, *The Coming Plague*, xvi.

45 "In 1989, Chin projected": Ibid., p. 481.

45 "Dismissed and even disparaged": There were, in fact, by the end of 1989 approximately 11.328 million global infections. UNAIDS data, provided by Karen Stanecki, March 13, 2003.

45 "After only a year and a half": Anil Soni, "From GPA to UNAIDS . . . ," p. 37.

46 "Mann found a fitting French phrase": Mark Schoofs, "Body & Soul: Human Rights = Public Health, Remembering AIDS Pioneer Jonathan Mann," *The Village Voice*, September 9, 1998.

46 " 'I'm not convinced that if someone' ": Ibid.

48 "Staff now numbered roughly": Anil Soni, "From GPA to UNAIDS . . . ," pp. 37, 38.

48 "His appeal led the UN": Laurie Garrett, *The Coming Plague*, p. 465.

48 "The U.S.'s senior most health official": Ibid., p. 459.

49 "GPA was working with over 80 percent": Anil Soni, "From GPA to UNAIDS . . . ," p. 37.

50 "Only half of the NAPs": Report of the External Review of the World Health Organization Global Program on AIDS. Geneva: World Health Organization, January, 1992. Comes from Anil Soni, "From GPA to UNAIDS . . . ," p. 73.

53 "Watching from the sidelines": According to Interview: Daniel Tarantola.

54 "He looked at his new colleagues": According to Interview: Daniel Tarantola.
54 " 'He didn't know anything about infectious diseases' ": Interview: Laurie Garrett.
54–55 "Nakajima was overheard": Bart Gellman, "The Belated Global Response . . ."
55 "Anil Soni observed": Anil Soni, "From GPA to UNAIDS . . . ," pp. 81, 82.
55 "Mann now needed documented permission": Interview: Daniel Tarantola.
57 " 'All those years lost!' ": Bart Gellman, "The Belated Global Response . . ."
57 "In that time 32.9 million people": UNAIDS data, provided by Karen Stanecki, March 13, 2003.

Quiescence (1990–1996)

CHAPTER FOUR. VOICES IN THE WILDERNESS, RACE AND SPACE

61 "At 3:30 P.M. on February 11, 1990": Nelson Mandela, *Long Walk to Freedom: The Autobiography of Nelson Mandela* (Boston: Little, Brown, 1994).
61 "South Africa's Nationalist President": Nelson Mandela, *Long Walk to Freedom*, p. 485.
62 " 'I was on to something' ": Interview: Princeton Lyman.
63 "But there were other issues": Ibid.
63 "By 1994 the number had soared": Department of Health, Republic of South Africa, "National HIV & Syphilis Antenatal Sero-Prevalence Survey in South Africa: 2002," p. 6. These figures are considered by UNAIDS to be the most accurate estimates available for the time period. Interview: Godfrey Sikipa, September 18, 2003.
63 "The CDC had deployed": Princeton Lyman, *Partner to History* (Washington, D.C.: United States Institute of Peace Press, 2002), p. 122. Lyman writes that the figure was $3.5 million. The USAID 1994 report entitled, "USAID Responds to HIV/AIDS," lists its FY 1994 obligation at $9,434,441 (p. 70). The USAID figure may include funds from population efforts, thereby inflating the reported figure.
63 "the CDC expert estimated back in 1994": Princeton Lyman, *Partner to History*, p. 122.
63 " 'Alas, he was too close' ": Ibid., p. 123. In fact, UNAIDS estimated that there were 5 million people living with HIV/AIDS in South Africa by the end of 2001. With 360,000 estimated deaths for that year, the country had probably reached 5 million cumulative infections (including deaths) shortly after the turn of 2000, making the earlier projection eerily accurate. UNAIDS, "2002: Epidemiological Fact Sheets on HIV/AIDS and Sexually Transmitted Infections," p. 2.
64 "Lyman watched aggrieved": In the late 1990s, in his postpresidency, Mandela would emerge as a forceful and vociferous activist for global AIDS causes.
65 "Lyman had indeed been a 'Partner' ": It's the title of his memoir-like account of his tenure as U.S. Ambassador to South Africa, from 1992 to 1996.
65 " 'We did not have the handle' ": Princeton Lyman, *Partner to History*, p. 123.
66 "He wrote of 'the withering away' ": Robert Kaplan, *The Coming Anarchy: Shattering the Dreams of the Post Cold War* (New York: Vintage Books, 2000), p. 9. "The Coming Anarchy" originally appeared in *The Atlantic Monthly* in February 1994.
66 "He described Conakry": Robert Kaplan, *The Coming Anarchy*, p. 17.
66 "President Clinton read it and passed the article around": Robert Rubin and Jacob Weisberg, *In an Uncertain World* (New York: Random House, 2003), p. 384.
67 "And than you have AIDS": Interview: Jack Chow.
67 "Bart Gellman explained that some": Bart Gellman, "The Belated Global Response . . ."
67 "Gellman cited a 1992 World Bank study": Ibid.
67 "Activist Jamie Love proferred": Ibid.
67 "If this would happen in the Balkans": Ibid.
68 "In the early 1990s, Russia": "On the Frontline of an Epidemic: The Need for Urgency in Russia's Fight Against AIDS," Transatlantic Partners Against AIDS (New York: East West Institute, 2003), p. viii. Source: Russian Federal AIDS Center, 2003.
68 " 'At the beginning of the epidemic' ": Interview: Patsy Fleming.
70 "Far from cresting, the epidemic": Interview: Paul Zeitz.

70 "In 1996, Zambia received": "USAID Responds to HIV/AIDS: A Report on the Fiscal Years 1995 and 1996 HIV/AIDS Prevention Programs of the United States Agency for International Development," p. 90.

71 "There were no nuclear weapons": After South Africa voluntarily gave up its nuclear arsenal in 1989. See Bill Keller, "The Thinkable," *The New York Times Magazine,* May 4, 2003.

71 " 'The end of the cold war' ": Somini Sengupta, "Liberia Seen as Icon of World's Neglect of Africa," *The New York Times,* May 16, 2003.

71 "Fourteen of the continent's countries": John Donnelly, "Development Aid to Africa Declines," *The Boston Globe,* February 16, 2001.

71 "Roughly sixty officer positions": Dr. J. Stephen Morrison and Jennifer Cooke, *A Review of U.S. Africa Policy* (Washington, D.C.: Center for Strategic and International Studies, December 2000), p. 7.

72 " 'We were shutting down missions' ": Interview: Stephen Morrison.

72 " 'Large stretches of the continent' ": Dr. J. Stephen Morrison and Jennifer Cooke, *A Review of U.S. Africa Policy,* p. 7.

72 "Through the 1990s the continent": James Dao, "In Quietly Courting Africa, U.S. Likes the Dowry: Oil," *The New York Times,* September 19, 2002.

72 "When asked if they think": Joshua Muravchik, "Affording Foreign Policy: The Problem Is Not Will, but Wallet," *Foreign Affairs,* Vol. 75, No. 2, March/April 1996.

73 "Helms used the tidbit": Interview: Paul DeLay.

75 "Every high-profile speech she gave": According to Shalala. Interview: Donna Shalala.

75 "there was a good deal of high-level": Interview: Patsy Fleming.

76 " 'You can't look at this issue' ": Interview: Donna Shalala.

77 "her official title changed no less": Interview: Helene Gayle.

78 "While there would be roughly": The actual amounts were $10.5 billion in 1999 and $11.6 billion in 2000. "Trends in Spending on HIV/AIDS," Henry S. Kaiser Family Foundation, July 2002.

78 "In that same period more than 40": UNAIDS estimates, provided by Karen Stanecki, March 13, 2003.

CHAPTER FIVE.
NO ADVOCACY FROM ABOVE, NO GROUNDSWELL FROM BELOW

80 " 'I had no direct involvement' ": Interview: Michael Merson.

81 "He was a 'technical' leader": Anil Soni, "From GPA to UNAIDS . . . ," p. 105.

81 "He traveled extensively": Interview: Michael Merson.

81 " 'He wasn't the same guy' ": Interview: Terje Anderson.

81 "Of his speech at Berlin": Interview: Michael Merson.

81 " 'I will attempt to show how we' ": Michael Merson, "The HIV/AIDS Pandemic: Global Spread and Global Response," IXth International Conference on AIDS, Berlin, World Health Organization, June 7, 1993, p. 1.

82 " 'Even when budgets are growing' ": Ibid., p. 5.

82 "he exclaimed that the world could prevent 10 million": From Mann's earliest estimations at GPA through the life of the program, predictions almost always fell short of reality. UNAIDS estimates that roughly 28.2 million were infected from 1993 to the end of 1999. UNAIDS data, provided by Karen Stenacki, March 13, 2003.

82 " 'So many lives saved' ": Michael Merson, "The HIV/AIDS Pandemic . . . ," p. 6.

82 "The plan would include: the promotion": Ibid., p. 6.

82 "It was barely enough to": Ibid., p. 6.

83 "The story made several major newspapers": Sheryl Stolberg, "AIDS Cases Could Triple by 2000, Meeting Is Told Science: Speaker in Berlin urges that $2.5 billion more be spent each year to fight the pandemic," *Los Angeles Times,* June 8, 1993.

83 "But, there was a critical caveat": Interview: Michael Merson.

83 "AIDS killed roughly 850,000 people": UNAIDS data, provided by Karen Stanecki, March 13, 2003.

84 "Tad Homer-Dixon likened the U.S.": Quote from Homer-Dixon in Robert Kaplan, *The Coming Anarchy*, p. 24.

84 "The stock market would increase": Haynes Johnson, *The Best of Times* (New York: Harcourt, 2001), p. 470.

84 "By 1999, 6.5 million had assets": Ibid., pp. 25, 26.

84 "Had Microsoft been a country": Ibid., p. 57.

84 "James Lindsay wrote in an article": James Lindsay, "The New Apathy: How an Uninterested Public is Reshaping Foreign Policy," *Foreign Affairs*, Vol. 79, No. 5. September/October 2000.

84 " 'Americans' interest in foreign policy' ": Henry Kissinger, *Does America Need a Foreign Policy?* (New York: Simon & Schuster, 2001), p. 18.

85 "Thus, when you 'see your 974th picture' ": Thomas de Zengotita, "The Numbing of the American Mind," *Harper's Magazine*, Vol. 304, No. 1823, April 2002, p. 36.

85 "By 1999, according to the survey": Haynes Johnson, *The Best of Times*, p. 492.

85 "This reflects the priority of being attached": Henry Kissinger, *Does America Need a Foreign Policy?*, p. 30.

86 "one of the students lamented": Haynes Johnson, *The Best of Times*, p. 506.

86 "and even a *Newsweek* cover story": Much of this detail on Rivers's background comes from Sandra Gregg, "Muddy Rivers," *Horizon*, October 1999.

88 "Leaders like Julian Bond, chairman of": Wil Haygood, "U.S. Black Leaders React," *The Boston Globe*, October 13, 1999.

88 "Through the twentieth century, both syphilis": Alan Brandt, *No Magic Bullet*, pp. 157, 158.

89 "Eventually, all U.S. government public health": Laurie Garrett, *Betrayal of Trust*, p. 325. Much of background on Tuskegee comes from pp. 324, 325.

89 " 'I believe AIDS is a form' ": Laurie Garrett, *The Coming Plague*, p. 384.

89 "Rivers explained, 'There was a sense' ": Jeffrey Bartholet, "The Plague Years," *Newsweek*, January 17, 2000.

90 " 'What verdict will our descendants render' ": "An Open Letter to the U.S. Black Religious, Intellectual, and Political Leadership Regarding AIDS and the Sexual Holocaust in Africa," The Twenty First Century Group, December 12, 1999. Rivers was one of 21 African-American leaders to sign the letter, and one of its key architects.

90 "the Pediatric AIDS Foundation": Started in 1988 as the Pediatric AIDS Foundation, it was renamed the Elizabeth Glaser Pediatric AIDS Foundation on December 1, 1997. Glaser spent much of the late 1980s and early 1990s educating Americans about pediatric AIDS after her children were infected with HIV, before she died of AIDS in 1994.

91 "For organizations like the National Council": Later renamed the Global Health Council.

CHAPTER SIX. THE CLINTON ENIGMA, BUNKER AND HUNKER DOWN

98 "The new president, whoever he may be": Interview: Jim McDermott.

98 "Gelb had counted the total": David Halberstam, *War in a Time of Peace* (New York: Scribner, 2001), p. 193.

98 "Clinton would tell voters that": Ibid, p. 58.

99 "They thought they had found one in Bosnia": David Halberstam, *War in a Time of Peace*; and Samantha Power, *A Problem from Hell* (New York: Basic Books, 2002).

99 " 'If the horrors of the Holocaust' ": Clifford Krauss, "U.S. Backs Away from Charge of Atrocities in Bosnia Camps," *The New York Times*, August 5, 1992. Quoted in Samantha Power, *A Problem from Hell*, p. xxi.

100 " 'The world economy, the world environment' ": Bill Clinton, "Presidential Inaugural Address," January 21, 1993.

100 " 'We will not shrink from the challenges' ": Ibid.

100 "Richard Holbrooke . . . and Colin Powell": The point is also made in David Halberstam, *War in a Time of Peace*, and Joe Klein, *The Natural*.

100 " 'the selection of a flaccid' ": Joe Klein, *The Natural*, p. 69.

100 "Clinton, in sharp contrast": David Halberstam, *War in a Time of Peace*, p. 242.

101 "The 1,300-page piece": For a good account of the "Healthcare Fiasco," see Joe Klein, *The Natural*, pp. 119–27.

101 "He sanctioned, with Colin Powell's consent": David Halberstam, *War in a Time of Peace*, pp. 260, 261, 263.

102 "As the genocide unfolded": See David Halberstam, *War in a Time of Peace*, and Samantha Power, *A Problem from Hell*, for excellent accounts of U.S. policy on Rwanda genocide.

102 "the Ryan White CARE Program": The program was named after a teenager in Indiana who had contracted HIV through a blood transfusion, and became a national spokesman for the fight against the disease before he died at nineteen years of age.

103 "the president pledged that the issue": Marlene Cimons, "Clinton Appoints AIDS Policy Director—Health: Patricia Fleming Sees Added Difficulties in Getting Ample Funds from Congress. President Vows to Make Fight Against Ailment a High Priority," *Los Angeles Times*, November 11, 1994.

103 "Eventually she would spend roughly": Interview: Patsy Fleming.

104 "The once aspiring artist": Ibid.

104 "In the bureaucratic underworld": Ibid.

104 "Officials at OMB responded": Ibid.

105 "It was 'a vehicle' ": Ibid.

105 "He was clearly 'sympathetic' ": Ibid.

105 "The Democrats lost ten seats": Joe Klein, *The Natural*, pp. 125, 126.

106 "They outlined the data": Interview: Donna Shalala.

106 " 'the message was that we have to move' ": Ibid.

106 "Clinton once pulled his nemesis": Haynes Johnson, *The Best of Times*, p. 348.

107 "The Clinton administration spent": Joe Klein, *The Natural*, p. 7.

107 " 'Bill Clinton operates by sonar' ": Ibid., p. 32.

108 "With his $2 million a year": Interview: Paul DeLay.

108 "With infection rates reaching 10 percent": Ibid.

109 "In 1993, USAID's official": "HIV/AIDS: The Evolution of the Pandemic, The Evolution of the Response," The U.S. Agency for International Development Program for Prevention and Control of HIV Infection, August 1993, p. 27.

109 "one of the undersecretary slots": Atwood did serve a brief stint as undersecretary of state for management.

110 "His own senior advisor Nils": Interview: Nils Daulaire.

110 "Pelosi and Atwood had a close": Interview: Brian Atwood.

111 "He once suggested that Helms's ideas": Ibid.

111 "The agency's budget would be lacerated": Ibid.

112 "demand management": The term "demand management" comes from some of Gellman's sources in Bart Gellman, "The Belated Global Response . . ."

112 " 'There was a concern that if we did' ": Interview: Paul DeLay.

112 "Then, as DeLay recounted": Ibid.

112 "Gillespie explained his position": Bart Gellman, "The Belated Global Response . . ."

112 "Gillespie summarized the agency's": Ibid.

113 "With $10,000, the bar graphs": Ibid.

113 "That translated into about": Interview: Paul DeLay. Total donor support from 1989 to 1998 was $180 million. Foreign donor contributions amounted to roughly 70 percent of that total. "What Happened in Uganda? Declining HIV Prevalence, Behavior Change, and the National Response," USAID, September 2002. Analysis by Elizabeth Marum, USAID/CDC HIV Program Director in Kampala.

113 "His government enlisted thousands": Tina Rosenberg, "On Capital Hill, Ideology is Distorting an African AIDS Success," editorial in *The New York Times*, April 28, 2003.

113 "In Jinja, incidence among": "A Measure of Success in Uganda," UNAIDS, May 1998, pp. 6, 8.

113 "Projections held that Thailand": Ushani Agalawatta, "Thai AIDS Drive Praised, but UN Policy Hit," *The Manila Times*, September 20, 2003.

114 "behavior modification among": "HIV Infections in Thailand: 1985–2000," UNAIDS.
115 "And because of the five-year contract cycle": Though some were extended.
116 " 'Given the resources they're given' ": Interview: RP Eddy.

An Awakening of Sorts (1996–1999)

CHAPTER SEVEN.
DRUGS CHANGE THE LANDSCAPE, A MISSION CRYSTALLIZES
122 " 'AIDS is not only a U.S. issue' ": Interview: Eric Sawyer.
123 " 'Look, we can't meet the needs' ": Ibid.
123 "Considerably less than 10 percent": Sawyer's estimate. Interview: Eric Sawyer.
123 "He exhorted the crowd": Interview: Paul Boneberg.
124 "One working group leader responded": Ibid.
125 "By the end of the proceedings": Interview: Eric Sawyer.
126 " 'It gives you an idea' ": Interview: Paul Boneberg.
127 "It was 1988 and Berkley's study": Interview: Seth Berkley.
127 "In 1994, the U.S. government": "U.S. Government Spending on AIDS Vaccine Research & Development," World Bank estimates provided by International AIDS Vaccine Initiative, October 3, 2003.
128 " '[The U.S. government] can't' ": Interview: Seth Berkley.
128 "The virus's lethal design and evasiveness": Interview: Jon Cohen.
128 "The insights gained from pursuing": Interview: Anthony Fauci.
129 "It wouldn't be easy": "Clinton's Challenge: Finds AIDS Vaccine by 2007," CNN, May 18, 2003.
130 "And some, like Congressman Elijah": Elijah Cummings. "Silence About AIDS Feeds the Destroyer of Lives," *Baltimore AFRO-American Newspaper,* May 22, 1999.
130 "The budget increased by an additional": "U.S. Government Spending on AIDS Vaccine Research & Development," World Bank estimates provided by International AIDS Vaccine Initiative, October 3, 2003.
130 "less than 10 percent of the overall U.S. research": Elijah Cummings, "Silence About AIDS Feeds the Destroyer of Lives."
130 "It would take the NIH one year": Hillary Stout, "Politics and Policy: President Sets AIDS Vaccine Goal of 10 Years," *The Wall Street Journal,* May 5, 1997. Also, AIDS Vaccine Advocacy Coalition, "Report Finds Clinton's 10-Year Goal in Jeopardy," *HIV Vaccine Handbook,* May 1998, p. 172.
130 "Funding and attention": U.S. government funding increased from $207 million in 1999 to $271 million in 2000. "U.S. Government Spending on AIDS Vaccine Research & Development," World Bank estimates for 1999, and IAVI estimates for 2000, provided by International AIDS Vaccine Initiative, October 3, 2003.
130 "Of greatest concern to AIDS expert Jon Cohen": Interview: Jon Cohen. Also see Jon Cohen, *Shots in the Dark* (New York: Norton, 2001).
130 "IAVI's advocacy notwithstanding": Ibid.
130 "In early 1996, the little that": All of the political forces driving vaccine development were domestic-centric. There is little evidence that prior to IAVI's creation, the emergence of the domestic AIDS activist community, and the upsurge in media attention in the late 1990s the international dimension was a key consideration driving vaccine efforts. Berkley agreed. Interview: Seth Berkley.
131 "If prevention and treatment": It is becoming increasingly clear that care, palliative care, and counseling, for example, aid in both prevention and treatment and are essential to a comprehensive approach.
132 "An estimated additional 26 million": UNAIDS data, provided by Karen Stanecki, March 13, 2003.
133 "As he finished, he began the chant": Eric Sawyer, "Remarks at the Opening Ceremony," at XI International AIDS Conference in Vancouver, Canada, July 7, 1996.
133 "The drug companies were refusing": Interview: Eric Sawyer.

133 " 'It was obvious to me' ": Interview: Laurie Garrett.

134 "By 1988 there had been a 70 percent": "HIV/AIDS Surveillance Report," CDC, Year end editions, December 1995, Vol. 7, No. 2; December 1996, Vol. 8, No. 2; December 1997, Vol. 9, No. 2; December 1998, Vol. 10, No. 2.

134 " 'in 1995 HIV was the number' ": From U.S. Vital Statistics website (www.hhs.gov). Laurie Garrett, *A Betrayal of Trust*, p. 473.

135 "At the time, many leading thinkers were buoyant": Francis Fukiyama, *The End of History and the Last Man* (New York: Avon, 1993).

135 "A *Newsweek* cover read": John Leland, "The End of AIDS?" *Newsweek*, December 2, 1996. The article's subtitle follows, "Not Yet, but New Drugs Offer Hope."

135 "Berkman, a 1960s radical": Gillian Murphy, "In Search of Solidarity," *Body Positive*, Vol. XV, No. 6, November 2002.

136 "At a village hospital, a flood": Ibid.

136 "Roughly 32 million people": UNAIDS data, provided by Karen Stanecki, March 13, 2003.

136 "Berkman agreed with Eric": Interview: Eric Sawyer.

136 " 'It was a very moving experience' ": Gillian Murphy, "In Search of Solidarity." Note that much of the background for Berkman comes from Murphy interview with Berkman detailed here.

136 "Their meeting in the late summer": Interview: Eric Sawyer.

137 "He and his fellow demonstrators": Ibid.

CHAPTER EIGHT. A CLASH, A FORUM

143 "Gore posed a personal, highly moralistic": David Halberstam, *War in a Time of Peace*, pp. 330–31.

143 "Fuerth estimated that the country's": Interview: Leon Fuerth.

144 "The United States also played a critical role": Bob Davis, "Gore Hopes New AIDS Pact Will Help Shake Protestors," *The Wall Street Journal*, August 12, 1999.

144 "The United States had 'waited too long' ": From an "authoritative" or "senior" source, as noted by Bart Gellman, in "A Conflict of Health and Profit," *The Washington Post*, May 21, 2000.

145 "Increasingly, the vice president": Interview: Leon Fuerth.

145 "The Americans suggested that by pursuing": Interview: Jamie Love.

146 "When the United States got wind": Ibid.

146 "The South African parliament": By the time it passed, it included parallel importing and compulsory licensing. Bob Davis, "Gore Hopes New AIDS Pact Will Help Shake Protestors."

146 "As early as May 1997": Bart Gellman, "A Conflict of Health and Profits."

146 "the industry had already donated": Most of this material from Bart Gellman, "A Conflict of Health and Profits." The pharma lobby would also contribute heavily to the Republican party.

147 " 'We are prepared to enter that fray' ": Ibid.

147 "South Africa would continue": Ibid.

147 "Gore 'urged Mbeki's' ": Ibid.

147 "By early 1998 roughly forty": Bob Davis, "Gore Hopes New AIDS Pact Will Help Shake Protestors."

147 "On February 5, 1998": Bart Gellman, "A Conflict of Health and Profit."

148 " 'I'm concerned that, without significant' ": Ibid.

148 " 'What for South Africa' ": Ibid.

148 "Pappas told Love that he": Interview: Jamie Love.

149 " 'You're all going to vote for Gore' ": Ibid.

150 " 'We get zero, bupkis' ": Interview: Jamie Love.

151 "None of them knew that just weeks": Bart Gellman, "A Conflict of Health and Profit."

151 "The deal called on South Africa": Ibid.

151 "Had they known about the proposal": Interview: Eric Sawyer.

152 " 'Now I'd like to have my say' ": Gore's remarks from both events from Charles Babcock, Charles and Cici Connelly, "AIDS Activists Badger Gore Again," *The Washington Post*, June 18, 1999.

153 "Gore continued: 'This epidemic' ": Ibid.

153 "A keen photographer": Ibid.

153 " 'In his first week or so' ": Interview: Bart Gellman.

153 "Fuerth said that Gore commanded": Interview: Leon Fuerth.

153 "Gore asked Fuerth how much longer": Ibid.

153 "The staffer told Fuerth": Ibid.

153 "Fuerth was 'incredulous' ": Fuerth continues to give little credence to the accusation. Love denies that Nader had anything to do with them and there is little evidence to suggest otherwise. Interview: Leon Fuerth, and interview: Jamie Love.

154 "A few days later, Donna Brazile": Bart Gellman, "A Conflict of Health and Profit."

154 "The next day the Gore camp": Bob Davis, "Gore Hopes New AIDS Pact Will Help Shake Protestors."

154 "Eric Sawyer now wanted": Interview: Eric Sawyer.

155 "Tipper said that she": Ibid.

156 " 'He was clearly pissed' ": Ibid.

156 " 'You know, I bet you do' ": Ibid.

156 "they began throwing out": "AIDS Activists Disrupt Gore's New Hampshire Campaign Stop," Act Up Philadelphia/Act Up New York Press Release, August 8, 1998.

157 " 'I'd like to talk to you' ": Norma Love, "AIDS Activists Disrupt Gore Speech," Associated Press, August 9, 1999.

157 "Gore replied that he would be glad": "AIDS Activists Disrupt Gore's New Hampshire Campaign Stop," Act Up Philadelphia/Act Up New York Press Release, August 8, 1998.

157 " 'They don't want to talk' ": Charles Babcock and Cici Connelly, "AIDS Activists Badger Gore Again," *The Washington Post,* June 18, 1999.

157 " 'I was certainly not aware' ": Bart Gellman, "A Conflict of Health and Profit."

157 "The same press release": Press Release 20508, Office of the United States Trade Representative, "U.S.-South Africa Understanding on Intellectual Property," September 17, 1999.

158 "In May 2000, the president": Bart Gellman, "A Conflict of Health and Profit."

159 " 'We are surrounded by' ": Steve Sternberg, "Former Diplomat Holbrooke Takes on Global AIDS," *USA Today,* June 10, 2002.

159 "The AIDS visits had become": Interview: RP Eddy.

159 "He asked for Secretary General": Holbrooke was also in telephone contact with Annan during the trip. He did an AIDS event in each one of the ten countries he visited. The idea to devote the U.S. presidency to Africa, and the first session of the new millennium to AIDS occurred to him during an AIDS visit to Harare, which Holbrooke remembered as yet "another horror show." Interview: Richard Holbrooke.

159 " 'It was at that point' ": Steve Sternberg, "Former Diplomat Holbrooke Takes on Global AIDS."

162 " 'If we get AIDS in the Security Council' ": Interview: RP Eddy.

162 " 'Everyone said you couldn't do' ": Interview: Richard Holbrooke.

163 "and had written a letter": Interview: Richard Holbrooke.

163 " 'This had us rolling' ": Mark Schoofs, "A New Kind of Crisis: The Security Council Declares AIDS in Africa a Threat to World Stability," *The Village Voice,* January 12–18, 2000.

164 " 'This meeting demands of us' ": Al Gore, "Opening Statement in the Security Council Meeting on AIDS in Africa," USUN Press Release, January 10, 2000.

164 " 'People always ask me' ": *Online NewsHour,* "Richard Holbrooke," July 13, 2000.

CHAPTER NINE. EVIDENCE-BASED ADVOCACY, START THE PRESS

167 " 'I didn't fully understand' ": Interview: Peter Piot.

167 " 'I wanted to switch' ": Ibid.

168 "A leading U.S. diplomat": James Walsh, "The UN at 50: Who Needs It?" *Time International,* October 23, 1995.

168 "U.S. Ambassador to the UN": Ibid.

168 "Upon UNAIDS's formation": Bart Gellman, "The Belated Global Response . . ."

169 "Hans Mulkirk, the Dutch": Anil Soni, "From GPA to UNAIDS . . ."
169 "According to Dr. Thierry Mertens": Ibid., pp. 83, 84.
169 " 'AIDS just happened to be there' ": Ibid.
169 " 'I would mark it there' ": Interview: Princeton Lyman.
169 " 'There's no question' ": Interview: Michael Merson.
171 "WHO's support dropped": Bart Gellman, "The Belated Global Response . . ."
171 " 'So, despite the fact' ": Interview: Sally Grooms Cowal.
172 " 'I see now that one' ": Interview: Peter Piot.
172 "After all, he says": Ibid.
172 " 'Tie the needs of the poor' ": Bart Gellman, "The Belated Global Response . . ."
173 " 'The evolution of my thinking' ": Interview: Peter Piot.
175 "There were 8 million AIDS orphans": "The Status of and Trends of HIV/AIDS Epidemics in the World," Monitoring AIDS Pandemic (MAP) Network, Geneva, Switzerland, June 26, 1998.
176. " 'That was really a pivotal' ": Interview: Todd Summers.
177 " 'Thirty years from now' ": Interview: Phil Bennett.
177 "Days later, Bart Gellman": Interview: Bart Gellman.
177 "Dean Arlene Notoro Morgan proclaimed": Arlene Morgan, Remarks at conference, "Covering HIV/AIDS: What's Next?" at Columbia School of Journalism, May 3–5, 2002.
178 " 'America was only interested' ": David Halberstam, *War in a Time of Peace*, pp. 160, 161.
178 "total foreign coverage on network": Garrick Utley, "The Shrinking of Foreign News: From Broadcast to Narrowcast," *Foreign Affairs*, Vol. 76, No. 2, March/April, 1997.
178 "new technologies such as cable": Ibid.
178 "As a result, the media sought": Ibid.
178 "Even cheaper still was": Haynes Johnson, *The Best of Times*, pp. 148–49, 431.
178 "a Harris poll indicated": Joe Klein, *The Natural*, p. 181.
179 "The title of the cover story": Jeffrey Bartholet, "The Plague Years," *Newsweek*, January 17, 2000.
180 "The pieces had the effect": Interview: Bart Gellman.
181 "The article reported that the Clinton": Bart Gellman, "AIDS Is Declared Threat to Security," *The Washington Post*, April 30, 2000.
181 "Whether the designation was in fact": The "national security" label is a discursive designation. A threat becomes a "national security" threat when the president, or someone on behalf of the president, clearly designates it as such.
181 "press secretary Joe Lockhart": Gellman recalled it, Interview: Bart Gellman.
181 "Senate Majority Leader Trent Lott": Trent Lott on *Fox News Sunday*, April 30, 2000.
182 "He learned that the government": Normally, Gellman considers his work his public service. When he won a $1,000 award for his coverage of global AIDS, immediately he wrote the check over to the Kaiser Family Foundation on condition that they would put it toward the outreach program in the Village of Hope. Kaiser matched Gellman's donation. The paper's company then matched the $2,000. Gellman went to friends to try to drum up more funds. All told, he raised $20,000, and it all went back to the Village of Hope. He continues to send several thousand dollars a year.
182–83 " 'The media is finally paying attention' ": *Jim Lehrer NewsHour*, PBS, July 13, 2000.
184 " 'The problem is not going to go away' ": Ibid.
184 "*The Washington Post* stayed with": There was a lull in the paper's coverage in the aftermath of 9/11. It picked up in the latter half of 2002 with a flurry of editorials.

Opportunities Squandered (1998–2000)

CHAPTER TEN. CONTINENTAL ABDICATION, THE ULTIMATE CRUTCH
190 "Boneberg explained that the protests": Interview: Paul Boneberg.
190 "Boneberg recalled him declaring: 'Americans need to realize' ": This episode recounted from interview: Paul Boneberg.

192 "Shalala was aghast": Interview: Leon Fuerth; and Interview: Donna Shalala.

192 " 'One of the reasons we are not' ": Interview: Leon Fuerth.

193 "Fuerth, who continued to follow": Ibid.

193 "a group of officials from the Department": Fuerth thought that the officials were from HHS, but was not certain. They were public health officials from the executive branch of the government at any rate. Interview: Leon Fuerth.

193 "China could still avert": Interview: Leon Fuerth.

194 " 'It requires all-out efforts' ": Shri Atal Bihari Vajpayee, "Address by Prime Minister," at meeting of National Program for Prevention and Control of HIV/AIDS, New Delhi, India, December 12, 1998.

194 "And there were patches of strong": "India: Stemming the AIDS Epidemic," The World Bank Group, 2003.

194 "Even in late 2002, when Bill Gates": In October 2003, Gates would announce another $100 million grant to India, bringing the sum to $200 million.

194 " 'That puts India in the seemingly' ": John Lancaster, "AIDS Begins to Widen Its Reach in India," *The Washington Post*, June 11, 2003.

195 "The region was home": Buki Ponle, "Meeting—Shy Leaders Send Wrong Signal on AIDS," The Panos Institute, September 17–30, 1999.

196 "Chiluba insisted to Piot": Interview: Peter Piot.

196 "The conference produced a ministerial": Buki Ponle, "Meeting—Shy Leaders Send Wrong Signal on AIDS."

196 "African leaders had passed no less": Gumisai Mutume, "Development: Are Africa's Leaders Really Up to the AIDS Challenge?" Inter Press Service, December 5, 2000.

196 "By the late 1990s, ten times more": Kurt Shillinger, "AIDS and the African: Denial, Most Leaders Won't Confront the Epidemic," *The Boston Globe*, October 12, 1999.

196 "In contrast, the United States spent": "Trends in U.S. Spending on HIV/AIDS," Henry S. Kaiser Family Foundation, July 2002.

197 " 'The funding has been going down' ": Peter Mwaura, "Governments Urged to Lead AIDS Fight," *Africa Recovery*, Vol. 12, No. 2, November 1998, p. 9.

197 "Zimbabwe spent roughly seventy times": Gumisai Mutume, "Development: Are Africa's Leaders Really Up to the AIDS Challenge?"

197 "defense expenditures among fourteen": Jeffrey Gow, "The HIV/AIDS Epidemic in Africa: Implications for U.S. Policy," *Health Affairs*, May/June 2002.

197 "the seventy-year-old leader": Kurt Shillinger, "AIDS and the African: Denial."

197 " 'It is reversing the gains' ": "Zimbabwe: 1,200 AIDS Deaths a Week," The Associated Press, April 18, 1999.

197 "Only a year prior": Judith Achieng, "Health—Kenya: President Moi Joins the Campaign Against HIV/AIDS," Inter Press Service, December 3, 1999.

198 "the Catholic Church, which wields strong": Ibid.

198 "Chiluba declared, 'So overwhelming' ": "Zambia: Chiluba Speaks of Devastation of AIDS," Integrated Regional Information Network, November 22, 2000.

198 "the oil-rich country had set aside": Ade Obisesan, "AIDS-Nigeria: Obasanjo to Lead War on AIDS, 2.6 million Nigerians Hit by HIV," Agence France-Presse, December 1, 1999.

199 "Mogae had already spoken": "Botswana's President Chides Rich Countries on AIDS, Debt," Reuters, November 15, 2000.

199 "during a United Nations General Assembly": Obasanjo even echoed Mogae's earlier remarks: "The future of our continent is bleak, to say the least, and the prospect of extinction of the entire population of a continent looms larger and larger."

199 "all making a strong case for": Judy Aita, "African Leaders Ask for Help with AIDS Crisis," U.S. State Department, International Information Programs, June 26, 2001.

199 " 'HIV/AIDS is one of those critical' ": Kurt Shillinger, "AIDS and the African: Denial."

199 "When Sheila Mitchell's NGO": Interview: Sheila Mitchell.

199 "Stephen Morrison said, 'These guys' ": Interview: Stephen Morrison.

200 "Zambia, for example, paid $170 million": Peter Mwaura, "Governments Urged to Lead AIDS Fight."

201 " 'By 1989,' remembered an ANC minister": Jon Jeter, "South Africa's Advances Jeopardized by AIDS," *The Washington Post,* July 6, 2000.

201 "An activist who attended remembered": Mark Schoofs, "AIDS: The Agony of Africa; Part Seven: Building a Movement on the Ruins of Apartheid," *The Village Voice,* December 22–28, 1999.

202 "Mandela reportedly proposed only": Jon Jeter, "South Africa's Advances Jeopardized by AIDS."

202 "Hein Marais, a South African journalist, wrote": Ibid.

202 "The apartheid government": Samantha Power, "The AIDS Rebel," *The New Yorker,* May 19, 2003.

202 " 'I get so angry' ": Mark Schoofs, "AIDS: The Agony of Africa; Part Seven: Building a Movement on the Ruins of Apartheid."

203 "From 1994 to 1999, the Health": Samantha Power, "The AIDS Rebel."

203 "Gore was pleased": Interview: Leon Fuerth.

203 "It soon became apparent": Samantha Power, "The AIDS Rebel."

204 "he stumbled onto a series": Ibid.

204 "He argued further that it was therefore": Ibid.

204 "he had come to espouse": Ibid.

204 "He would be careful to avoid": At a luncheon in New York City on October 1, 2003, the author asked Mbeki pointedly, "You have spoken about the relationship between poverty and the disease. Would you say, scientifically speaking, that the HIV virus causes AIDS?" Mbeki's reply did not include a direct answer to the question.

205 "In May 2000, he convened": Samantha Power, "The AIDS Rebel."

205 "Mbeki—too proud and too": Interview: Princeton Lyman.

205 "Mbeki refused to take an AIDS test": *State of Denial,* documentary directed by Elaine Epstein, 2003.

206 " 'it would have stirred' ": Interview: Stephen Morrison.

CHAPTER ELEVEN. A FAILURE TO RECALIBRATE, TURF AND NEGLECT

207 "Born into a prominent": Martha Brant, "Into Africa," *Stanford Magazine,* January/February 2000.

208 "A gleeful Albright": Ibid.

209 "*New York Times* journalist James Bennett": James Bennett, "Clinton Declares the U.S. and World Failed Rwandans," *The New York Times,* March 26, 1998.

210 "He expressed contrition": Ibid.

210 "A few days into the trip": R. W. Apple, "Clinton's Motley Entourage Plays to Different Audiences," *The New York Times,* March 27, 1998.

210 "He listened to stories": James Bennett, "Clinton Declares the U.S. and World Failed Rwandans."

210 "During the genocide": Samantha Power, *A Problem from Hell,* p. 335.

210 "And later, the administration": Ibid., p. 335.

210 " 'He said that he not only' ": James Bennett, "Clinton Declares the U.S. and World Failed Rwandans."

210 "One in five adults": Botswana's infection rate was nearing one in three; Uganda's was descending having exceeded one in five; South Africa was nearing one in five; Rwanda was nearing one in five; Ghana's was escalating, but below one in five, and Senegal's had been kept in the single digits.

211 "Clinton was 'going through the motions' ": Interview: Sally Grooms Cowal.

211 "Two hundred people were dead": Martha Brant, "Into Africa."

211 "Rice had buoyantly declared": "Rice Says, 'New Paradigm for U.S. Policy Can Help Boost African Take-Off," allAfrica.com, October 22, 1997.

211 "In the case of conflict": Interview: Susan Rice.

211   "The natural proclivity": The State Department is divided into both regional and functional bureaus. Given the tumult and crises in Africa in 1998, leadership from the issue might have come from the apposite functional bureau—the Office of Environment and Science Affairs (OES). Nobody at the bureau was championing the pandemic though. Rice doesn't remember her counterpart, or anybody for that matter, at OES engaging her on the issue or pushing her to act during her entire tenure at State. Interview: Susan Rice. Rice's counterpart at OES, Nancy Carter Foster, had, as Stephen Morrison remembered it, "no standing on the issue."

212   "Decreasing steadily over the preceding several years, the tally": Paula Hoy, *Players and Issues in International Aid* (West Hartford, CT: Kumarian Press, 1998), p. 29.

212   "Her budget request asked for": Interview: Susan Rice.

213   "In a sense, Rice was still": Martha Brant, "Into Africa."

214   "Measured against the plethora": Albright devoted roughly one page of her 512-page memoir to global AIDS. She wrote: "Probably the most striking example of where we did much more (but still not nearly enough) was in the fight against HIV/AIDS." Madeleine Albright, *Madam Secretary* (New York: Miramax Books, 2003), p. 452.

215   "Atwood was close to Gore": Interview: Donna Shalala.

216   "As a Cabinet secretary": Interview: Brian Atwood.

216   "According to Shalala": Interview: Donna Shalala.

CHAPTER TWELVE. A FOILED PLAN, "TOO LITTLE, TOO LATE"

218   "Her reaction: 'I hit the roof!' ": Interview: Sandy Thurman.

221   " 'This is just unacceptable' ": Ibid.

221   "But when Thurman entered": Ibid.

223   "A poll suggested that a month": Haynes Johnson, *The Best of Times*, p. 373. Media Studies Center Survey conducted by the Freedom Forum.

223   "140 newspapers would call": Ibid, p. 378.

223   "According to David Halberstam": David Halberstam, *War in a Time of Peace*, pp. 374, 375.

224   " 'By his conduct,' Haynes Johnson": Haynes Johnson, *The Best of Times*, p. 439.

225   " 'Even in 1998 and 1999' ": Joe Klein, *The Natural*, p. 156.

226   "There he spent his days": Interview: Daniel Tarantola.

229   " 'The alternative,' he wrote": Leon Fuerth, "Revisiting the End of History: The Coming of a New Historical Era," Elliot School Shapiro Lecture, George Washington University, November 6, 2001.

230   " 'And remember, all else being equal' ": Interview: Ken Bernard; and Interview: RP Eddy.

231   "They were formulating a plan": Interview: Ken Bernard.

233   " 'By the end of the decade' ": In the late 1990s some experts spoke of 40 million orphans in 2010. Now the 40 million estimate refers to the world's orphans at large. UNAIDS estimates that there will be 25 million AIDS orphans in 2010.

233   " 'they just didn't know . . .' ": Interview: Sandy Thurman.

234   " 'If that's true, then Jesse' ": Ibid.

234   "On one trip she traveled": Ibid.

237   "Typically, Joe Gannon": In fact, the NIC had just released, though still in classified form, a landmark report, authored by David Gordon, exploring the impact of AIDS and other global infectious diseases on U.S. national security. The report was widely circulated and had significant impact in getting the foreign policy and political communities to consider the global AIDS-security nexus.

237   "They were skeptical": Interview: Ken Bernard.

238   "She threw Bernard's memo": Ibid.

240   " 'lost the stomach for battle' ": Ibid.

240   "Brainstorming, the two": Eddy and Bernard approached Princeton Lyman about the position. The bureaucratic jostling had rendered the post's mandate uncertain, repelling Lyman and other bona fide statesmen. Interview: RP Eddy; and Interview: Princeton Lyman.

240   "Ashamed, it scalded him": Though it should be noted that the king's own efforts, as with most of his contemporaries in Southern Africa, were negligible.

241   " 'One quarter of you' ": Interview: Ken Bernard.

241   "They seemed relieved": Ibid.

241   "Nearly 9 *million* people": UNAIDS data, provided by Karen Stanecki, March 13, 2003.

A Great Awakening? (2001–2003)

CHAPTER THIRTEEN. A BLEAK OUTLOOK, FINALLY — A VEHICLE

246   " 'We should not send our troops' ": "Stretched Out," From *Nightline*, ABCNews.com, July 7, 2003.

246   "Bush said, 'While Africa' ": "Newsmaker: George W. Bush," *Online NewsHour*, February 16, 2000. In the course of the interview with Lehrer, Bush said that Africa fell under U.S. economic interests, but seemed to carve the continent out of U.S. strategic or military interests.

246   "Some of the activists who had": Interview: Ken Bernard.

248   "When pressed further, Fleischer said": Carter Yang, "Open for Business?" ABCNews.com, February 7, 2001.

248   "According to the *The Washington Post*": Mike Allen, "Bush Acts to Quell Flap on AIDS, Race," *The Washington Post*, February 8, 2001.

249   "His reaction upon learning": Interview: Scott Evertz.

250   "Also in attendance was": John Donnelly, "The New Crusade," *The Boston Globe*, June 3, 2001.

251   " 'I propose the creation of' ": "The Secretary General Address to the African Summit of HIV/AIDS, Tuberculosis and Other Infectious Diseases," Abuja, Nigeria, April 26, 2001.

251   " 'If you call for a global fund' ": John Donnelly, "The New Crusade," *The Boston Globe*, June 3, 2001. Much of the detail from the Abuja Conference and Sachs's participation comes from Donnelly's article. Also from Interview: Jeffrey Sachs.

253   "An in-depth analysis revealed": Amir Attaran and Jeffrey Sachs, "Defining and Refining International Donor Support for Combating the AIDS Pandemic," *The Lancet*, Vol. 357, January 6, 2001.

254   " 'I'm not a legislator' ": Interview: Jeffrey Sachs.

254   "Finally, there would be an expert": Jeffrey Sachs, "HIV Non-Intervention: A Costly Option—A New Framework for Globalization," Comments at International AIDS Conference in Durban, South Africa, July 13, 2000.

255   " 'Sub-Saharan Africa will require": Ibid. Sachs's $10 billion figure included the global effort to combat not only HIV/AIDS, but also tuberculosis, malaria, and "other major killer diseases."

255   " 'He has gotten people thinking' ": Foege quoted in John Donnelly, "The New Crusade."

255   " 'If we didn't have Jeff Sachs' ": John Donnelly, "The New Crusade."

256   "Bush later said that at that March meeting": "Remarks by the President During the Announcement of Proposal for Global Fund to Fight HIV/AIDS, Malaria and Tuberculosis," The White House, May 11, 2001.

257   "In a point he would come to regret": From Andrew Natsios, testimony before the International Relations Committee of the House of Representatives, June 7, 2001.

257   " 'I'm sorry,' the world's leading diplomat": Interview: RP Eddy.

258   "Rice was 'noncommittal' ": Interview: Jeffrey Sachs.

258   "The president called it a 'beginning' ": "Remarks by the President During the Announcement of Proposal for Global Fund to Fight HIV/AIDS, Malaria and Tuberculosis," The White House, May 11, 2001.

259   "Jeffrey Sachs's response was measured": Comments by Frist, Booker, and Sachs, and account of activist from John Donnelly, "U.S. Commits $200M to AIDS Fund—UN, Nigeria Say More Is Needed," *The Boston Globe*, May 12, 2001.

261   "UN Special Envoy for HIV/AIDS Stephen Lewis remarked": Interview: Anil Soni.

261   "By then, the fund had already received": Ibid.

264   "Without missing a beat Powell responded": "Transcript: Colin Powell Interview on ABC-TV's 'This Week' Sunday Talk Show," U.S. Department of State International Information Programs, February 5, 2001.

264 "In an interview on the *The Jim Lehrer NewsHour*": Powell's answer mirrored his earlier response: "It is a very serious issue. You can call it a national security issue; you can call it a pandemic; you can call it a destroyer of families and cultures. . . . And what we need is a full-scale assault not just from the United States but from the rest of the world to deal with this." *The Jim Lehrer NewsHour*, April 23, 2001.

265 " 'I was a one-man show' ": Interview: Jack Chow.

265 "He highlighted the issue": Interview: Walter Kansteiner.

265 "When Sachs spoke of the need": Interview: Jeffrey Sachs.

265 "While Powell publicly called": Comments on *The Jim Lehrer NewsHour*, April 23, 2001.

265 "On the flight from Washington to Mali": Ben Barber, "Tough Love for Africa," Salon.com, May 28, 2001.

265 " 'As [the secretary] traveled' ": Ibid.

266 "The child, Powell was told": "Powell Takes on Killer," ABC.com, May 27, 2001.

266 "The Powells watched as young girls": Ben Barber, "Tough Love for Africa."

266 " 'It was difficult to see the young boy' ": Ibid.

266 "When they finally told her, they castigated her": Ibid.

266 " 'I see you as a role model' ": Ibid.

266 " 'I can assure you that Africa' ": Jim Lobe, "Powell Picks Republican Businessman for Top African Post," Inter Press Service, March 9, 2001.

266 " 'Even though there are wars' ": Michael Phillips, "While in Africa, Powell Tours AIDS Center, Hears Stories of Its Victims, Promises Action," *The Wall Street Journal*, May 29, 2001.

266 "Powell pledged that he": "Remarks by Secretary of State Colin L. Powell at the AIDS Support Organization (TASU), Mulago Hospital," U.S. Department of State, May 27, 2001.

266 "there is 'no enemy in war' ": "Powell promises continued U.S. support in AIDS fight," CNN.com, June 25, 2001.

267 "But 'Powell has certainly had his successes' ": Joanna McGeary, "Odd Man Out," *Time* magazine, September 10, 2001.

267 " 'We thought we were riding' ": Interview: Paul Zeitz.

267 "The issue was gaining momentum": Interview: Terje Anderson.

268 " 'Regardless of what happened last week' ": Interview: Jack Chow.

CHAPTER FOURTEEN. RIGHTING THE RESPONSE, GETTING RELIGION

270 " 'I'm so ashamed I've done so little' ": Jim Fisher-Thompson, "Senator Helms Pledges More Attention to HIV/AIDS in Africa," U.S. Department of State International Information Programs, February 22, 2002.

270 " 'In the end,' Helms concluded": Jesse Helms, "We Cannot Turn Away," *The Washington Post*, March 24, 2002.

270 "There was one more, though": Ibid.

271 "After the concert, Bono and his wife": Josh Tyrangiel, "Bono's Mission," *Time*, February 23, 2002.

271 " 'I thought it was the guy from downstairs' ": Interview: Jamie Drummond.

272 "He requested a meeting": Josh Tyrangiel, "Bono's Mission."

272 " 'Jeffrey Sachs not only let me' ": Bono, "Class Day Address," at Harvard University, June 6, 2001.

272 "Bono set his sights on Washington": Interview: Bobby Shriver.

272 "Bono's activism": "The Debt Crisis," www.data.org/whyafrica/issuedebt.php.

272 "$20–30 billion in poor country debt": DATA website put this figure at $100 billion, but much of this was nominal debt already written off or down in value.

272 "Late in 2000, Bono, Shriver, and Drummond founded": Along with help from key financial backers.

272 "Just as his hero had mobilized": Josh Tyrangiel, "Bono's Mission."

273 "Bono 'is also a Christian' ": Interview: Jamie Drummond.

273 "The team was armed not only": Ibid.

273 "Helms said later, in his February 2002 luncheon speech": Jim Fisher-Thompson, "Article: Senator Helms Pledges More Attention to HIV/AIDS in Africa."

273 " 'It's an extraordinary thing' ": Dana Bush, "U2 Singer, Jesse Helms Discuss AIDS," CNN.com, June 13, 2001.

273 "He wasn't necessarily a big fan": John Donnelly, "Helms's Reversal on U.S.A. Reverberates," *The Boston Globe*, March 27, 2002.

274 "Rice chided those who": Condoleezza Rice, "Promoting the National Interest," *Foreign Affairs*, Vol. 79, No. 1, January/February 2000.

274 "Terrorists had secured harbor": "The National Security Strategy of the United States of America," The White House, September 2002.

275 "They form an important part": Nicholas Lemann, "The Controller," *The New Yorker*, May 12, 2003, p. 81.

275 "Bush told Bono that": Interview: Jamie Drummond.

276 " 'Bono, I appreciate your heart' ": "Remarks by the President on Global Development Inter-American Development Bank," Washington, D.C., March 14, 2002.

276 "Not since Elvis Presley": David Corn, "Bush Backtracking on AIDS a Slap in the Face for Bono," *The Philadelphia Inquirer*, July 1, 2002.

276 " 'We [felt] like we extracted' ": Interview: Jamie Drummond.

276 " 'I think Paul O'Neill' ": Adam Zagorin, "On the Road with Bono and O'Neill," *Time*, May 28, 2002.

277 "Bono had his own explanation": Bono, Class Day Address at Harvard University, June 6, 2001.

278 "Frist—whose nickname": David Grann, "The Ascent of Bill Frist: The Price of Power," *The New York Times Magazine*, May 11, 2003.

278 "The tactic helped deliver": Ibid.

278 " 'History is going to record' ": John Donnelly, "U.S. Urged to Fund AIDS War in Africa," *The Boston Globe*, March 16, 2001.

279 " 'Our actions will show the world' ": "Frist and Helms Seek $500 Million Increase for AIDS," Press Release Senator Bill Frist's Office, March 24, 2002.

279 "It would have 'had to have been' ": Interview: Paul Zeitz.

281 "One possible explanation": "Senator Frist Backs Down," editorial in *The Washington Post*, Page A30, June 12, 2002.

281 "With $200 million already approved": David Corn, "Bush Backtracking on AIDS a Slap in the Face for Bono."

281 " 'The White House is taking the wrong' ": "Retreat on Fighting Global AIDS," editorial in *The New York Times*, June 21, 2002.

282 "Frist had two words": Interview: Paul Zeitz.

282 " 'No other Secretary [of Health]' ": Mark Schoofs and Rachel Zimmerman, "Activists' Chants Drown Out Thompson's Speech on AIDS," *The Wall Street Journal*, July 10, 2002.

284 "Placards read: 'Bush and Thompson' ": Sanjay Gupta, "Bush's Thompson Booed at AIDS Conference," CNN.com, July 9, 2002.

284 " 'Secretary Thompson probably was surprised' ": "U.S. Under Fire at AIDS Conference," CBSNews.com, July 9, 2002.

284 " 'We will meet the objectives' ": Schoofs and Zimmerman, "Activists' Chants Drown Out Thompson's Speech on AIDS."

285 "He told the secretary that ten years earlier": Recalled in interview: Terje Anderson.

CHAPTER FIFTEEN. BEHIND CLOSED DOORS, COALESCENCE

288 "Running CARE, O'Neill had overseen": "Biography of Director Joseph O'Neill," from the White House website, www.whitehouse.gov.

289 " 'This is a great start' ": According to Interview: Anthony Fauci.

289 " 'OK, we're going to go' ": Ibid.

289–90 "The group came to include": John Donnelly, "Big Spending on AIDS Seen as Go-It-Alone Plan," *The Boston Globe*, January 30, 2003.

290 " 'Just stop right there' ": Interview: Jack Chow.

291 "Stealthily, they would assemble": Interview: Ken Thomas.

292 " 'They thought I was crazy' ": Interview: Jeffrey Sachs.

292 "Fauci and O'Neill directed the group": Tina Rosenberg, "On Capitol Hill, Ideology Is Distorting an African AIDS Success," *The New York Times*, April 28, 2003.

292 "By the end of the decade": James Dao, "In Quietly Courting Africa, U.S. Likes the Dowry: Oil," *The New York Times*, September 19, 2002.

293 "One of the key questions": John Donnelly, "Big Spending on AIDS Seen as Go-It-Alone Plan." Quote from Eric Goosby, a former Clinton administration official and AIDS expert who attended the meeting.

293 " 'Our biggest problem,' he explained": Sheryl Gay Stolberg and Richard Stevenson, "The President's Proposals: AIDS Policy; Bush AIDS Effort Surprises Many, But Advisers Call It Long Planned," *The New York Times*, January 30, 2003.

294 " 'If in fact what we've said' ": Interview: Ken Thomas.

294 " 'Well, we'll consider it": Interview: Jack Chow.

295 " 'The time is not right' ": Ibid.

295 "Tight-lipped to the end": Ibid.

295 "The World Bank estimated": Christof Ruhl, Vadim Pokrovsky, and Viatchslav Vinogradav, "The Economic Consequences of HIV in Russia," The World Bank Group, May 15, 2002. Rounded up from "pessimistic" estimate of 14.53 million.

295 "Many doctors still refused": Anna Badkhen, "Global Pandemic—Fear, Ignorance Lead to Limited Patient Care," *The San Francisco Chronicle*, July 29, 2002.

296 "Yanhai, whose activist group": BBC News, "China Releases AIDS Activist," September 20, 2002.

296 "It seemed emblematic": Elisabeth Rosenthal, "China's Top AIDS Activist Missing; Arrest is Suspected," *The New York Times*, August 28, 2002.

296 "Combining the next-wave": National Intelligence Council, prepared under auspices of David F. Gordon, "The Next Wave of HIV/AIDS: Nigeria, Ethiopia, Russia, India, and China" Intelligence Community Assessment, September 2002, p. 4.

297 " 'The rise of HIV/AIDS' ": Ibid., p. 5.

298 " 'China is facing a decisive moment' ": BBC News, "Annan Highlights China's AIDS Problem," October 14, 2002.

298 "the Microsoft mogul came across": Geoffrey Cowley, "Bill's Biggest Bet Yet," *Newsweek*, February 4, 2002.

298 " 'Trey [Gates's boyhood nickname]' ": Ibid.

299 " 'Much of this progress' ": Bill Gates, "Slowing the Spread of AIDS in India," *The New York Times*, November 9, 2002.

300 "Yet Moscow, New Delhi, and Beijing": Nicholas Eberstadt, "The Future of AIDS: Grim Toll in Russia, China and India."

302 " 'If George Bush spent more time' ": Jeffrey Sachs, "Weapons of Mass Salvation," *The Economist*, October 24, 2002.

302 "It was not an easy thing": Bob Woodward, *Bush at War* (New York: Simon & Schuster, 2002). Idea germinated from interview: Stephen Morrison.

302 "There was a keen desire": Interview: Stephen Morrison.

303 "They were promptly arrested": Manny Fernandez, "Protestors Take AIDS Message to White House," *The Washington Post*, November 27, 2002.

304 "The title of the piece": Melissa Fay Greene, "What Will Become of Africa's AIDS Orphans?" *The New York Times Magazine*, December 22, 2002.

304 " 'The Bush administration is preparing' ": Editorial entitled, "Denial Here at Home," in *The Washington Post*, December 23, 2002.

305 "The secretary general spoke": Kofi Annan, "In Africa, AIDS Has a Woman's Face," *The New York Times*, December 29, 2002.

305 "It's a chance to show what America": Bono, "Mr. President, Africa Needs Us," *The Washington Post*, January 27, 2003.

305 "Up until the final days": Interview: Anthony Fauci.

306 " 'Fifteen billion dollars' ": Colin Powell, "Address to Global Business Coalition Against AIDS at 2003 Awards for Business Excellence," June 12, 2003. Kennedy Center, Washington, D.C.

307 "The cost of AIDS drugs had fallen": By the end of 2003, it was still not clear whether the United States would endorse generics. Pharma prices had continued to decrease, and U.S. Global AIDS coordinator Randall Tobias was noncommittal.

307 " 'You know, I believe God' ": John Donnelly, "Africa Tour, Africa Awaits Bush Action," *The Boston Globe*, July 13, 2002.

308 "the administration pledged only $2.1 billion": Congress forced through a final appropriation of $2.4 billion. The administration claimed it needed time to scale up.

308 " 'You were right,' Sachs told him": Interview: Jeffrey Sachs.

311 "In the months following": In the fall of 2003, Donnelly moved to South Africa to cover Africa for the *Globe*.

312 "He couldn't help but notice": Later amended, so that the plan would include a fifteenth country.

Acknowledgments

I have always known Africa to be a land of contrasts. When my parents immigrated to the United States in 1972, they left behind apartheid, and its attendant inhumanity and miseries. But they also left a continent of unmatched splendor, rich in natural bounty and flush with life.

Thirty years after my parents had departed, I was casting around for a thesis topic while reading for an M.Phil in International Relations at Oxford. I was very interested in "new" security issues, and Oxford afforded me the opportunity to think about big global issues. During the course of my research, I came across some news stories on the AIDS crisis in Africa. Digesting the statistics for the first time, I was stunned. The pandemic was consuming Southern Africa. I decided to write my thesis on the emergence of the pandemic as a threat to U.S. national security. As the project progressed, a more general underlying question lingered: "What had the United States done to address this crisis?"

While I was writing my thesis, my father, Darryl Behrman, passed away unexpectedly of a heart attack, at fifty-one years of age, while on holiday with my mother. Having left Africa at twenty-two, not knowing a soul in his new country, my father was an emblem of the American ideal. He lived his dreams. He was a visionary entrepreneur and a passionate conservationist. An accomplished adventurer and outdoorsman, he held eight fly-fishing world records, completed a marathon, and competed in triathlons. Mostly, he was my best friend.

Through the course of my research on global AIDS, I had become deeply impassioned about the crisis. It was clear to me that this was our Holocaust, the defining moral challenge of our time. I grew resolute to do my part, however small. There seemed to me to be no more pressing question than how we had responded to this crisis. Well before I could give it faces, places, and contours, I felt deeply that this was a story that had to be told. Personally, it was also to be a paean to my father, a spotlight for the continent that never left his soul, and a challenge to the America he loved and believed in.

It was a labor of deep passion. And it could not have been done without the generosity of many, who deserve much more than a short mention of thanks.

Acknowledgments must start with the roughly one hundred policy makers and thinkers who have played a part in the U.S. response over the last twenty years and agreed to be interviewed for this book. Each agreed to take time out of a demanding schedule to probe his or her memory for details and insights—often painful—that were invaluable to the construction of this story. Bravely, they hazarded critical portrayal, undoubtedly, in the service of a cause much greater than any one of the players in its drama. For my part, I have done my very best to put forth an accurate and measured account. Where I have fallen short, I hope that anyone with differing views will express them. History, it has been said, is argument without end. It is my hope that this book constitutes one of the first chapters in the historical discourse on this matter, not the last.

This book benefited handsomely from the work of John Donnelly, Laurie Garrett, and Bart Gellman. They have all been gracious and supportive of this book, and it is deeply appreciated. Alan Batkin, Nils Daulaire, John Donnelly, RP Eddy, Laurie Garrett, Eliza Griswold, Princeton Lyman, Joshua Cooper Ramo, and several others kindly agreed to read manuscripts. They saved me from errors in fact and judgment. I am very grateful. Needless to say, the responsibility for the shortcomings that remain is mine alone.

I am indebted to Gershon Kekst for his abiding support, counsel, and generosity. Rich Friedman, Terry O'Toole, Beth Cogan, and Henry Cornell, a friend and mentor, all at Goldman Sachs, have been extremely kind and generous. My incredible friends never failed to offer the right words of encouragement at the right times. I am so grateful to Georg, Marquez, John, Oliver, Bobby and Mary, Kate, Charlotte, Katy, Stephen, Pamela, Zach, Colm, Matt, Glen and Lynn, Alex, Betsy, Andrew, and Nat and Sara. Rachel Laitala has been a source of great warmth and encouragement.

I am so lucky to have such an extraordinary extended family. Fay, Shelley, Doug, and Kimmie Behrman; and Gloria, Felicia, Craig, and Gary

Stern have provided steadfast support. Colin Stern has been a sage. Grant Behrman has stood shoulder to shoulder with me every step of the way. My late grandfathers, Errol Behrman and Leonard Stern, would have enjoyed sharing in this project very much.

Two ladies made this book possible. To my super-agent, Jennifer Joel, at ICM, I promised adventure. In return, she lent me her unflagging commitment and her prolific talents, and, what's more, her friendship. Elizabeth Stein's attentive and judicious pen marks every page. Though an incredible editor, she has been much more than that. She has been a partner, a friend, and a champion, and I was very lucky to have her in my corner. To both, I will be forever grateful. Maris Kreizman was immensely helpful and Linnea Johnson provided spectacular copyediting.

Amanda Behrman Zeitlin has always been much more than a sister. Wise beyond her years, she is my most trusted advisor and cherished friend. Her husband, Zac, has been a deeply valued friend and brother.

My mother, Janine Behrman, ever a study in elegance, courage, and dignity, has always been my biggest supporter. I could not be prouder, nor could I admire her more.

As always, my thoughts turn to my father. If heaven looks like a place, then it is the Okavango Delta. It is just before dawn. A fire has begun to crackle and Dad is smiling, thinking of what might be.

Index

ABC, 178, 264
"ABC" approach, 113
abortion, 35
abstinence, 28, 286
Abubakar, Hajara, 184–85
Abuja Summit (2001), 250–51, 256–57, 258
activist community, 25, 220, 222; advent of efficacious ARV treatment and, 132–35; aggressive, "in your face" tactics adopted by, 121–22; Bush II and, 247–48, 249, 280–82, 284–86, 290, 302–3; candlelight vigils and, 119; Clinton candidacy and, 99; conservatives' displeasure with, 285–87; decline of U.S. death rates and, 134–35; emergence of global awareness in, 119–26, 132–35, 179; focused on domestic front, 90–91, 123–25, 233; global drug access and, 133–34, 136–40, 148–58; Gore as target for, 148–57, 179, 247, 248; high-profile advocacy and, 26–27, 90–91, 270–77; pharmaceutical companies as target for, 136–37, 139; religious convictions and, 248, 270, 272–73; State Summit and, 123–25; Thompson's Barcelona address and, 284–86, 290; Thurman's relations with, 234; USTR as target for, 149, 157–58; vaccine vs. treatment agenda and, 128–29. See also specific organizations and activists
ACT UP (AIDS Coalition to Unleash Power), 25, 29, 121–23, 124, 137, 149–50, 248, 282, 284

Afghanistan, 269, 302
Africa: American mind-set about, 66–68, 71; cutbacks in U.S. foreign aid to, 72–74; Ebola outbreaks in, 4–5, 8, 9–10; economic growth in, 71; end of Cold War and, 71; first longitudinal study of AIDS in, 41–42; inflated estimates of AIDS in, 15–16; negligence ascribed to national leaders in, 195–206; sensitivity of political leaders in, 15–16; statistics on AIDS in, xi–xii, 65, 195, 196, 200; strategic importance of, 246, 292–93. *See also specific countries*
African-American community, 86–90, 233, 248; Bush II and, 247–48, 304; mute on AIDS in Africa, 87–90; rise of AIDS in, 130; tensions between U.S. public health establishment and, 88–89; weakness of links to mother continent and, 90
African Summit on HIV/AIDS, Tuberculosis and Other Infectious Diseases (2001), 250–51, 256–57, 258
"Agony of Africa, The" (Schoofs), 179, 180
Aidid, Mohammed Farah, 101, 102
AIDS: discovery of HIV and, 14; HIV testing and, 15, 292; initial outbreaks of, 3–13; latency factor and, 83–84, 91, 200; prevention of (*see* prevention); statistics on, xi, 15, 17, 25, 30, 32, 44–45, 65, 83, 134, 173–75, 176, 195, 196, 200; stigma attached to, 25–26, 46, 69, 158, 162, 233; transmission of, 6, 10, 11–12;

341

Global Program on AIDS (GPA) (*cont.*)
79–80, 176, 227; Mann's strategy for,
44–47, 80; Merson's leadership at,
79–83, 92–96; Nakajima/Mann
conflict and, 52–57, 80; originally
known as Special Program on AIDS,
40–48; shortcomings of, 50–51, 80–81
"Global Strategy for the Prevention and
Control of AIDS," 44–47
Godwin, Ronald, 27
gonorrhea, 25, 88
Goosby, Eric, 293
Gore, Al, 94, 97, 109, 110, 141–57, 181,
195, 215, 216; candidacy of, 11–142,
146–49, 151–57, 163–64, 229,
239–40, 245–46, 278; Chinese health
issues and, 193; formal position on
drug pricing policy of, 154; issues of
interest to, 142–43; Republican
National Platform and, 245–46;
Russian health issues and, 143–44,
191–93; South African mobilization
against AIDS and, 144–48, 150, 151,
153–54, 203; as target for activists,
148–57, 179, 247, 248; UN Security
Council session chaired by, 163–64
Gore, Al, Sr., 141
Gore, Tipper, 142, 150, 153, 154–55, 156
Graham, Franklin, 270
Graham, Rev. Billy, 270
Greater Involvement of People with AIDS
(GIPA), 75–76
GRID (gay-related immunodeficiency
disease), 6
G7, 176

HAART (Highly Active Anti-Retroviral
Therapy), 131–32. *See also* AIDS
drugs
Haiti, 6, 65, 293
Halberstam, David, 143, 178, 223–24
Harper's Magazine, 85
Harris, Jeffrey, 20, 22–24, 34–39, 48, 51,
74, 93, 108–9, 113
Harris, Judy, 22–23, 24, 34, 39
Harvard University, 173, 175, 272, 277,
303; AIDS Institute at, 199; Bagnoud
Center for Health and Human Rights
at, 226; Institute for International
Development at, 252
Haygood, Wil, 179
HBO, 298
Head Start, 225
Health and Human Services Department,

U.S. (HHS), 11–12, 13–14, 18–19,
20, 37, 39, 91, 93, 281, 286, 287;
Cabinet-level task force and, 282–83;
funding for global AIDS and, 215,
216, 235; Shalala's activism at, 74–76
Health Care Task Force, 101
HealthGap Coalition, 136, 137, 139–40,
142, 148–49
Heart of America Tour, 303
Heckler, Margaret, 13–14, 128
Helms, Jesse: Bono's advocacy and, 273,
275, 276; Emergency Supplemental
Bill co-sponsored by, 273, 279–81,
285; foreign assistance opposed by,
72–73, 76, 212, 213, 214, 225, 234;
halting of payments to UN and, 160;
reversal of, on AIDS issues, 269–70,
273, 279; USAID attacked by, 73,
110–11
hemophiliacs, 6
heterosexual transmission of AIDS, 10,
11–12
Heymann, David, 127
Ho, David, 135
Holbrooke, Richard, 100, 158–65, 182–83,
184, 240, 299; Africa tour of, 158–59,
161; UN Security Council session on
global AIDS and, 159, 161–65
Homer-Dixon, Tad, 84
homosexuals, 5–6, 10, 25, 26, 27
human rights, 46–47

Idoko, John, 184, 185
immigration policy, 30–31
"In Africa, AIDS Has a Woman's Face"
(Annan), 305
India, 76, 138; burgeoning AIDS crisis in,
xii, xiii, 32, 75, 191, 193–95,
296–927, 298–99, 300–301; Gates's
philanthropy in, 194, 298–99
intellectual property rights, 138, 145–46,
157
Interagency Working Group, 230–32,
236–37, 238
Inter-American Development Bank, 275
international AIDS conferences: of 1985
(Atlanta), 14–15; of 1987
(Washington, D.C.), 29; of 1988
(London), 48–49; of 1990 (San
Francisco), 30; of 1992 (Amsterdam),
30–31, 122, 123; of 1993 (Berlin), 79,
81–83, 94–95; of 1996 (Vancouver),
131–34; of 1998 (Geneva), 136, 175,
176; of 1999 (Lusaka), 195–96; of

About the Author

Greg Behrman is the coordinator for the Council on Foreign Relations Roundtable on Improving U.S. Global AIDS Policy. He graduated magna cum laude from Princeton and received his M.Phil in International Relations from Oxford. He is a member of the Brookings Council and the Explorers Club. He lives in New York City.